NURSING THEORISTS *and* THEIR WORK

NURSING THEORISTS and THEIR WORK

Ann Marriner, Ph.D., R.N.

Professor, Indiana University School of Nursing,
Indianapolis, Indiana

The C. V. Mosby Company

St. Louis • Toronto • Princeton   1986

A TRADITION OF PUBLISHING EXCELLENCE

Editor: David P. Carroll
Assistant Editor: Megan Thomas
Project Editor: Teri Merchant
Manuscript Editor: Clifton B. Metcalf, Jr.
Design: J. Rokusek
Production: Ginny Douglas

Printed in the United States of America

The C.V. Mosby Company
11830 Westline Industrial Drive, St. Louis, Missouri 63146

Library of Congress Cataloging-in-Publication Data

Marriner, Ann, 1943-
    Nursing theorists and their work.
    Includes bibliographies and index.
    1. Nursing—Philosophy. I. Title. [DNLM: 1. Models,
Theoretical. 2. Nursing. 3. Philosophy, Nursing.
WY 86 M359n]
RT84.5.M37 1986   610.73'01   85-15471
ISBN 0-8016-3162-9

C/VH/VH 9 8 7 6 5 4 3   04/C/531

Contributors

Mary Lee Ackermann

OB/GYN Nurse Practitioner,
Louisville, Kentucky

Sr. Judith Alexander

Doctoral Student and Research Assistant,
    March of Dimes Birth Defects Foundation,
Indiana University School of Nursing,
Indianapolis, Indiana

Jill K. Baker

Patient Care Coordinator of Plastic Surgery
OR and Allied Areas—Long Surgery,
Indiana University Medical Center,
Indianapolis, Indiana

Carolyn J. Beagle

Clinical Charge Nurse at St. Vincent's Hospital,
Indianapolis, Indiana

Sarah J. Beckman

Patient Care Coordinator, University Hospitals,
Indianapolis, Indiana

Sue Marquis Bishop

Associate Professor and Chair,
Graduate Department of Psychiatric/Mental
    Health Nursing,
    Indiana University School of Nursing,
    Indianapolis, Indiana

Carolyn L. Blue

Assistant Professor, School of Nursing,
Purdue University,
West Lafayette, Indiana

Debra A. Borchers

Educational Nurse Specialist,
Children's Hospital,
Medical Center,
Cincinnati, Ohio

Sallie Anne Brink

Charge Nurse, Coronary Care Unit,
Sts. Mary and Elizabeth Hospital,
Louisville, Kentucky

Karen M. Brubaker

Staff Development Instructor/Critical Care,
Wishard Memorial Hospital,
Indianapolis, Indiana

Pam Butler

Staff Nurse, Mental Health,
St. Vincent's Stress Center,
Indianapolis, Indiana

Jane A. Caldwell-Gwin

Assistant Manager, Nursing Unit,
Adult Burn Unit,
Wishard Memorial Hospital,
Indianapolis, Indiana

Elizabeth T. Carey

Instructor, ADN Program,
Parkland College,
Champaign, Illinois

Patricia Chapman-Boyce

Hemodialysis Home Training Coordinator,
Indiana University,
Indianapolis, Indiana

Elizabeth Chong Choi

Assistant Professor,
Pediatrics, Family, and Women's Health,
Indiana University School of Nursing,
Indianapolis, Indiana

Debra Trnka Cochran

PNA Student at Indiana University,
Indianapolis, Indiana

Sydney Coleman-Ehmke

Graduate Student,
Indiana University School of Nursing,
Indianapolis, Indiana

Sharon S. Conner

Psychiatric Staff Nurse,
Ball Memorial Hospital,
Hartford City, Indiana

Terri Creekmur

Patient Care Coordinator, Burn Unit,
James Whitcomb Riley Hospital,
Indiana University Medical Center,
Indianapolis, Indiana

Joann Sebastian Daily

Instructor, Educational Services,
Bartholomew County Hospital,
Columbus, Indiana

Marguerite D. Danko

Lecturer, Indiana University School
of Nursing,
Indianapolis, Indiana;
Pediatric Nurse Associate,
Marion Community Health Center,
Marion, Indiana

Janet DeFelice

Staff R.N., ICU,
Winona Memorial Hospital,
Indianapolis, Indiana

Karen R. deGraaf

Health Care Coordinator,
Jewish Hospital,
Louisville, Kentucky

Deborah Wertman DeMeester

Cardiology Coordinator,
Metro Health/Health America,
Indianapolis, Indiana

Deborah A. Dougherty

Nursing Service Supervisor,
Johnson County Memorial Hospital,
Franklin, Indiana

Dorothy Kay Dycus

Family Nurse Practitioner,
Lake County Health Department of Lake
County, Indiana,
Crown Point, Indiana

Jeanne Donohue Eben

Staff Development Instructor,
Emergency Nursing,
Wishard Memorial Hospital
Indianapolis, Indiana

Karen J. Foli

Director, Continuing Care Center,
Lakeview Medical Center,
Danville, Illinois

Alta J.H. Gochnauer

Graduate Student,
Indiana University School of Nursing,
Indianapolis, Indiana

S. Brook Gumm

Patient Care Coordinator,
Children's Hospital,
Cincinnati, Ohio

Cheryl A. Hailway

Medical Search Specialist,
Midwest Medical Consultants,
Indianapolis, Indiana

DeAnn M. Hensley

Supervisor,
University Heights Hospital
Indianapolis, Indiana

Mary E. Hermiz

Student,
Indiana University School of Nursing,
Indianapolis, Indiana

William H. Hobble

Staff Nurse,
V.A. Medical Center,
Indianapolis, Indiana

Anne Hodel

Education Coordinator,
Visiting Nurse Services,
Indianapolis, Indiana

Nancy E. Hunt

Major, U.S. Army Nurse Corps

Connie Rae Jarlsberg

Manager, Nursing Unit,
Adult Burn Unit,
Wishard Memorial Hospital,
Indianapolis, Indiana

Tamara Johnson

Assistant Manager, ICUs,
Community Hospital of Indianapolis,
Indianapolis, Indiana

Cathy Greenwell Jones

Staff Nurse II, ICU,
Sts. Mary and Elizabeth Hospital,
Louisville, Kentucky

Juanita Fogel Keck

Assistant Professor,
Nursing of Adults with Biodissonance,
Indiana University School of Nursing,
Indianapolis, Indiana

Kimberly A. Kilgore

Student,
Indiana University School of Nursing,
Indianapolis, Indiana

Jill Vass Langfitt

Student,
Indiana University School of Nursing,
Indianapolis, Indiana

Theresa Lansinger

Nursing Instructor, Department of Education,
Lakeview Medical Center,
Danville, Illinois

Tamara Lauer

Clinical Nurse,
Indiana University Hospitals,
Indianapolis, Indiana

Judith E. Marich

Manager, Labor and Delivery,
St. Vincent's Hospital,
Indianapolis, Indiana

Ann Marriner

Professor,
Indiana University School of Nursing,
Indianapolis, Indiana

Judy Sporleder Maupin

Assistant Director, Nursing Service,
Bartholomew County Hospital,
Columbus, Indiana

Judy McCormick

Staff Nurse,
Indiana University Medical Center,
Clinical Research Center,
Indianapolis, Indiana

Cynthia A. McCreary

Chief Nurse, Children and Youth Project,
University of Texas Health Science Center at
   Dallas,
Dallas, Texas

Mary Meininger

Staff Nurse—Renal Intensive Care Unit,
Indiana University Hospital,
Indianapolis, Indiana

Kathleen Millican Miller

Post-Anesthesia Care Unit,
St. Elizabeth Hospital,
Lafayette, Indiana

Deborah I. Mills

Instructor,
Parkview Methodist School of Nursing,
Fort Wayne, Indiana

Sandra L. Moody

Staff Nurse,
St. Vincent Hospital,
Indianapolis, Indiana

Cynthia L. Mossman

Staff Nurse, Special Care Nursery,
University Hospital,
Indianapolis, Indiana

Margaret J. Nation

Nurse Auditor,
Wishard Memorial Hospital,
Indianapolis, Indiana

Susan E. Neal

Public Health Nurse,
Marion County Bureau of Public Health
   Nursing,
Indianapolis, Indiana

Kathryn W. Noone

Staff Nurse,
Cardiac Intensive Care,
Indiana University Hospital,
Indianapolis, Indiana

Sherry B. Nordmeyer

Instructor,
Indiana University School of Nursing,
Indianapolis, Indiana

Nancy Orcutt

Pediatric Nurse Associate, Metro Health
Indianapolis, Indiana

Katherine R. Papazian

Professor, School of Nursing,
Ball State University,
Muncie, Indiana

Gwynn Lee Perlich

Nursing Supervisor,
St. Vincent Hospital and Health Care Center,
Indianapolis, Indiana

Kim Tippey Peskoe

Faculty,
Ball State University School of Nursing,
Muncie, Indiana

LaPhyllis Peterson

Student,
Indiana University School of Nursing,
Indianapolis, Indiana

Cheryl Y. Petty

Graduate Student,
Indiana University School of Nursing,
Indianapolis, Indiana

Mary Carolyn Poat

Staff RN,
Indiana University Hospital,
Indianapolis, Indiana

LaDema Poppa

Manager, Outpatient Transfusion and Pheresis,
Methodist Hospital of Indiana,
Indianapolis, Indiana

Beverly D. Porter

Research Nurse,
Indiana University Hospital,
Indiana University Medical Center,
Indianapolis, Indiana

Beth Bruns Prusinski

Staff Nurse,
St. Vincent's Hospital,
Indianapolis, Indiana

Rosalyn A. Pung

Graduate Student,
Indiana University School of Nursing,
Indianapolis, Indiana

LyNette Rasmussen

Staff Nurse,
Parkview Memorial Hospital,
Fort Wayne, Indiana

Cynthia M. Riester

Patient Care Coordinator,
St. Francis Hospital,
Indianapolis, Indiana

Karen D. Andrews Robards

Department Manager, CCU and Telemetry,
Johnson County Memorial Hospital,
Franklin, Indiana

Martha Carole Satterly

Head Nurse, Ambulatory Surgery,
Bartholomew County Hospital,
Columbus, Indiana

Marcia K. Sauter

Instructor,
Parkview Methodist School of Nursing,
Fort Wayne, Indiana

Donna N. Schmeiser

Student,
Indiana University School of Nursing,
Indianapolis, Indiana

Larry P. Schumacher

Director, Critical Care Nursing,
Research Medical Center,
Kansas City, Missouri

Bryn Searcy

Staff Nurse,
St. Vincent's Hospital,
Indianapolis, Indiana

Maribeth Slebodnik

Staff Nurse, Special Care Nursery,
Wishard Memorial Hospital,
Indianapolis, Indiana

Rebecca S. Sloan

Research Nurse,
Indiana University Medical Center,
Indianapolis, Indiana

Nancy L. Stark

Staff Nurse, Intensive Care Unit,
St. Vincent's Hospital,
Indianapolis, Indiana

Margery Stuart

Instructor,
Lakeview Medical Center School of Nursing,
Danville, Illinois

Elizabeth Godfrey Terry

Certified Pediatric Nurse Associate,
Metro Health Care,
Indianapolis, Indiana

Judith K. Watt

Coordinator, Communicable Disease Control,
Marion County Health Department,
Indianapolis, Indiana

Cynthia A. Wesolowski

Educational Nurse Specialist,
Children's Hospital,
Medical Center,
Cincinnati, Ohio

Roseanne Yancey

Lecturer,
Indiana University School of Nursing,
Indianapolis, Indiana

Susan T. Zoretich

Staff Nurse,
St. Vincent's Hospital,
Indianapolis, Indiana

Theorists

Faye Glenn Abdellah

Dept. Surgeon General and Chief Nurse
  Officer
U.S. Public Health Service
Dept. of Health & Human Services
Room 18-67 Parklawn Building 5600 Fisher
  Lane
Rockville, MD 20857
(301) 443-4000

Evelyn Adam

Faculty of Nursing University of Montreal
  P.O. Box 6128
Station A
Montreal, Quebec H3C-3J7
(514) 343-7154

Kathryn E. Barnard

University of Washington
Mail Stop WJ-10
Seattle, WA 98195
(206) 543-9200

Helen C. Erickson

University of Michigan
1325 Catherine Rd.
Med. Science #1
School of Nursing
Fundamentals Area
Ann Arbor, MI 48109
(313) 764-5503

Joyce J. Fitzpatrick

Case Western Reserve University
Frances Payne Bolton School of Nursing
2121 Abington Road
Cleveland, OH 44106
(216) 368-2544

Lydia E. Hall

Deceased

Virginia Henderson

(retired)
164 Linden Street
New Haven, CT 06511
(203) 624-1272

Dorothy E. Johnson

(retired)
715 Grouper Lane
Key Largo, FL 33037
(305) 852-3149

Imogene King

University of Southern Florida
4202 Flower Avenue
Tampa, FL 33620
(813) 974-2011

Madeleine Leininger

Wayne State University
5557 Cass
Detroit, MI 48202
(313) 577-4085

Myra Estrin Levine

University of Illinois
Chicago Health Science Center
College of Nursing
845 S. Damen Avenue
Chicago, IL 60612
(312) 996-7900

Betty Neuman

Box 488
Beverly, OH 45715
(614) 749-3322

Margaret A. Newman

University of Minnesota
School of Nursing
5-104 Unit F
308 Howard Street
Minneapolis, Minnesota 55455
(612) 376-7299

Florence Nightingale

Deceased

Dorothea E. Orem

Orem & Shields, Inc.
4820 Morgan Drive
Chevy Chase, MA 20015
(301) 656-0930

Rosemarie Rizzo Parse

Discovery International
P.O. Box 633
Pittsburgh, PA 15230

Ida Jean Orlando Pelletier

80 Hawthorne
Belmont, Mass. 02178
(617) 489-0348

Hildegard E. Peplau

(retired)
14024 Ostego Street
Sherman Oaks, CA 91403
(818) 783-2272

Martha E. Rogers

The Division of Nursing
New York University
429 Shimkin Hall
Washington Square
New York, NY 10003
(212) 598-3921

Sister Callista Roy

Dept. of Physiological Nursing
School of Nursing
N611Y University of California
San Francisco, CA 94143
(415) 666-5150

Joan Riehl Sisca

Harrisburg Area Community College
Harrisburg, PA
(717) 780-2316

Mary Ann P. Swain

Office of Academic Affairs
University of Michigan
Ann Arbor, MI 48109
(313) 764-0151

Evelyn M. Tomlin

University of Michigan
1325 Catherine Rd.
Med. Science #1
School of Nursing
Fundamentals Area
Ann Arbor, MI 48109
(313) 764-5503

Joyce Travelbee

Deceased

Jean Watson

University of Colorado
Health Sciences Center
School of Nursing
4200 E. Ninth Avenue
Denver, CO 80262

Ernestine Wiedenbach

(retired)
926 Eastridge Village Drive
Miami, FL 33157
(305) 235-5931

Preface

This book is a tribute to nursing theorists. It identifies major thinkers in nursing, reviews some of their important ideas, and lists their publications, what has been written about them, and the major sources they used. The first chapter is a brief overview of the book and is appropriate for the baccalaureate level. The other chapters in Unit I define terminology and discuss history and philosophy of science, logical reasoning, the theory development process, and the evolution of nursing theory development at a graduate level.

The theorists are clustered into four categories according to major themes. The categories are not mutually exclusive. Nightingale, Henderson, Abdellah, Hall, Orem, Adam, Leininger, Watson, and Parse have written about the art and science of humanistic nursing. Peplau, Travelbee, Orlando, Wiedenbach, King, Riehl-Sisca, Erickson, Tomlin, Swain, and Barnard have all dealt with interpersonal relationships. Johnson, Roy, and Neuman have written about systems. Levine, Rogers, Fitzpatrick, and Newman are associated with energy fields.

Credentials and background of the theorist, theoretical sources for the theory development, use of empirical data, major concepts and definitions, assumptions, theoretical assertions, logical form, acceptance by the nursing community, further development, and a critique are identified for each theorist. Baccalaureate students may be most interested in the concepts, definitions, and theoretical assertions. Graduate students will be interested in logical form, acceptance by the nursing community, the theoretical sources for theory development, and the use of empirical data. The extensive bibliographies should be particularly useful to graduate students for locating primary and secondary sources.

Many of the scholars identified in this book do not consider themselves theorists and never intended to develop theory. Is it fair to evaluate them as theorists and their work as theory? Probably not, but their thoughts are important contributions to the development of nursing theory. It is now our responsibility to analyze and synthesize their work, generate new ideas, and continue theory development.

I would like to thank the theorists for critiquing the chapters about themselves so the content could be current and accurate. So that their omission does not appear to have been an oversight, the work of Paterson and Zderad has not been included in this volume at their request. Thanks are expressed to the following graduate students for assistance with data collection: Jeanette Adam, Cythia J. Allen, Fatmah Arafat, Judy K. Cowling, Sharon Evick, Kathy McGregor, Catherine Martin, Glenda Mitchell, Janet Pezelle, Nancy Preuss, Larry P. Schumacher, and Anthony G. Smith. Appreciation is expressed to the following: Shirley Bastin helped obtain audiotapes for the learning laboratory. Ann Van Camp ran computer searches while Terry Brenner, Beth Gruenwald, and Marilyn Wacker obtained materials through interlibrary loans. Lynn Smith and Mary Thomson purchased library acquisitions that I recommended. The reference librarians—Fran Brahmi, Sandra Brown, Linda Bennett, and Lori Klein—helped us locate the theorists and their work. Harold Shaffer, Janine Orr, Stephanie Ogle, Kenn Tolle, and Beth Gibson worked the circulation desk, controlled the reserved books, and searched for missing materials. Dorothy Pock did an outstanding job of typing the manuscript as she patiently worked her way through several drafts, repairing format and noting problems. Lisa Mount provided secretarial services for the many contracts and correspondence necessary for this project. I would also like to thank my family—Jerry, Natasha, and David—for their assistance at home, and my mother, Arlene Clawson, for caring for me when I was ill.

Ann Marriner

Contents

UNIT
I

Analysis of Nursing Theories

Introduction to Analysis of Nursing Theories

Ann Marriner

1

REASONS FOR THEORY

Theory helps provide knowledge to improve practice by describing, explaining, predicting, and controlling phenomena. Nurses' power is increased through theoretical knowledge because systematically developed methods are more likely to be successful. Nurses also know why they are doing what they are doing if challenged. Theory provides professional autonomy by guiding the practice, education, and research functions of the profession. The study of theory helps develop analytical skills, challenge thinking, clarify values and assumptions, and determine purposes for nursing practice, education, and research.[7, 8, 12, 44:4-9]

MAJOR CONCEPTS AND DEFINITIONS OF THEORY DEVELOPMENT

Philosophy

Philosophy is "the science comprising logic, ethics, aesthetics, metaphysics, and epistemology." It is the "investigation of causes and laws underlying reality" and is "inquiry into the nature of things based on logical reasoning rather than empirical methods."[34:985]

Science

Science is "the observation, identification, description, experimental investigation, and theoretical explanation of natural phenomena."[34:1162] It is a "body of knowledge."[7:72]

Knowledge

"Knowledge is an awareness or perception of reality acquired through learning or investigation."[7:72]

Fact

A fact is "something known with certainty."[34:469]

Model

"A model is an idea that explains by using symbolic and physical visualization."[54:62] Symbolic models may be verbal, schematic, or quantitative. They no longer have a recognizable physical form and are a higher level of abstraction than physical models. Verbal models are worded statements. Schematic models may be

3

diagrams, drawings, graphs, or pictures. Quantitative models are mathematical symbols. Physical models may look like what they are supposed to represent, for example, body organs, or they may become more abstract while still keeping some of the physical properties, like ECG.[24] Models can be used "to facilitate thinking about concepts and relationships between them"[5] or to map out the research process.[6]

Paradigm

A paradigm is "a conceptual diagram."[54:62] It can be a large structure used to organize theory.*

Theory

A theory is "a set of concepts, definitions, and propositions that project a systematic view of phenomena by designing specific interrelationships among concepts for purposes of describing, explaining, predicting, and/or controlling phenomena."[7:70]

Concept

A concept is a "complex mental formulation of an object, property, or event that is derived from individual perceptual experience."[7:53] It is "an idea; a mental image; a generalization formed and developed in the mind."[1:116] Concepts label phenomena.

ABSTRACT CONCEPT. Abstract concepts are completely independent of time or place. Temperature, for example, is an abstract concept.[44:49]

CONCRETE CONCEPT. A concrete concept is specific to time and place, such as the body temperature of a specific person at a specific time on a specific day.[44:49]

Phenomenon

A phenomenon is "any occurrence or fact that is directly perceptible by the senses."[34:983] It is reality on "what exists in the real world."[21:7]

*References 7:76; 33:70-71; 44:21-33.

Definitions

Definitions are statements of the meaning of a word, phrase, or term.[34:346]

CONNOTATIVE DEFINITIONS. Connotative definitions "imply or suggest accompaniments."[7:113]

DENOTATIVE DEFINITIONS. Denotative definitions specify what something is by naming "the object, properties, or events the concept represents such that particulars are clearly assigned to the term."[7:113]

THEORETICAL DEFINITIONS. "Theoretical definitions convey the general meaning of the concept in a manner that fits the theory and projects empirical indicators for concepts."[7:92]

OPERATIONAL DEFINITIONS. Operational definitions specify "the activities or 'operations' necessary to measure a construct or a variable."[54:62]

Assumptions

Assumptions are statements supposed to be true without proof or demonstration.[34:80] They may be explicit or implicit.[7:119]

Theoretical Statements

Theoretical statements describe a relationship between two or more concepts.

LAW. A law is "a statement that describes a relationship in which scientists have so much confidence they consider it an absolute 'truth.' "[44:78]

AXIOMS. Axioms are "a basic set of statements, each independent of the others (they say different things), from which all other statements of the theory may be logically derived."[44:78] Axioms are often associated with plane geometry.

PROPOSITIONS. Propositions are theorems or statements derived from axioms. The term is often used interchangeably with hypotheses to mean "any idea or hunch that is presented in the form of a scientific statement."[44:78]

HYPOTHESIS. An hypothesis is a relationship statement to be tested.[44:78]

EMPIRICAL GENERALIZATIONS. Empirical generalizations are patterns "of events found in a number of different empirical studies."[44:79]

EXISTENCE. Existence statements establish a typology by indicating a concept exists.[44:76]

RELATIONAL STATEMENTS. Relational statements indicate that values of one concept are associated or correlated with values of another. Relationships may be linear or curvilinear. Linear relationships may be either positive ("when one concept occurs, or is high, the other concept occurs, or is high, or vice versa") or negative ("when one concept occurs or is high, the other concept is low, and vice versa") or no relationship may exist (when "the occurrence of one concept gives no information about the occurrence of the other concept and vice versa").[44:70] Curvilinear relationships are characterized by curved lines (when one concept is high and low, the other concept is high or low).

CAUSAL. One concept is believed to cause the occurrence of another concept if they have a causal relationship.[44:71] Correlation is not necessarily causation.

DETERMINISTIC. Dependent variables are determined by independent variables.[44:74]

PROBABILISTIC. Probability predicts both nonoccurrence and occurrence of something.[44:75]

Research

"Research is a rigorous application of the method of science to obtain reliable and valid knowledge about reality."[7:73] Research may

generate theory with an inductive approach or test it by a deductive approach.

Range of Theories

"Subject matter for a theory may be very broad and all inclusive or very narrow and limited."[21:13]

GRAND THEORY. Grand theories are broad in scope and complex. "In most instances, grand theories require further specification and partitioning of theoretical statements for them to be empirically tested and theoretically verified. Grand theorists state their theoretical formulations at the most general level of abstraction, and it is often difficult to link these formulations to reality."[21:13] Grand theories contain summative concepts that incorporate smaller range theories.

MIDDLE RANGE THEORY. Middle range theory has a narrower focus than grand theory and a broader focus than micro theory. The scope is not so large as to be relatively useless for summative concepts and not so narrow that it cannot be used to explain complex life situations.[33:68]

MICRO THEORY. Micro theories are the least complex and most specific. They are "a set of theoretical statements, usually hypotheses, that deal with narrowly defined phenomena."[21:13]

DEVELOPMENT OF THEORY
Theory Development Process

Theory development is a process that primarily involves induction, deduction, and retroduction.

INDUCTION. Induction is "a form of reasoning that moves from the specific to the general. In inductive logic, a series of particulars is combined into a larger whole or set of things. In inductive research, particular events are observed and analyzed as a basis for formulating general theoretical statements, often called grounded 'theory.' "[7:202] This is a research to theory approach.

DEDUCTION. Deduction is a form of logical reasoning that progresses from general to specific. This process involves a sequence of theoretical statements derived from a few general statements or axioms. Two or more relational statements are used to draw a conclusion. Abstract theoretical relationships are used to derive specific empirical hypotheses. This is a theory to research approach.[7:202]

RETRODUCTION. Retroduction combines induction and deduction.[7:205] It uses analogy to devise theory. Theorists may gain insight from a theory in another field. They advance theory development when they move content or structural aspects of that theory to their own field to form a new theory. This is more than borrowing from another field.[53]

Forms of Theory

Theories may be organized according to their form into three categories. These categories include set-of-laws, axiomatic, and causal process.

SET-OF-LAWS. This is an inductive approach that seeks patterns in research findings. Research findings are selected and sorted according to degree of empirical support into categories of laws, empirical generalizations, and hypotheses. It may be difficult to organize and interrelate these generalizations. Because the statements are not interrelated, support for one statement does not support another statement. Consequently, research efforts must be extensive.[44]

AXIOMATIC. The axiomatic form is an interrelated logical system of concepts, definitions, and relationship statements arranged in hierarchical order. Abstract axioms are at the top of the hierarchy with derived propositions being lower. Required research is less extensive because empirical support for one relational statement also supports the theory.[44]

CAUSAL PROCESS. The causal process increases understanding through relationship statements that specify cause between independent and dependent variables. This form also requires concepts, definitions, and relationship statements. It explains how something happens.[44,52]

CRITERIA FOR EVALUATION OF THEORY

Although many authors use different terms to describe criteria for evaluating theory, issues often discussed are clarity, simplicity, generality, empirical precision, and derivable consequences.

Clarity

Semantic and structural clarity and consistency are important. To assess this, one should identify the major concepts and subconcepts and identify definitions for them. Denotative definitions provide the most clarity, but connotative definitions are better than none. Words should be invented only if necessary, and they should be carefully defined. Sometimes words have multiple and competing meanings within and across disciplines. Therefore, words should be borrowed cautiously and defined carefully. Diagrams and examples may provide more clarity and should be consistent. The logical development should be clear, and assumptions should be consistent with the theory's goals.[6:133-137]

Reynolds refers to intersubjectivity when he says, "there must be shared agreement of the definitions of concepts and relationships between concepts within a theory."[44:13] Hardy refers to meaning and logical adequacy when stating that "concepts and relationships between concepts must be clearly identified and valid."[16:106] Stevens also speaks of clarity and consistency.[49] Ellis refers to the criterion of terminology to evaluate theory and addresses the danger of lost meaning when terms are borrowed from other disciplines and used in a different context.[10:221] Walker and Avant say, "logical adequacy of a theory is the logical structure of the concepts and statements independent of the meaning of those concepts or statements."[53:119]

Simplicity

Chinn and Jacobs state, "In nursing, practitioners need simple theory to guide practice."[6:138] Argyris indicates that a theory "should be maximally comprehensive and concrete . . . and it should do so with the fewest concepts and the simplest relations of concepts."[3:198] In contrast, Ellis believes a theory must have complexity to be significant.[10:219] Reynolds suggests that simply counting the number of concepts is not sufficient. He says the most useful theory provides the greatest sense of understanding.[44:135] Walker and Avant refer to parsimony as ". . . elegant in its simplicity, even though it may be broad in content."[53:130]

Generality

To determine the generality of a theory, the scope of concepts and goals within the theory are examined. The more limited the concepts and goals, the less general the theory. Ada Jacox says, "There is no pressing need to develop a 'grand theory' that supposedly includes everything that nurses need to know."[49:65] Chinn and Jacobs believe situations to which the theory applies should not be limited.[6:139-140] Ellis says, "The broader the scope . . . the greater the significance of the theory."[10:219] Stevens suggests that both broad and narrow scopes are necessary and that the complexity or simplicity should be determined by the complexity of the subject matter.[49:65-66]

Empirical Precision

Empirical precision is linked to the testability and ultimate use of a theory and refers to the "extent that the defined concepts are grounded in observable reality."[6:144] Hardy states that "how well the evidence supports the theory is indicative of empirical adequacy" and agrees there "should be a match between theoretical

claims and the empirical evidence."[16:105] Reynolds refers to empirical relevance and the trait that "anyone be able to examine the correspondence between a particular theory and the objective empirical data."[44:18] He notes that other scientists should be able to evaluate and verify results for themselves. Walker and Avant say, "If a theory cannot generate hypotheses, it is not useful to scientists and does not add to the body of knowledge."[53:131] In contrast, Ellis states, testability of a theory can be sacrificed in favor of scope, complexity, and clinical usefulness. Elegance and complexity of structure are preferred to precision in the meaning of concepts.[10:220] She maintains that theories should be clearly recognized as tentative and hypothetical. Chinn and Jacobs believe "if research, theory, and practice are to be united, then theory in nursing should lend itself to research testing, and research testing should guide practice."[7:142]

Derivable Consequences

Chinn and Jacobs state, "Nursing theory ought to guide research and practice, generate new ideas, and differentiate the focus of nursing from other professions."[7:142] Ellis indicates that to be considered useful, "it is essential for theory to develop and guide practice . . . theories should reveal what knowledge nurses must, and should, spend time pursuing."[10:220] Hardy believes the nursing profession should "make use of existing theory to predict certain outcomes and control events in such a way that desired outcomes are achieved."[16:106]

NURSING THEORISTS
Art and Science of Humanistic Nursing

Nightingale, Henderson, Abdellah, Hall, Orem, Adam, Leininger, and Watson are grouped together because of their views about humanistic nursing as an art and science.

Florence Nightingale believed every woman

would be responsible for someone's health at sometime and consequently would be a nurse. She thought disease was a reparative process, and the nurse should manipulate the environment to facilitate the process. Her directions regarding ventilation, warmth, light, diet, cleanliness, and noise are recorded in her *Notes on Nursing*.[38]

Virginia Henderson has made enormous contributions to nursing in more than 60 years of service as a nurse, teacher, author, and researcher. She has published prolifically throughout those years. Her definition of nursing first appeared in the fifth edition of *Textbook of the Principles and Practice of Nursing* in 1955.[17] Henderson indicates, "The unique function of the nurse is to assist the individual, sick or well, in the performance of those activities contributing to health or its recovery (or to peaceful death) that he would perform unaided if he had the necessary strength, will, or knowledge and to do this in such a way as to help him gain independence as rapidly as possible."[19:7] In *The Nature of Nursing,* she also identified 14 basic needs of patients that comprise the components of nursing care: (1) breathing, (2) eating and drinking, (3) elimination, (4) movement, (5) rest and sleep, (6) suitable clothing, (7) body temperature, (8) clean body and protected integument, (9) safe environment, (10) communication, (11) worship, (12) work, (13) play, and (14) learning.[19:16-17] She identified three levels of nurse-patient relationships: being a (1) substitute for the patient, (2) helper to the patient, and (3) partner with the patient.[19:16] She supports empathetic understanding and says the nurse needs to "get inside the skin of each of her patients in order to know what he needs."[18:63] Henderson believes many nurses' and physicians' functions overlap. She says the nurse works in interdependence with other health professionals and compares the health team to wedges on a pie graph. The sizes of pie vary depending on the patient's needs. The goal is to have the patient represented by most of the pie as he gains independence.[19:22-23]

Faye Glenn Abdellah has written prolifically about a variety of subjects since the early 1950s. She and others conceptualized 21 nursing problems based on systematic use of research data to teach and evaluate students. The typology of 21 nursing problems first appeared in the 1960 edition of *Patient-Centered Approaches to Nursing*.[2]

Lydia E. Hall used her philosophy of nursing to design and develop the Loeb Center for Nursing at Montefiore Hospital in New York. She served as Administrative Director of the Loeb Center from its opening in 1963 until her death in 1969. Most of her work was published in the 1960s. Her model for nursing was presented in "Nursing: What is it?" in *The Canadian Nurse* in 1964[14] and discussed in "The Loeb Center for Nursing and Rehabilitation" in the *International Journal of Nursing Studies* in 1969.[15] She believed nursing functions differently in the three interlocking circles that constitute aspects of the patient. She labeled the circles the body (the care), the disease (the cure), and the person (the core). Nursing functions in all three circles but share them with other providers to different degrees. She believed that more professional nursing care and teaching are needed as less medical care is needed and that professional nursing care will hasten recovery.

Dorothea E. Orem had a spontaneous insight about the concept of nursing in 1958. She has been publishing since the 1950s about nursing practice and education. She identifies her self-care deficit theory of nursing as a general theory composed of three related theories: (1) the theory of self-care, (2) the theory of self-care deficit, and (3) the theory of nursing systems. Orem identifies three types of nursing systems: (1) wholly compensatory—doing for the patient, (2) partly compensatory—helping the person do for himself, and (3) supportive-educative—helping the person learn to do for himself. The theories are discussed more fully in her book, *Nursing: Concepts of Practice*. She believes nurses share some functions with other health care providers.[39]

Evelyn Adam started publishing in the mid 1970s. Much of her work focuses on developing models and theories on the concept of nursing. She uses a model she learned from Dorothy Johnson. In her book, *To be a Nurse,*[1] she applies Virgina Henderson's definition of nursing to the model and identifies the assumptions, beliefs and values, and major units. In the latter category she includes the goal of the profession, the beneficiary of the professional service, the role of the professional, the source of the beneficiary's difficulty, the intervention of the professional, and the consequences.

Madeleine Leininger has published prolifically about a variety of topics since 1960. Although she has written several books about transcultural nursing and caring, the most complete account of transcultural care theory is found in *Transcultural Care Diversity and Universality: A Theory in Nursing.*[25] Some of the major concepts are care, caring, culture, cultural values, and cultural variations. Leininger has generated many hypotheses and hopes to stimulate further ethnoscience research by nurses in ethnonursing.

Jean Watson started publishing in the mid 1970s. Her book, *Nursing: The Philosophy and Science of Caring,* was published in 1979.[54] The content was further refined in *Nursing: Human Science and Health Care* in 1985.[55] In an effort to reduce the dichotomy between theory and practice, Watson proposed a philosophy and science of caring. She identified 10 carative factors: (1) the formation of a humanistic-altruistic system of values; (2) the instillation of faith-hope; (3) the cultivation of sensitivity to self and to others; (4) the development of a helping-trust relationship; (5) the promotion and acceptance of the expression of positive and negative; (6) the systematic use of the scientific problem-solving method for decision making; (7) the promotion of interpersonal teaching-learning; (8) the provision for a supportive, protective, or corrective mental, physical, sociocultural, and spiritual environment; (9) assistance with the gratification of human needs; and (10) the allowance for existential-phenom-enological forces. Watson believes nurses should develop health promotion through preventive actions such as recognizing coping skills and adaptation to loss, teaching problem-solving methods, and providing situational support.

Rosemarie Rizzo Parse drew from the work of Martha Rogers and the existential-phenomenologists for the development of *Man-Living-Health: A Theory of Nursing.*[42] Major concepts include imaging, valuing, languaging, revealing-concealing, enabling-limiting, connecting-separating, powering, originating, and transforming. Parse stresses humanism.

Interpersonal Relationships

Peplau; Travelbee; Orlando; Wiedenbach; King; Riehl-Sisca; Erickson, Tomlin, and Swain; and Barnard all address interpersonal relationships.

Hildegard E. Peplau's contributions to nursing in general and the specialty of psychiatric nursing specifically have been enormous. She has been publishing prolifically since the early 1950s, beginning with her book, *Interpersonal Relations in Nursing.*[41] She teaches psychodynamic nursing and stresses the importance of the nurse understanding his or her own behavior in order to help others identify perceived difficulties. She identifies four phases of the nurse-patient relationship: (1) orientation, (2) identification, (3) exploitation, and (4) resolution. Peplau describes six nursing roles: (1) stranger, (2) resource person, (3) teacher, (4) leader, (5) surrogate, and (6) counselor. She discusses four psychobiological experiences—needs, frustrations, conflicts, and anxieties—that compel destructive or constructive responses.

Joyce Travelbee published predominantly in the mid 1960s. She died in 1973 at a relatively young age. Travelbee promoted her Human-to-Human Relationship Model in her book, *Interpersonal Aspects of Nursing.*[50,51] She wrote about illness, suffering, pain, hope, communication, interaction, therapeutic use of self, empathy, sympathy, and rapport. She believed nursing was accomplished through human-to-human relationships that began with (1) the original encounter and then progressed through stages of (2) emerging identities, (3) developing feelings of empathy, and (4) later of sympathy, until (5) the nurse and patient attained a rapport in the final stage.

Ida Jean Orlando (Pelletier) first described her Disciplined Professional Response Theory in *The Dynamic Nurse-Patient Relationship*[40] and related research is reported in *The Discipline and Teaching of Nursing Process.*[41] Her theory stresses the reciprocal relationship between the nurse and the patient. Each is affected by what the other says and does. Orlando emphasizes the importance of exploring perceptions, thoughts, and feelings with the other party for verification. This process discipline or exploration validates the patient's need for help, which the nurse then meets directly or indirectly. Deliberative nursing actions purposefully identify and meet the patient's immediate need for help. If nursing actions are not deliberative, they are automatic and may not meet the patient's need for help.

Ernestine Wiedenbach, a maternity nurse, was stimulated by Orlando to think about the use of self and how thoughts and feelings affect a nurse's actions. She identifies and defines many concepts in her book, *Clinical Nursing: A Helping Art.*[56] Concepts and subconcepts include: patient, need-for-help, nurse, purpose, philosophy, practice (knowledge, judgment, and skills), ministration, validation, coordination (reporting, consulting, conferring), and art (stimulus, preconception, interpretation, and actions—rational, reactionary, and deliberative). Nurses need to identify the patient's need-for-help by (1) observing behaviors consistent or inconsistent with comfort, (2) exploring the meaning of patient's behavior with him, (3) determining the cause of the discomfort or incapability, and (4) determining if the person can resolve his problem or has a need-for-help. Next the nurse administers the help needed and validates that the need-for-help was met.

Imogene King has been publishing since the mid 1960s. *Toward a Theory for Nursing* was published in 1971,[22] and *A Theory for Nursing* was published in 1981.[23] Many of her publications have dealt with conceptual framework, models, theory, and specifically her theory of goal attainment. Her major concepts are interaction, perception, communication, transaction, role, stress, growth and development, and time and space. She suggests that the patient's and the nurse's perceptions, judgments, and actions lead to reaction, interaction, and transaction.

Joan Riehl Sisca began publishing in the mid 1970s. Her work on symbolic interactionism is presented in Riehl and Roy's book, *Conceptual Models for Nursing Practice.*[45] According to symbolic interactionism theory, people interpret each other's actions based on the meaning attached to the action before reacting. Human interaction is mediated by symbols, interpretation, and meaning, and is a process of interpretation between the stimulus and response.

Helen C. Erickson, Evelyn M. Tomlin, and *Mary Ann P. Swain's* book, *Modeling and Role-Modeling: A Theory and Paradigm for Nursing* was published in 1983.[11] Modeling is developing an understanding of the client's world. Role-modeling is the nursing intervention or nurturance that requires unconditional acceptance. Erickson, Tomlin, and Swain believe that while people are alike because of their holism, lifetime growth and development, and their affiliated individualism, they are also different because of inherent endowment, adaptation, and self-care knowledge.

Kathryn E. Barnard is an active researcher who has published prolifically about infants and children since the mid 1960s. She started by studying mentally and physically handicapped children and adults, moved into studying activities of the well child, and then expanded her work to include methods of evaluating growth and development of children and mother-infant relationships. She was also concerned about disseminating research and consequently developed the Nursing Child Satellite Training Project. While Barnard never intended to develop theory, the longitudinal nursing child assessment study provided the basis for her child health assessment interaction model. Barnard believes that the parent-infant system is influenced by individual characteristics of each member and that those characteristics are modified to meet the needs of the system by adaptive behavior.[4]

Systems

Johnson's, Roy's, and Neuman's works deal with systems.

Dorothy E. Johnson published from the mid 1940s to the early 1970s, with most of her work published during the 1960s. Johnson presented her Behavioral System Model in Riehl and Roy's book, *Conceptual Models for Nursing Practice*.[20] She identified six subsystems of the behavioral system: (1) attachment-affiliation, (2) achievement, (3) sexual, (4) ingestive-eliminative, (5) aggressive, and (6) dependency. Each subsystem can be analyzed in terms of structure and functional requirements. The four structural elements are: (1) drive or goal; (2) set, a predisposition to act; (3) choice, alternatives for action; and (4) behavior. The functional requirements are protection, nurturance, and stimulation. A need for nursing intervention exists if there is a state of instability in the behavioral system. The nurse needs to identify the source of the problem in the system and take appropriate nursing actions to maintain or restore the behavioral system balance.

Sister Callista Roy has been publishing prolifically since the late 1960s. She developed her adaptation model after being challenged by Johnson to develop a conceptual model for nursing. It is discussed at length in Roy's book, *Introduction to Nursing: An Adaptation Model*.[47,48] Major concepts include system, adaptation, stimuli, regulator, cognator, and adaptive modes—physiological, self-concept, role performance, and interdependence. Man's self and his environment are sources of focal, residual, and conceptual stimuli that create

needs for adaptaton. The four interrelated adaptive modes are physiological needs, self-concept, role function, and interdependence. The adaptation mechanisms are the regulator and the cognator. Adaptation maintains integrity. Roy believes people constantly scan the environment for stimuli so they can respond and adapt. The nurse is to help the person adapt by managing the environment.

Betty Neuman developed her first teaching/practice model for mental health consultation in the late 1960s. She designed the Systems Model in 1970 to help graduate students evaluate nursing problems. It was first published in *Nursing Research* in 1972[36] and further refined in the *Neuman Systems Model* in 1982.[35] Major concepts include total persons approach, holism, open-system, stressors, energy resources, lines of resistance, lines of defense, degree of reaction, interventions, levels of prevention, and reconstitution. Neuman believes the nurse should use purposeful interventions and a total person approach to help individuals, families, and groups reach and maintain wellness.

Energy Fields

Levine wrote about conservation of energy during the 1960s. Fitzpatrick's, Neuman's and Parse's work has been stimulated by Rogers.

Myra Estrin Levine started publishing in the mid 1960s. She has written about numerous topics. Never intending to develop theory, she wrote *Introduction to Clinical Nursing*[31,32] as a textbook to teach medical-surgical nursing to beginning students. Journal articles containing information about holism and the four conservation principles of nursing include "Adaptation and Assessment: A Rationale for Nursing Intervention,"[26] "The Four Conservative Principles of Nursing,"[27] "For Lack of Love Alone,"[28] "The Pursuit of Wholeness,"[29] and "Holistic Nursing."[30] More recently, Levine has given presentations about the conservation principles at nurse theory conferences, some of which have been audiotaped. Wholism, holism, integrity, and conservation are major concepts.

The nurse is to use the principles of conservation of (1) energy, (2) structural integrity, (3) personal integrity, and (4) social integrity to keep the holism of the individual balanced. Levine also identified four levels of organismic response—fear, inflammatory response, response to stress, and sensory response—and recommended trophicognosis, a scientific approach to determine nursing care, as an alternative to nursing diagnosis.

Martha E. Rogers is considered one of the most creative thinkers in nursing. She has published prolifically since the early 1960s. Her work regarding Unitary Human Beings is published in *An Introduction to the Theoretical Basis of Nursing*.[46] She characterizes life process by wholeness, openness, unidirectionality, pattern and organization, sentience, and thought. She also works with energy fields, open systems, and four-dimensionality. Her theory's principles were derived from the four concepts of energy fields, openness, pattern and organization, and four-dimensionality. The principles are: (1) complementarity, mutual and simultaneous movement of human and environmental fields; (2) resonancy, wave patterns that change from low frequency to higher frequency patterns; and (3) helicy, field changes characterized by increasing diversity of field patterns. Rogers has stimulated a number of other scholars including Fitzpatrick, Newman, and Parse.

Joyce J. Fitzpatrick derived her Life Perspective Model from Rogers' work. The major concepts are nursing, person, health, environment, temporal patterns, motion patterns, consciousness patterns, and perceptual patterns. She began publishing in 1970 and has written about aging, suicidology, temporal experience, and motor behavior.[13]

Margaret Newman started publishing in the mid 1960s. She has drawn from several fields of inquiry and was influenced by Johnson and Rogers. Her model appeared in *Theory Development in Nursing*[37] and has been explained further in subsequent chapters of various books. The major concepts in her model of health are movement, time, space, and consciousness.

They are all interrelated. "Movement is a reflection of consciousness. Time is a function of movement. Time is a measure of consciousness. Movement is a means whereby space and time become a reality."[37:60] Health is viewed as the expansion of consciousness and can encompass pathology.

EVALUATION OF THEORY DEVELOPMENT

Early nursing scholars dealt with the philosophy, definition, and art of nursing. Interpersonal communications received considerable attention during the 1960s. By the end of the decade the focus had shifted to the science of nursing. Humanism and nursing as an art and a science are gaining popularity during the 1980s.

The published works share some common themes. There is also evidence that scholars use the same or similar terms differently and have divergent views of nursing, environment, health, and person. Authors have also changed their views over time as their historical perspective changed. It is appropriate to analyze the previous work for themes, similarities, and differences to generate more ideas. Several middle and micro range theories are needed to direct our nursing practice. If, in fact, we develop generalizable theories about humanism, other disciplines should be able to borrow theory from nursing as we have borrowed theories from other disciplines.

REFERENCES

1. Adam, E. (1980). *To be a nurse.* New York: W.B. Saunders.
2. Abdellah, F.G., et al. (1960). *Patient-centered approaches to nursing.* New York: Macmillan.
3. Argyris, C., & Schon, D. (1974). *Theory in practice.* San Francisco: Jossey-Bass.
4. Barnard, K.E. (1978). Nursing child assessment and training: Learning resource manual.
5. Bush, H.A. (1979). Models for nursing. *Advances in Nursing Science, 1*(2):13-21.
6. Chinn, P., & Jacobs, M.K. (1979). A model for

theory development in nursing. *Advances in Nursing Science, 1*(1):1-11.

7. Chinn, P.L., & Jacobs, M.K. (1983). *Theory and nursing: A systematic approach.* St. Louis: C.V. Mosby.

8. DeTornyay, R. (1977, Nov.-Dec.). Nursing research: The road ahead. *Nursing Research, 26:*404-407.

9. Dickoff, J., James, P., & Wiedenbach, E. (1968). Theory in a practice discipline, Part I. Practice oriented theory. *Nursing Research, 17*(5):415-435.

10. Ellis, R. (1968). Characteristics of significant theories. *Nursing Research, 17*(5):217-222.

11. Erickson, H.D., Tomlin, E.M., & Swain, M.A. (1983). *Modeling and role-modeling: A theory and paradigm for nursing.* Englewood Cliffs, N.J.: Prentice-Hall.

12. Fawcett, J. (1980, June). A declaration of nursing independence: The relation of theory and research to nursing practice. *Journal of Nursing Administration, 10:*36-39.

13. Fitzpatrick, J., & Whall, A. (1983). *Conceptual models of nursing: Analysis and application.* Bowie, Md.: Robert J. Brady.

14. Hall, L.E. (1964, Feb.). Nursing: What is it? *The Canadian Nurse, 60:*150-154.

15. Hall, L.E. (1969). The Loeb Center for nursing and rehabiliation. *International Journal of Nursing Studies, 6:*81-95.

16. Hardy, M.E. (1978). Perspectives on nursing theory. *Advances in Nursing Science, 1:*37-48.

17. Hauner, B., & Henderson, V. (1955). *Textbook of the principles and practice of nursing.* New York: Macmillan.

18. Henderson, V. (1964, Aug.). The nature of nursing, *American Journal of Nursing, 64:*62-68.

19. Henderson, V. (1966). *The nature of nursing: A definition and its implications for practice, research, and education.* New York: Macmillan.

20. Johnson, D.E. (1980). The behavioral system model for nursing. In J.P. Riehl, & C. Roy (Eds.), *Conceptual models for nursing practice* (2nd ed.). New York: Appleton-Century-Crofts.

21. Kim, H.S. (1983). *The nature of theoretical thinking in nursing.* Norwalk, Conn.: Appleton-Century-Crofts.

22. King, I. (1971). *Toward a theory for nursing: General concepts of human behavior.* New York: John Wiley & Sons.

23. King, I. (1981). *A theory for nursing: Systems, concepts, process.* New York: John Wiley & Sons.

24. Lancaster, W., & Lancaster, J. (1981). Models and model building in nursing. *Advances in Nursing Science, 3:*31-42.

25. Leininger, M. (1985). *Transcultural care diversity and universality: A theory of care and nursing.* New York: Grune & Stratton.

26. Levine, M.E. (1966). Adaptation and assessment: A rationale for nursing intervention. *American Journal of Nursing, 66*(11):2450-2453.

27. Levine, M. (1967). The four conservation principles of nursing. *Nursing Forum, 6:*45.

28. Levine, M. (1967, Dec.). For lack of love alone. *Minnesota Nursing Accent, 39:*179.

29. Levine, M.E. (1969, Jan.). The pursuit of wholeness. *American Journal of Nursing, 69:*93.

30. Levine, M.E. (1971, June). Holistic nursing, *Nursing Clinics of North America, 6:*253.

31. Levine, M.E. (1969). *Introduction to clinical nursing.* Philadelphia: F.A. Davis.

32. Levine, M.E. (1973). *Introduction to clinical nursing* (2nd ed.). Philadelphia: F.A. Davis.

33. Merton, R. (1968). *Social theory and social structure.* New York: The Free Press.

34. Morris, W. (Ed.) (1978). *The American heritage dictionary of the English language.* Boston: Houghton Miffin.

35. Neuman, B. (1982). *The Neuman systems model: Application to nursing, education, and practice.* Norwalk, Conn.: Appleton-Century-Crofts.

36. Neuman, B.M., & Young, R.J. (1972, May-June). A model for teaching total person approach to patient problems. *Nursing Research, 21:*264-269.

37. Newman, M. (1980). *Theory development in nursing.* Philadelphia: F.A. Davis.

38. Nightingale, F. (1957). *Notes on nursing.* Philadelphia: Lippincott. (Originally published in 1859.)

39. Orem, D. (1985). *Nursing: Concepts of practice.* New York: McGraw-Hill.

40. Orlando, I. (1961). *The dynamic nurse-patient relationship.* New York: G.P. Putnam's Sons.

41. Orlando, I. (1972). *The discipline and teaching of nursing process.* New York: G.P. Putnam's Sons.

42. Parse, R.R. (1981). *Man-living-health: A theory of nursing.* New York: John Wiley & Sons.

43. Peplau, H. (1952). *Interpersonal relations in nursing.* New York: G.P. Putnam & Sons.

44. Reynolds, P.D. (1971). *A primer for theory construction.* Indianapolis: Bobbs-Merrill.

45. Riehl, J.P., & Roy, C. (Eds.). (1980). *Conceptual models for nursing practice* (2nd ed.). New York: Appleton-Century-Crofts.

46. Rogers, M.E. (1970). *An introduction to the theoretical basis of nursing*. Philadelphia: F.A. Davis.

47. Roy, C. (1976). *An introduction to nursing: An adaptation model*. Englewood Cliffs, N.J.: Prentice-Hall.

48. Roy, C. (1984). *An introduction to nursing: An adaptation model* (2nd ed.). Englewood Cliffs, N.J.: Prentice-Hall.

49. Stevens, B.J. (1984). *Nursing theory: Analysis, application, evaluation*. Boston: Little, Brown.

50. Travelbee, J. (1966). *Interpersonal aspects of nursing*. Philadelphia: F.A. Davis.

51. Travelbee, J. (1971). *Interpersonal aspects of nursing* (2nd ed.). Philadelphia: F.A. Davis.

52. Turner, J.H. (1982). *The structure of sociological theory*. Homewood, Ill.: The Dorsey Press.

53. Walker, L., & Avant, K. (1983). *Strategies for theory construction in nursing*. Norwalk, Conn.: Appleton-Century-Crofts.

54. Watson, J. (1979). *Nursing: The philosophy and science of caring*. Boston: Little, Brown.

55. Watson, J. (1985). *Nursing: Human science and health care*. Norwalk, Conn.: Appleton-Century-Crofts.

56. Wiedenbach, E. (1964). *Clinical nursing: A helping art*. New York: Springer.

Terminology of Theory Development

Juanita Fogel Keck

2

INTRODUCTION

Terms associated with theory and theory development have been used inconsistently in the nursing literature. Establishing the meanings of terms used in this book will enable the reader to gain a better understanding of the material covered. The definitions of terms used in this chapter represent those definitions accepted by a consensus of nursing theorists and noted philosophers of science.

In the interest of professionalism nursing leaders have suggested the discipline needs an identified body of knowledge that can be used to guide nursing practice. The terms *science, philosophy, theory,* and *paradigm* all relate to the development of an identified body of knowledge that can be recognized as associated with a particular scientific discipline.

SCIENCE

Science is defined both as a unified body of knowledge concerned with specific subject matter and as the skills and methodologies necessary to provide such knowledge. Therefore, nursing science is that knowledge germane to the discipline of nursing, plus the processes and methodologies used to gain that knowledge. A goal of science is the identification of truths or facts about the subject matter of a discipline—ascertaining the what, where, when, who, and how of phenemena of interest to that discipline.

KNOWLEDGE

The term *knowledge* suggests that science is composed of what one knows about the subject matter of a discipline. A distinction is made between what is known to be (fact) and what is believed to be. Knowledge is based on factual information. One derives a fact through the use of sound logic or empirical testing. Fact is truth supported by repeated observation and replication.[1]

Science is empirically based. Feigl[3] suggested a characteristic of science is that it is replicable by scientists within a discipline using the appropriate scientific methodologies. Replication requires that the components of phenomena studied to provide knowledge be observable and measureable. One acquires knowledge about things and events comprising the subject matter of interest through experience. Experiencing things or events requires the involvement of one or more of the human senses of sight, hearing, touch, taste, and smell. An empirical entity

15

is that which can be experienced through the human senses.

PHENOMENA

Phenomena comprise the subject matter of a discipline. *Webster's New Collegiate Dictionary* defines a phenomenon as "an object or aspect known through the senses rather than by thought or intuition, a fact or event of scientific interest susceptible to scientific description and explanation."[13:860] Science is composed of facts about phenomena of interest to a discipline. Facts are truths supported by empirical evidence.

PHILOSOPHY

Philosophy is concerned with judgments about components of science. Philosophical concerns are not empirically based. Components of a discipline that are not amenable to empirical testing are within the realm of philosophy. The "this we believe" statements associated with nursing practice contribute to the philosophy of the discipline. Statements that reflect values, goals, or opinions contribute to philosophy. It is the philosopher who suggests the methodologies by which scientific knowledge is obtained. Philosophical statements are based on opinion. They are by their very nature untestable because there is no definitive truth about them to discover. They cannot be tested for their correctness. They are accepted in a discipline through public affirmation. The prevailing philosophy of a discipline is the one shared by the greatest number of members in terms of accepting the beliefs, values, goals, and opinions of the philosophy.

THEORY

Although it is facts about phenomena of interest to the discipline that comprise the knowledge germane to the discipline, a mass of uncollated facts provides little guidance to the members of the discipline as they attempt to use that knowledge. The facts need to be ordered in a cohesive entity that will result in an organized body of knowledge. This will allow one to explain past events, provide a sense of understanding about current events, predict future events, and provide the potential for controlling them. If one can predict events, one has the basis for control of those events. Nursing intervention is served through the ability to predict and ultimately to control phenomena associated with health and health care.

It is through the construction of theories that such ordering occurs. Theories are models of empirical real world phenomena that identify the components or elements of the phenomena and the relationships between them. The functions of theory include summarization of knowledge, explanation of phenomena of interest to the discipline employing the theory, and provision of the means to predict and ultimately to control phenomena.[8] In fact, Theobald[11] suggested that only through theory is explanation or prediction possible.

Numerous definitions of theory exist in the literature. Most reflect an understanding of theory consistent with the following: Theory is a logically consistent set of propositions that presents a systematic view of a phenomenon. A proposition is composed of the elements of the phenomenon and the relationships between them. The elements or components of a phenomenon are the concepts necessary to understand the phenomenon. The concepts are linked by specific statements identifying how two or more concepts are related to each other to provide understanding about the phenomenon. Therefore theories are composed of statements that state specific relationships between two or more concepts.

CONCEPTS

Concepts are the subject matter of theory. They are symbolic representations of the things or events of which phenomena are composed. Concepts represent some aspect of reality that can be quantified. An example of concepts nec-

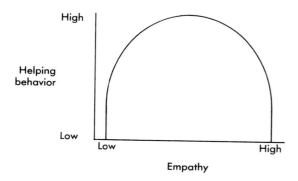

essary to explain a phenomenon is found in Hoffman's beginning theory of altruism.[5] Altruism is the phenomenon Hoffman has attempted to explain. One of the propositions of the theory is that helping behavior and empathy are related in a curvilinear manner. Both low and high levels of empathy are associated with low levels of helping behavior. Moderate empathy is associated with high level of helping. *Helping behavior* and *empathy* are the concepts comprising the proposition. To be able to ultimately explain altruism by means of this theory one must include empathy and helping behavior.

Dubin[2] categorized concepts into five groups—enumerative, associative, relational, statistical, and summative.

Enumerative Concepts

Enumerative concepts are characteristics of a phenomenon that are always present. The concept of *age* is an enumerative unit. Everyone to whom a theory incorporating age is generalizable is characterized by an age. The concept is universal to all persons in the population to which the theory applies. Age is always present in the phenomenon being explained. An enumerative concept cannot have a zero value. There is no such thing as an individual with zero age. As soon as an individual exists, his or her age can be ascertained.

Associative Concepts

Associative units are those concepts that can exist in only some conditions within the phenom-

enon.[2] Associative concepts can have a zero value. Persons to whom a theory composed of the concepts applies can exist with none of the concepts. Examples include income, presence of disease, and anxiety. It is possible to identify persons with no income in the population to which a theory incorporating income applies. Associative and enumerative units are the simplest, least complex forms of concepts.

Relational Concepts

Relational concepts are those characteristics of a phenomenon that can be understood only through the combination or interaction of two or more enumerative or associative concepts.[2] *Elderly* is a concept that cannot be understood without an understanding of the combination of age and *longevity*. *Mother* cannot exist without the interaction of *man, woman* and *birth*. Therefore both *elderly* and *mother* are relational concepts.

Statistical Concepts

Statistical concepts are those that relate the property of the thing being represented in terms of its distribution in the population.[2] *Average blood pressure* is an example of a statistical unit.

Summative Concepts

Summative concepts are the most complex. Dubin[2] suggested summative concepts were global units that represented an entire complex entity or phenomenon. Four concepts—nursing, man, health, and environment—have been identified by numerous nurse authors and theorists as the concepts of primary concern for the discipline of nursing. They are readily identifiable as summative concepts because each represents a global and extremely complex entity.

Dubin[2] suggested many problems exist when summative concepts are used within a theory. An entire phenomenon is explained by the use of one or two words. Each summative concept is composed of numerous enumerative, associative, and relational concepts and their interactions, but none are named or defined. One can only assume which of these less complex concepts contribute to the summative unit, how they interact, and under what conditions they contribute to the phenomenon.

Dubin[2] said that summative concepts have little utility in theory development because the concepts cannot be adequately defined and the interactions between them are not readily ascertainable. For a theory to be useful in aiding the attainment of the goals of science, it must contribute to understanding, explanation, prediction, and ultimately control. Before prediction and control are possible, the theory must be testable. One can only predict future events if the proposed relationships between concepts have been repeatedly supported by empirical findings. In other words, the real world correlates of the concepts have been measured and the relationships between them verified. If such relationships have been repeatedly verified in the past, one can predict the relationship between the concepts will hold true in the future. Summative units are not measureable. How would one measure environment as a totality? One is usually interested in individual components of environment and their interactions with some specific attributes of human beings. One may be interested in a theory that states a person's recovery from illness is related to environment. However, the theory is not useful to one concerned with a specific attribute of humans, such as *recovery,* unless specific aspects of the environment that influence recovery and their interactions are stated. A useful theory then would be composed of the less complex concepts that refer to the specific environmental attributes rather than the totality of the environment. Concepts must be clearly definable and measureable to be of use to the practicing nurse in the clinical setting.

DEFINITIONS

Concepts are abstract symbols of the real world. They are mental representations constructed in language terms. The concepts of a theory reflect the theorist's own individual perception and definition of reality that the concept is supposed to represent. The concept may be open to many interpretations. Different individuals may hold differing understandings of the meanings of the words used to convey conceptual aspects of the real world. Definitions supplied by the theorist are needed so the user of theory can know what the theorist means by the concept. It is the theorist's meaning that must be used in the theory he or she developed. Therefore, the user of theory must know the meaning intended by the author.

Two classifications of definitions are associated with theory. *Conceptual definitions* relate the general meaning of the concept. *Operational definitions* identify an empirical referent for the concept. For example, *pain* may be conceptually defined as a subjective experience perceived as unpleasant initiated by potentially damaging stimuli but influenced by affective variables. It may be operationally defined as the score obtained on a 10 cm visual analogue scale in which zero represents no pain and ten represents the worst pain imaginable.

0	10
No pain	Worst pain imaginable

Scores are obtained by asking subjects to place a mark on the line to represent the severity of their pain. The resulting score is observable and is therefore an empirical referent for the subject's pain. The score is the operational definition for pain.

An additional classification of definitions may be considered. Definitions may be classified as either denotative or connotative. *Denotative definitions* define concepts in terms of what the concept is or represents. A denotative definition of father is *male parent.* Father is the male parent. A *connotative definition* suggests or implies associations one might make with the concept. A connotative definition suggests what one might think of when considering the term *father.* A connotative definition of father is *strong, provider, disciplinarian,* that is, terms that are associated with *father.*

RELATIONSHIP STATEMENTS

Concepts alone do not create theory. A theory does not exist until the specific relationships between concepts comprising the theory are expressed in relationship statements. Several labels for relationship statements may be found in the literature related to theory. Relationship statements may be classified as propositions, hypotheses, empirical generalizations, laws, axioms, or theorems. Nursing and philosophical theorists essentially agree that all relationship statements, regardless of classification, indicate specific relationships between two or more concepts. Examples of relationship statements include the following:

If one has a family history of Alzheimer's disease *then there is a specific probability that* one will develop Alzheimer's disease.

Tissue damage *is the antecedent of* pain perception.

Learning ability *varies* with anxiety *in a curvilinear relationship.*

Job satisfaction *is a function of* the fit between the job environment and the individual's personality.

Anxiety and accurate information about a diagnostic procedure *are negatively related.*

The goals of science are to aid in understanding, explaining, predicting, and controlling phenomena. These goals are achieved through the relationships proposed by theory. Meeting these goals requires that *specific* relationships between concepts be clearly stated. Simply stating that anxiety and learning ability are related is insufficient. For the theory to be useful one needs to understand how and under what conditions they are related. Stating there is a curvilinear relationship between anxiety and learning provides the practitioner with information that may allow the prediction of situations in which one is most or least able to learn. The practitioner responsible for developing and implementing a teaching program for home care following myocardial infarction would be directed to implement the program during periods of moderate anxiety for the recipients of the program rather than during periods of low or high anxiety.

Laws

Differences between classifications of relationship statements appear to reflect the abstractness of the concepts included in the statements and the amount of empirical support derived through testing the proposed relationship. Laws, empirical generalizations, and hypotheses are classifications of statements that include relatively concrete concepts.[4,9,12] The concepts incorporated in these statements represent things or events observable in the real world. Because they are observable, they can provide measures that are valid indicators of the concept. Laws and empirical generalizations are found primarily in disciplines, such as chemistry and physics, that deal with readily observable and measureable phenomena. They differ in the amount of empirical support that has been generated for the proposition. Boyle's law states that when temperature is held constant, the volume of a gas is inversely proportional to the pressure exerted on it. The statement suggests volume is influenced by the variables of temperature and pressure. To determine the influence of pressure alone, one must control for the influence of temperature. Because current technology makes temperature and pressure readily manipulatable, a researcher can control for the influence of temperature by holding temperature constant. Then by measuring volume and pressure he or she determines the influence of pressure changes on volume. If volume repeatedly and invariably decreases when pressure is increased, a law regarding the influence of pressure upon gas volume becomes tenable. A great deal of empirical support can be generated for the proposition.

Empirical Generalizations

Empirical generalizations differ from laws only in the amount of empirical support generated for the proposed relationship statements. Laws have overwhelming support; empirical generalizations have moderate support. The problem in classifying statements is deciding when moderate support becomes overwhelming support. The decision is a philosophical one and is arrived at through agreement among scientists in a discipline.

Hypotheses

Hypotheses differ from empirical generalizations and laws again in the amount of empirical support generated. Hypotheses are the first tentative suggestions a specific relationship exists. As a hypothesis is repeatedly confirmed, it progresses to an empirical generalization and ultimately to a law. The words used in the proposition may not change. Boyle's law was Boyle's hypothesis and Boyle's empirical generalization before being accepted as a law within disciplines using the relationship.

Axioms and Theorems

Axioms and theorems are relationship statements that include abstract concepts—concepts that relate mental images of entities not readily observable. Theories emanating from the social sciences contain primarily axioms and theorems. Concepts such as anxiety, job satisfaction, learning ability, and personality are abstractions in the real world. They are neither directly observable nor measureable. Therefore they would be amenable to incorporation in either a theorem or axiom.

Axioms and theorems differ in the degree of generality incorporated in the relationship. Axioms state the most general relationship between concepts. Theorems emanate from axioms. An example of a statement that could be an axiom is "Anxiety is negatively related to accurate information about a diagnostic procedure." The statement allows for the full range of possible values associated with each concept.

A theorem suggests that a specific range of values of one concept is associated with a specific range of values of the other. An example of a possible theorem would be "Low levels of anxiety are associated with a high degree of accurate information about a diagnostic procedure."

Relationship statements become an axiom or theorem through the mechanism of empirical support. A statement is not referred to as an axiom unless it has been subjected to considerable testing and repeatedly supported. However, neither axioms nor theorems are directly testable. They have no directly observable empirical referent to be measured. Hypotheses provide the mechanism for testing them. Previously it was suggested that a hypothesis is a statement of relationship between concrete measurable entities for which little empirical support has been generated. Hypotheses must also be the antecedents of axioms and theorems. The abstract concepts must be operationalized to provide an empirical referent for each. Relationships are then tested by means of the empirical referent. A previous example included a visual analogue scale to measure pain. The scale and the resulting score provide an empirical referent for the abstract concept *pain*. One cannot directly observe pain, but one can see the scale and the score used to represent it. Hypotheses are used to test propositions incorporating abstract concepts regardless of the previous empirical support for the proposed relationships among concepts.

The discussion concerning differing classifications of relationship statements is provided to explain terms often used in the literature germane to theory development. They differ primarily in degree of abstractness and amount of empirical support. The components of the statements, concepts, and specified relationships between them may not differ. One can conclude that although the classification of relationship statements may differ among scientists, there is general agreement as to the structure of the statements. Relationship statements must include appropriate concepts that have been clearly defined, and the specific relationships among those concepts must also be clearly stated.

ASSOCIATIONAL OR CAUSAL STATEMENTS

Relationship statements are generally considered to be of two types, associational and causal process.

Associational Relationship Statements

Associational relationship statements assert that values of one concept are associated with values of another. Linear and curvilinear are the two general types of associational relationships. If the relationship is linear, three possibilities exist. There may be a positive relationship, a negative relationship, or no relationship among the concepts.[9] In a linear relationship, the direction of the relationship is established in the relationship statement. If the relationship is curvilinear, such is stated in the relationship statement. An example of an associational relationship statement is "Anxiety is negatively related to the degree of accurate information one has about a diagnostic procedure." If one knows a category of values for one variable, one can infer a category of values for another. Relationship statements found in the social sciences are primarily of the associational form.

Causal Relationship Statements

Causal relationship statements state that one concept is the cause of another. Boyle's law is an example of a causal relationship statement. When temperature is held constant, a change in pressure causes an inverse change in the volume of gas. For every value of pressure there is an exact value for volume. If one knows the value for pressure, one can determine the exact value for volume.

ASSUMPTIONS

Assumptions are beliefs about phenomena one must accept as true in order to accept a theory about the phenomena as true. They are not tested but are assumed to represent reality. An example of assumptions can be found in Selye's theory of human stress.[10] Selye proposed a theory of stress based on animal studies. The theory was to operate within the realm of human stress and was to reflect the totality of the stress experience. The theory requires several assumptions before one can accept it as an explanation of the totality of human stress. One must first accept the assumption that results of animal studies are completely generalizable to humans and that the stress measured in rodents is the same as the stress experienced by humans. In addition, the theory suggests that human stress is mediated by stress energy that enables one to handle that stress. A major assumption of the theory is that everyone is born with a finite amount of stress energy and death ensues when the energy is depleted. The assumption is not testable because the amount of stress energy one might have throughout life is not measureable; it is a belief one must accept before accepting Selye's theory as an appropriate and adequate explanation of total human stress.

MODEL

The term *model* is often used in nursing literature. A model is a schematic representation of some aspects of reality. Theories are models of some phenomenon. Models fall into two broad classifications, theoretical and empirical. *Empirical models* are replicas of observable reality. A plastic model of the heart is an empirical model. *Theoretical models* are representatives of the real world expressed in language or mathematical symbols. Theories are theoretical models of reality, often a reality that is not directly observable. Models are useful in theory development because they aid in the selection of relevant concepts necessary to represent a phenomenon of interest and the determination of the relationships among the concepts. Models also allow manipulation of concepts on paper before testing in the real world. In addition, models aid theory users by providing an observable explanation of theory components. Although all theories are models, not all models are theories.

RANGE OF THEORIES

Theories differ in complexity and scope along a continuum from micro theories to grand theories. *Micro theories* are the least complex. They contain the least complex concepts and refer to specific, easily defined phenomena. They are narrow in scope because they attempt to explain a small aspect of reality. They are primarily composed of enumerative or associative concepts. *Grand theories* are the most complex and broadest in scope. They attempt to explain broad areas within a discipline. They are composed of summative concepts and incorporate numerous narrower range theories. Middle range theories fall somewhere between. They are primarily composed of relational concepts. The domain represented by mid range theory is not so large as to be useless to the user as summative concepts are useless. But neither do middle range theories represent such a narrow aspect of reality that they cannot be used in the more complex realm of real life.

Partial theories are theories in the developmental stage. In a partial theory some concepts necessary to explain a phenomenon have been identified and some relationships have been identified between them, but the theory is not complete. A criterion of a complete theory is that the concepts and proposed relationships must be exhaustive. That is, every thing or event comprising the phenomenon is represented in the theory. Theories derived from the social sciences, including nursing, are probably exclusively partial theories because there are few, if any, phenomena that have been totally and completely explained.

PARADIGM

Science, philosophy, and theory are all components of the domain of any scientific discipline. *Paradigm* is a term used to denote the prevailing network of science, philosophy, and theory accepted by a discipline. Current interest in paradigmatic issues stems from the work of Kuhn.[6] Kuhn defined a paradigm to reflect his belief that a paradigm was synonymous with the scientific community or community of individuals comprising discipline. The term was meant to refer to what members of the community have in common.[7] Included in the matrix shared by the scientific community are the knowledge, philosophy, theory, educational experience, practice orientation, research methodology, and literature identified with the discipline. The prevailing paradigm directs the activities of a discipline. As such, it is accepted by the majority of individuals within the discipline and suggests the areas of study of interest to the discipline and the means to study them. Nursing literature includes numerous references to conceptual models and conceptual frameworks. I believe these terms are synonymous with *paradigm.*

SUMMARY

This chapter has been concerned with the terminology associated with theory development. Science, theory, philosophy, and paradigm have been addressed. In addition, terms necessary for a clearer understanding of these terms have been included. Fact, phenomenon, concepts, definitions, categories of concepts, relationship statement, law, empirical generalization, theorem, axiom, hypothesis, associational relationship statement, causal process relationship statement, assumption, model, and range of theories have been considered. I hope this discussion will allow a clearer understanding of the theoretical work addressed on the following pages.

REFERENCES

1. Brodbeck, M. (1953). The nature and function of the philosophy of science. In H. Feigl & M. Brodbeck (Eds.), *Readings in the philosophy of science.* New York: Appleton-Century-Crofts.
2. Dubin, R. (1978). *Theory building* (Rev. ed.). New York: The Free Press.
3. Feigl, H. (1953). The scientific outlook: naturalism and humanism. In H. Feigl and M. Brodbeck (Eds.) *Readings in the philosophy of science.* New York: Appleton-Century-Crofts.
4. Hardy, M.E. (1973). The nature of theories. In M. Hardy (Ed.), *Theoretical foundation for nursing.* New York: MSS Corp.
5. Hoffman, M.L. (1981). Is altruism part of human nature? *Journal of Personality and Social Psychology, 40:*126-131.
6. Kuhn, T.S. (1970). *The structure of scientific revolutions.* Chicago: University of Chicago Press.
7. Kuhn, T.S. (1974). Second thoughts on paradigms. In F. Suppe (Ed.), *The structure of scientific theories.* Urbana: University of Illinois Press.
8. Mehlberg, H. (1962). The theoretical and empirical aspects of science. In E. Nagel, P. Suppes and A. Tarski (Eds.), *Logic, methodology and philosophy of science.* Stanford: Stanford University Press.
9. Reynolds, P.D. (1971). *A primer in theory construction.* Indianapolis: Bobbs-Merrill.
10. Selye, H. (1956). *The stress of life.* New York: McGraw-Hill.
11. Theobald, D.W. (1968). *An introduction to philosophy of science.* London: Methuen.
12. Wartofsky, M.W. (1968). *Conceptual foundations of scientific thought and introduction to the philosophy of science.* New York: MacMillan.
13. *Webster's New Collegiate Dictionary* (1976). Springfield, Mass.: Merriam.

History and Philosophy of Science

Sue Marquis Bishop

3

Modern science is a relatively new intellectual activity. Established as recently as 400 years ago, it has occupied only a short span of time in the history of humankind.[2] Scientific activity has persisted because it has improved the quality of life while satisfying human needs for creative work, a sense of order, and the desire to understand the unknown.[2,8,16] If we are interested in understanding, predicting, or controlling a given phenomenon, or in describing what we know in science, we are seeking a theory.[19,29] The development of science thus requires the *formalization* of the phenomena and events with which each science is concerned.[27] The construction of nursing theories is the formalization of attempts to describe, explain, predict, or control states of affairs in nursing.

HISTORICAL VIEWS OF THE NATURE OF SCIENCE

If we are interested in formalizing the science of nursing, we must consider such basic questions as: What is science? What is to be regarded as knowledge? What is truth? What are the methods by which scientific knowledge can be produced? These are philosophical questions. The term *epistemology* is concerned with the theory of knowledge in philosophical in-

quiry. The particular philosophical perspective selected to answer these questions will influence how scientists choose to carry out scientific activities, how they interpret outcomes, and even what they regard as science and knowledge.[3:8] Although philosophy as an activity has been documented for 3000 years, formal science is a relatively new human pursuit.[8] Only recently has scientific activity itself become the object of investigation.[3]

Two competing theories of science have evolved (with several variations) in the era of modern science: *rationalism* and *empiricism*.[8] Gale[8] labeled these alternative epistemologies as centrally concerned with the "power of reason" and the "power of sensory experience." He noted some similarity in the divergent views of science in the time of the classical Greeks. For example, Aristotle believed advances in biological science would develop through systematic observation of objects and events in the natural world, whereas Pythagorus believed knowledge of the natural world would develop from mathematical reasoning.

Rationalism

Rationalist epistemology emphasizes the importance of a priori reasoning as the appropriate method for advancing knowledge. The scientist in this tradition approaches the task of scientific inquiry by developing a systematic explanation (theory) of a given phenomenon.[8] This conceptual system is analyzed by addressing the logical structure of the theory and the logical reasoning involved in its development. Theoretical assertions, derived by deductive reasoning, are then subjected to experimental testing to corroborate the theory. Reynolds[19] labeled this approach the "theory-then-research" strategy. If the research findings fail to correspond with the theoretical assertions, additional research is conducted or modifications are made in the theory and further tests devised, or the theory is discarded in favor of an alternative explanation.[8,29]

Popper[17] argued that science would evolve more rapidly through the process of conjectures and refutations in which new ideas are formulated and research devised to attempt to refute them.

The rationalist view is most clearly evident in the work of the theoretical physicist, Einstein, who made extensive use of mathematical equations in developing his theories. The theories Einstein constructed offered an "imaginative framework," which has directed research in numerous areas.[4] As Reynolds[19] noted, if one believes that science is a process of *"inventing* descriptions of phenomena," the appropriate strategy for theory construction is the theory-then-research strategy. In Reynolds' view:[19:145]

> As the continuous interplay between theory construction (invention) and testing with empirical research progresses, the theory becomes more precise and complete as a description of nature and, therefore, more useful for the goals of science.

Empiricism

The empiricist view is based on the central idea that scientific knowledge can only be derived from sensory experience. Francis Bacon (c. 1620) is given credit for popularizing the basis for the empiricist approach to inquiry.[8] Bacon believed scientific truth was discovered by the generalization of observed facts in the natural world. This approach, which has been called the *inductive* method, is based on the idea that collection of facts precedes attempts to formulate generalizations—the "research-then-theory" approach.[19]

The strict empiricist view is reflected in the work of the behaviorists, Watson and Skinner. In a 1950 paper, Skinner[21] asserted that advances in the science of psychology could be expected if scientists would focus on the collection of empirical data. He cautioned against the drawing of premature inferences and proposed a moratorium on theory building until further facts were collected. Skinner's approach to theory construction was clearly an inductive one. His view of science and the popularity of behaviorism have been credited with influencing the shift in emphasis in psychology during the 1950s to 1970s from theory construction to fact gathering.[22] The difficulty with the inductive mode of inquiry is the world presents an infinite number of possible observations. Therefore the scientist must "bring ideas to experiences" to decide what to observe and what to exclude.[23] Although Skinner disclaimed in his early writings to be developing a theory, Bixenstine[1:465] noted:

> Skinner is startlingly creative in applying the conceptual elements of his—let's be frank—*theory* to a wide variety of issues, ranging from training pigeons in the guidance of missiles, to developing teaching machines, to constructing a model society.

During the first half of this century, philosophers focused on the analysis of the structure of theories, while scientists focused on empirical research. There was minimal interest in the history of science, the nature of scientific discovery, or the similarities between the philosophic view of science and scientific methods.[3] Positivism, a term first used by Comte, emerged as the dominant view of modern science.[8] Modern logical positivists believed empirical research and logical analysis were the two approaches that would produce scientific knowledge. The system of symbolic logic, published in 1910-1913 by Whitehead and Russell, was hailed by the logical positivists as an appropriate approach to discovering truth.[3]

The logical empiricists, offering a more lenient view of logical positivism, argued that theoretical propositions must be able to be tested through observation and experimentation.[3] This perspective is rooted in the idea that empirical facts exist independently of theories and offer the only possible basis for objectivity in science.[3] In other words, objective truth exists in the world, independent of the researcher; the task of science is to discover it. The empiricist view shares similarities with Aristotle's view of biological science and Bacon's inductive method as the true method of scientific inquiry.[8] Gale[8] argued that this view of science is often presented in methodology courses as the "single orthodox view" of the scientific enterprise. In his words, this view is taught in the following manner:

> The scientist first sets up an experiment; observes what occurs . . . ; reaches a preliminary hypothesis to describe the occurrence; runs further experiments to test the hypothesis (and) finally corrects or modifies the hypothesis in light of the results.[8:13]

The increasing use of computers permitting the analysis of large data sets may have contributed to the acceptance of the positivist approach to modern science.[22] In the 1950s however, the literature began to reflect an increasing challenge to the positivist view, thereby ushering in a new view of science.[2]

EMERGENT VIEWS OF SCIENCE AND THEORY

In recent years, several authors have presented analyses challenging the positivist position, thus offering the basis for a new perspective of science.[7,10,13,25] In 1977, Brown[3] argued there was a new intellectual revolution in philosophy

that emphasized the *history of science,* replacing formal logic as the major analytical tool in philosophy of science. One of the major perspectives in the new philosophy was the focus on science as a *process of continuing research,* as opposed to the emphasis on accepted findings. In this emergent epistemology, the emphasis was on understanding scientific discovery and the processes involved in changes in theories over time. In 1966, Foucault[7] published his analysis (in French) of the epistemology of human sciences from the seventeenth to the nineteenth centuries. His major thesis was that empirical knowledge was arranged in different patterns at a given time and in a given culture. He found changes over time in the focus of inquiry, in what was regarded as scientific knowledge, and in how knowledge was organized. Further, he concluded that humans only recently emerged as objects of study. Schutz[20] in his *Phenomenology of the Social World,* argued that scientists seeking to understand the social world cannot cognitively know an external world, independent of their own life experiences.

Empiricists argue that in order for science to maintain objectivity, data collection and analysis must be independent of theory.[3] This assertion is based on the position that objective truth exists in the world, waiting to be discovered. Brown[3] argued that the new epistemology challenged the empiricist view of perception by acknowledging that theories play a significant role in determining what the scientist will observe and how it will be interpreted. A story related to me by my grandmother illustrates Brown's thesis that observations are "concept-laden," that is, what one observes is influenced by ideas in the mind of the observer:

> A husband and wife are sitting by the fire silently watching their firstborn son asleep in the cradle. The mother looks at her infant son and imagines him learning to talk and then to walk. She continues her reverie by imagining him playing with friends, coming home from school, then going to college. She ends her daydreaming by visualizing him elected President of the United States. She

smiles and glances up at her husband who also had been staring intently at their son, "What are you thinking, honey?" The husband replies, "I was just thinking that I can't imagine how anyone could build a fine cradle like this and sell it for $5.98 and still make a profit."

Brown[3] presented the example of a chemist and a child walking together past a steel mill. The chemist perceived the odor of sulfur dioxide, while the child smelled rotten eggs. Each of them responded to the same observable data with distinctly different cognitive interpretations. In teaching nurses to be family therapists, I frequently use videotapes of family therapy sessions for students to analyze as we progress through the study of different approaches to family therapy. Novice student therapists tend to focus on the content of family interaction (what one member says to another) or the behavior of individual family members. Following the study of the *systems view* of families, and pointing out examples of patterned transactions among family members, during the second viewing students can "see" and describe transactions among family members they did not perceive during the first viewing (the son withdrawing when his parents argue or the wife gritting her teeth when her husband talks, for example). Concepts and theories create boundaries for selecting phenomena to observe and for reasoning about specific patterns. For example, the concept *social network* may be more fruitful for studying social relations than the concept *group* because it focuses attention on a more complex set of relationships beyond the boundaries of any one setting.[12]

If, however, scientists perceive patterns in the empirical world based on their presupposed theories, how can new patterns ever be perceived or new discoveries formulated? Gale[8] answers by arguing that the scientist is able to perceive "forceful intrusions" from the environment that challenge his or her "a priori mental set," thus raising questions in regard to the current theoretical perspective. Brown[3] maintained

that while a presupposed theoretical framework influences perception, theories are not the single determining factor of the scientist's perception. He identified three different views of the relationships of theories to observation:

1. Scientists are merely passive observers of occurrences in the empirical world. Observable data are objective truth, waiting to be discovered.
2. Theories structure what the scientist perceives in the empirical world.
3. Presupposed theories and observable data *interact* in the process of scientific investigation.

Brown's argument for an interactionist's perspective coincides with scientific consensus in the study of pattern recognition in human information processing. Two distinct mini theories have directed research efforts in this area: the data-driven or bottom-up theory and the conceptually driven or top-down theory. In the former, cognitive expectations (what is known or ways of organizing meaning) are used to select input and process incoming information from the environment. The second theory asserts that incoming data are perceived as unlabeled input and analyzed as raw data with increasing levels of complexity until all the data are classified. Current research evidence suggests human pattern recognition progresses by an interaction of both data-driven and conceptually driven processes, using sources of information in both currently organized cognitive categories and stimuli from the sensory environment.[15] The interactionist's perspective also is clearly reflected in Piaget's theory of human cognitive functioning:

Piagetian man actively selects and interprets environmental information in the construction of his own knowledge rather than passively copying the information just as it is presented to his senses. While paying attention to and taking account of the structure of the environment during knowledge seeking, Piagetian man reconstrues and reinterprets that environment [according to] his own

ork. . . . The mind neither copies
nor does it ignore the world [by]
: mental conception of it out of
. . . The mind meets the environ-
. in an extremely active, self-directed way.[6:6]

If we are to accept the thesis that no objective truth exists, and that science is an interactive process between "invented" theories and empirical observations, how are scientists to determine truth and scientific knowledge? In the new epistemology, science is viewed as an ongoing process and much importance is given to the idea of consensus among scientists. As Brown[3] concluded, we must forego the myth that science can establish "final truths," and accept the notion that tentative consensus based on reasoned judgments about the available evidence is the most that can be expected. In this view of science, scientific knowledge is what the community of scientists in any given historical era regard as such. The truth of a given theoretical statement is determined by current consensus among scientists as to whether it presents an "adequate description of reality."[3] This consensus is possible through the collaboration of many scientists, in making their work available for public review and debate and building on previous inquiries.[18] "The individual (scientist) *introduces* ideas, the scientific community *appraises* them" by its objective criteria.[18:59]

Science in any given era and in any given discipline is structured by an accepted set of presuppositions that define the phenomena to study and the appropriate methods for data collection and interpretation.[3] These presuppositions set the boundaries for the scientific enterprise. In Brown's view of the transactions between theory and empirical observation:

> Theory determines what observations are worth making and how they are to be understood, and observation provides challenges to accepted theoretical structures. The continuing attempt to produce a coherently organized body of theory and observation is the driving force of research, and the prolonged failure of specific research projects leads to scientific revolutions.[3:167]

The presentation and acceptance of a revolutionary theory may alter the existing presuppositions and theories, thereby creating a different set of boundaries and procedures. The result is a new set of problems or a new way to interpret observations, that is, a new picture of the world.[13] It is crucial that the emphasis in this view of science be on ongoing research rather than on established findings.

THEORY AND RESEARCH

Traditionally, theory building and research have been presented to students in separate courses. This separation has often resulted in problems for students in understanding the nature of theories and in comprehending the relevance of research efforts.[28] The acceptance of the positivist view of science may have influenced the sharp distinction between theory and research methods.[8] Although theory and research can be viewed as distinct operations, they are more appropriately regarded as interdependent components of the scientific process.[5] In constructing a theory, the theorist must be knowledgeable about available empirical findings and attempt to take these into account, since theory is, in part, concerned with the formalization of available knowledge.[29] The theory also is subject to revision if the hypotheses fail to correspond to empirical findings, or the theory may be abandoned in favor of an alternative explanation that accounts for the new information.[3,5,19]

In contemporary theories of science, the scientific enterprise has been described as a series of phases, with emphasis on the *discovery* and *verification* (or acceptance) phases.[8,9] Gale[8] described these phases as primarily concerned with the presentation and testing of new ideas. Discovery is the phase during which new ways of thinking about phenomena or new data are introduced to the scientific community. The focus during this time is on presenting a persuasive argument that the new conceptions represent an improvement over previous conceptions.[8] Verification is characterized by efforts in the scientific community to critically analyze and test the new conceptions in an attempt to refute them. During this time the new views are "put through the trial by fire."[8] Brown[3] argued, however, that discovery and verification cannot really be viewed as sharply distinct phases because a new conception is not usually accepted by the scientific community until it has "passed enough tests" to warrant acceptance as a new discovery.

At this point it should be clear that it is not appropriate in a scientific discipline to judge a theory on the basis of "authority, faith, or intuition," rather than on the basis of *scientific consensus.*[18] For example, if a specific nursing theory is to be determined acceptable, this judgment should not be made because a respected nursing leader advocates the theory. Neither should personal feelings about the theory, such as, "I like this theory" or "I don't like this one," provide the basis for the judgment. The only defensible reason for judging a theory acceptable is on the basis of logical and conceptual or empirical grounds. These judgments are made by the scientific community.[2]

The advancement of science is a collaborative endeavor in which many researchers evaluate and build upon one another's work. In order for evidence to be cumulative, theories, procedures, and findings from empirical studies must be made available for critical review by scientists. In this way, the same procedures can be used to support or refute a given analysis or finding.[18] A theory is accepted when the consensus among scientists is the theory provides an "adequate description of reality."[3] The acceptance of a scientific hypothesis depends on the appraisal of the *coherence* of theory, which involves questions of logic, and the *correspondence* of the theory, which involves efforts to relate the theory to observable phenomena through research.[24] Gale[8] labeled these criteria as epistemological and metaphysical concerns. The consensus of correspondence of the theory with reality is not based on a single study. Repeated testing is crucial, replicating the study

under the same conditions and exploring the theoretical assertions under different conditions, or with different measures. Consensus is therefore based on accumulated evidence.[9] Even when the theory does not appear to be supported by research, it is not necessarily rejected by the scientific community. Rather than an automatic agreement there is a problem with the theory itself, there may be judgments made about the validity or reliability of the measures used in testing the theory or in the appropriateness of the research design. These possibilities are considered in critically evaluating attempts to test a given theory.

Dubin[5] identified three areas in which scientific consensus is necessary in regard to any given theory: (1) agreement on the boundaries of the theory (the phenomenon it addresses and the phenomena it excludes), (2) agreement on the logic used in constructing the theory so meanings can be understood from a similar perspective, and (3) agreement that the theory fits the data collected and analyzed through research. Consensus in these three areas essentially constitutes agreement among scientists to "look at the same 'things,' to do so in the same way, and to have a level of confidence certified by an empirical test."[5:13] Therefore the theory must be capable of being operationalized for testing in order to check the theory against reality. In the process of science, retroductive, deductive, and inductive forms of reasoning may be used as science progresses by building theoretical descriptions and explanations of reality, attempting to account for available findings, deriving testable hypotheses, and evaluating theories from the perspective of new empirical data.[24]

Most research can be considered to be in the category Kuhn[13] described as *normal science.* Scientific inquiry in normal science involves testing a given theory, developing new applications of theory, or extending a given theory. Occasionally a new theory with different assumptions is developed that seeks to replace previous theories. Kuhn[13] described this as *rev-*

olutionary science, and the theory with different presuppositions as a revolutionary theory.

A change in the accepted presuppositions creates a different set of boundaries and procedures that suggest a new set of problems or a new way to interpret observations.[13] Currently, there is some challenge in the social and behavioral sciences to the assumptions underlying accepted methods of experimental design, measurement, and statistical analysis that emphasize the search for universal laws and the use of procedures for random assignment of subjects across contexts.[14] Mishler[14] argues that scientists should develop methods and procedures for studying behavior as dependent on context for meaning, rather than eliminating context by searching for laws that hold across contexts. This critique of the methods and assumptions of research is emerging from phenomenological and ethnomethodological theorists who view the scientific process from a very different paradigm.[11,14,26]

The proper focus of research is not to attempt to prove a theory or hypothesis, but to attempt to set up research to refute a given hypothesis.[17] Failure of repeated attempts at refutation lend support to the theory and acceptance of the theory by the scientific community.[5] The emphasis, however, is always on ongoing research rather than established findings.[3] In the future new information or a new compelling way to view the same evidence may lead to a reappraisal of the theory. One previously accepted theory may be abandoned for another theory if it fails to correspond to empirical findings or if it no longer presents clear directions for further research. The theory selected as an alternative is judged by the scientific community to account for available data and to suggest further lines of inquiry.[3]

Popper[17] observed that, unfortunately, refutations of a given theory are frequently viewed as a failure of the theorist or of the theory. In his view:

> Every refutation should be regarded as a great success; not merely as a success of the scientist who refuted the theory, but also of the scientist who created the refuted theory and who thus . . . suggested, if only indirectly, the refutation experiment.[17:243]

If a theoretical hypothesis fails to account for the observed facts in the world, one explanation is eliminated and science is thus advanced.[26]

Finally, the process of scientific inquiry may be viewed as a social enterprise.[14] In Gale's words, "Human beings *do* science."[8:290] It therefore might be anticipated that the scientific enterprise may be influenced by social, economic, or political factors.[3] For example, the popularity of certain ideologies may influence how phenomena are viewed and what problems are selected for study.[11] In addition, the availability of funds for research in a specified area may precipitate a flurry of research activity in that area. Science, however, does not depend on the "personal characteristics" or persuasions of any given scientist, or group of scientists, but is powerfully self-correcting within the community of scientists.[18] Science thus progresses by "reasoned judgments on the part of scientists and through debate within the scientific community."[3:167]

REFERENCES

1. Bixenstine, E. (1964). Empiricism in latter-day behavioral science. *Science,* 145:465.
2. Bronowski, J. (1979). *The visionary eye: Essays in the arts, literature and science.* Cambridge, Mass.: The MIT Press.
3. Brown, H. (1977). *Perception, theory and commitment: The new philosophy of science.* Chicago: The University of Chicago Press.
4. Calder, N. (1979). *Einstein's universe.* New York: Viking.
5. Dubin, R. (1978). *Theory building.* New York: The Free Press.
6. Flavell, J.H. (1977). *Cognitive development.* Englewood Cliffs, N.J.: Prentice-Hall.

7. Foucault, M. (1973). *The order of things: An archaeology of the human sciences.* New York: Vintage Books.

8. Gale, G. (1979). *Theory of science: An introduction to the history, logic and philosophy of science.* New York: McGraw-Hill.

9. Giere, R.N. (1979). *Understanding scientific reasoning.* New York: Holt, Rinehart & Winston.

10. Hanson, N.R. (1958). *Patterns of discovery.* Cambridge: Cambridge University Press.

11. Hudson, L. (1972). *The cult of the fact.* New York: Harper & Row.

12. Irving, H.W. (1977). Social networks in the modern city. *Social Forces, 55:*867-880.

13. Kuhn, T.S. (1962). *The structure of scientific revolutions.* Chicago: The University of Chicago Press.

14. Mishler, E.G. (1979). Meaning in context: Is there any other kind? *Harvard Educational Review, 49:*1-19.

15. Norman, D.A. (1976). *Memory and attention: An introduction to human information processing.* New York: John Wiley & Sons.

16. Piaget, J. (1970). *The place of the sciences of man in the system of sciences.* New York: Harper & Row.

17. Popper, K. (1962). *Conjectures and refutations.* New York: Basic Books.

18. Randall, J.H. (1964). *Philosophy: An introduction.* New York: Barnes & Noble.

19. Reynolds, P. (1971). *A primer in theory construction.* Indianapolis: Bobbs-Merrill.

20. Schutz, A. (1967). *The phenomenology of the social world.* Evanston, Ill.: Northwestern University Press.

21. Skinner, B.F. (1950). Are theories of learning necessary? *Psychological Review, 57:*193-216.

22. Snelbecker, G. (1974). *Learning theory, instructional theory, and psychoeducational design.* New York: McGraw-Hill.

23. Steiner, E. (1977). *Criteria for theory of art education.* Monograph presented at Seminar for Research in Art Education, Philadelphia. Unpublished.

24. Steiner, E. (1978). *Logical and conceptual analytic techniques for educational researchers.* Washington, D.C.: University Press.

25. Toulmin, S. (1961). *Foresight and understanding.* New York: Harper & Row.

26. Turner, J. (1978). *The structure of sociological theory.* Homewood, Ill.: The Dorsey Press.

27. Werkmeister, W. (1959). Theory construction and the problem of objectivity. In L. Gross (Ed.), *Symposium on sociological theory.* Evanston, Ill.: Row, Peterson, & Co.

28. Winton, C. (1974). *Theory and measurement in sociology.* New York: John Wiley & Sons.

29. Zetterberg, H.L. (1966). *On theory and verification in sociology.* Totowa, N.J.: The Bedminster Press.

Logical Reasoning

Sue Marquis Bishop

4

A theory may be evaluated by using the criterion of logical development. This requires that the development of the series of theoretical statements follow a logical form of reasoning, that is, the premises justify the conclusions. Logic is a branch of philosophy concerned with the analysis of inferences and arguments.[9] An *inference* involves the forming of a conclusion based on some evidence. Although the common meaning of argument implies a disagreement, in logic, an *argument* consists of a conclusion and its supportive evidence. The evidence supporting a conclusion may involve one or more theoretical statements, or premises. The tools of logic permit the analysis of the reasoning from the premises to the conclusion.[7]

Theories can be developed and tested through deductive, inductive, or retroductive forms of reasoning. These approaches have been explicitly presented in the literature as systematic procedures for devising theory. An in-depth discussion of these forms is beyond the scope of this chapter and the reader is referred to Geach,[1] Giere,[2] Pospesel,[7] Salmon,[8,9] and Steiner[14] for further study. It is important, however, to grasp the basic differences between these forms of reasoning in order to understand how a given theorist may choose to approach the task of theory building.

DEDUCTION

Deduction is a form of logical reasoning in which specific conclusions are inferred from more general premises or principles. Reasoning thus proceeds from the general to the particular.[13] The deductively developed theory usually involves a lengthy sequence of theoretical statements derived from a relatively few broad axioms or general statements. Conclusions thus derived may offer predictions that can be tested empirically. The deductive argument usually takes the form of a syllogism with general premises and a conclusion. In logical analysis, letters may be substituted for concepts, since emphasis on the analysis of the argument is focused on the *form of the argument*. Example A presents a valid deductive argument with letter notation.

EXAMPLE A

Premise: All victims of abuse have low self-esteem. (All S are M)
Premise: Martha and Tom are victims of abuse. (All P are S)
Conclusion: Therefore, Martha and Tom have low self-esteem. (*Ergo,* All P are M)

In Example A, the conclusion follows from, or was deduced from the general premises. There may be a lengthy number of premises in a given argument preceding the conclusion. Note in the above example there is no new information presented in the conclusion that is not at least implied in the premises. The deductive form of reasoning is defined as:

1. If A were true, then B would be true.
2. A is true.
3. Hence, B is true.[14:9]

As you study the nursing literature, you will not often find arguments presented in the form in Example A with the premises and conclusions placed in order and clearly labeled. But with practice you can sharpen your skills in identifying arguments and labeling the premises and conclusions from your reading of narrative text. You may find the conclusion may be presented at the beginning or end, or even in the middle of an argument.[9] Salmon[9] suggests that certain words or phrases are clues that specific statements are offered as premises or conclusions. Examples of terms that often precede a premise include *since, for,* and *because.* Examples of terms that often precede a conclusion are *therefore, consequently, hence, so,* and *it follows that.*

Arguments may be evaluated in two different ways: (1) the validity of the argument may be assessed as to whether the conclusion logically follows from the premises, and (2) the content of the premises may be assessed in terms of the truth or falsity of the statements.[7] The validity of a deductive argument refers to the logic involved in reasoning from the premises to the conclusion in such a way that if the premises are true, the conclusion must necessarily be true.[7,9,14] A deductive argument may contain all true statements or one or more false statements and be considered either valid or invalid. This judgment is made on the basis of whether the conclusion is supported by the premises. For example:

	Premise: All victims of abuse have low self-esteem.
EXAMPLE B	*Premise:* Martha has low self-esteem.
	Conclusion: Therefore, Martha is a victim of abuse.

Although Martha may very well be the victim of abuse, the truth or falsity of the conclusion (or any of the statements) is not at issue when evaluating the validity of an argument. In Example B, the conclusion that Martha is a victim of abuse is not established by the supporting evidence in the premises. The conclusion goes beyond the explicit and implicit information in the premises. This is not a valid argument. (Compare the reasoning in Examples A and B.)

Whereas *validity* refers to the form of the deductive argument, *truth* refers to the content of a given theoretical statement. It is therefore inappropriate to label a single theoretical statement valid or an argument true.[9]

In a valid deductive argument, if the premises are true, it necessarily follows that the conclusion must be true. (This combination is marked [R] in Figure 4-1.) It is therefore impossible for the conclusion to be false. (This combination is marked [S] in Figure 4-1.) If, however, one or more of the premises are false, two outcomes are possible: the conclusion may be either true or false.

Example C presents a deductively valid argument that leads from false premises to a false conclusion. (This combination is marked [X] in Figure 4-1.)

		The conclusion is:	
		True	False
If the premises are:	All true	Necessary (R)	Impossible (S)
	Not all true	Possible (Y)	Possible (X)

(R) If the premises are true, it *necessarily follows* that the conclusion be true.

(S) If the premises are true, it is therefore *impossible* for the conclusion to be false.

(Y), (X) If one or more of the premises are false, it is *possible* the conclusion may be *either* true or false.

Figure 4-1. Potential outcomes of a valid deductive argument.

Adapted from Giere, R.N. (1979). *Understanding scientific reasoning.* New York: Holt, Rinehart & Winston.

EXAMPLE C

Premise: The dime is larger than the nickel. (FALSE)
Premise: The nickel is larger than the Susan B. Anthony dollar. (FALSE)
Conclusion: Thus, the dime is larger than the Susan B. Anthony dollar. (FALSE)

As Figure 4-1 suggests, and Example D illustrates, it is also possible that a valid argument can lead from one or more false premises to a true conclusion. (This combination is marked [Y] in Figure 4-1.)

EXAMPLE D

Premise: The nickel is larger than the Susan B. Anthony dollar. (FALSE)
Premise: The Susan B. Anthony dollar is larger than the dime. (TRUE)
Conclusion: Thus, the nickel is larger than the dime. (TRUE)

It may be helpful to study Examples C and D to understand how the conclusions are derived from the information given in the premises. (Note in these examples that "larger than" refers to physical size, not the value of the coins.) In science, deductive arguments can be a powerful form of reasoning for deriving new conclusions by making explicit the implied information contained in what is known. These derived conclusions can then be subjected to empirical test.

INDUCTION

Induction is a form of logical reasoning in which a generalization is induced from a number of specific observed instances. Inductive reasoning has been less well developed than deductive reasoning.[7] The form of the inductive argument is:

1. A is true of $b_1, b_2 \ldots b_n$.
2. $b_1, b_2 \ldots b_n$ are some members of class B.
3. Hence, A is true of all members of class B.[14:9]

The inductive form is based on the assumption that members of any given class share common characteristics. Therefore what is true of any randomly selected members of the class is accepted as true for all members of the class.[14] Suppose a sample of the population of victims of abuse has been selected for study. Example E presents an argument in the inductive form that may be developed based on this hypothetical study:

EXAMPLE E

Premise: Every victim of abuse that has been observed has low self-esteem.
Conclusion: All victims of abuse have low self-esteem.

The premise in Example E states observations from a number of instances, that is, a limited number of subjects. The conclusion states a generalization extending beyond the observations to the whole class of victims of abuse.

The inductive generalization also may be stated in terms of a mathematical quantity.[9] For example, assume a researcher decides to survey a sample of 400 nurses to determine their opinions as to whether nurses should establish independent private practices. Results indicate sixty-five percent of nurses in the sample support independent private practice activities in nursing. The inductive statement may be stated as:

EXAMPLE F

Premise: Sixty-five percent of nurses in the sample support independent private practice activities in nursing.
Conclusion: Sixty-five percent of all nurses support independent private practice in nursing.

Whereas, in a deductive argument, if the premises are true, the conclusion must necessarily be true, the inductive argument can have true premises and yet produce a false conclusion.

An inductive conclusion based on limited or biased evidence can clearly lead to a fallacious argument and perhaps a false conclusion.[9] Suppose the argument in Example E was developed by one nurse's experience with observing five victims of abuse. The conclusion that victims of abuse have low self-esteem may or may not be true. However, this conclusion is not warranted based on the number of observed instances. There is too little evidence in this case to justify the conclusion about all victims of abuse.

Even if the sample size is appropriately sufficient (or based on several studies), the sample may be biased. Assume in Example F that the sample of nurses was drawn from faculty in schools of nursing. The opinions of this select group of nurses may be expected to be different in some respects and may not reflect the opinions of all nurses. It may be that a greater proportion of nursing faculty members are engaged in private practice activities than the proportion of all nurses. Considering a number of factors in selecting representative samples can help avoid introducing bias into observations. This reasoning is the basis for the random selection of subjects in research projects. Descriptive and inferential statistics are used to characterize the sample and population and help with decisions about the strength of the evidence. The inductive inference thus has been termed the statistical inference.[14,17]

A distinguishing characteristic of inductive arguments is that the inferred conclusion goes beyond the implicit and explicit information in the premises. In Example E not all victims of abuse have been observed. This conclusion is inferred on the basis of selected instances. In a deductive argument the conclusion can be considered true if the argument is structured so that implicit information in the premises is made explicit.[9] The inductive argument, on the other hand, goes beyond the information in the premises. The inductive argument thus expands on the information presented. Giere[2] has argued this characteristic permits the justification of scientific conclusions that may not be justifiable by deductive reasoning, since they contain information beyond the premises. An example would be a scientific hypothesis about the future based on observations in the present.

Whereas deductive arguments are considered

to be either valid or invalid, the concept of validity does not apply to inductive arguments. The correctness of inductive arguments is not viewed in either/or terms, but on degrees of strength, measured in terms of the *probability* with which the premises lead to a given conclusion. The inferred conclusion then can be determined to have low, medium, or high probability.[9] Statistical procedures can be used for making these judgments.

In Example A, the only possibility for the conclusion being false is if one or more of the premises are false, that is, if all victims of abuse do not have low self-esteem, or if Martha and Tom are not victims of abuse. If these are true, the conclusion must necessarily be true. However, in Example E the reasoning suggests that all victims of abuse have low self-esteem. But the premises state only selected victims of abuse have been observed. The premises may lend some support for the conclusion. The fact that no victims of absue without low self-esteem have been observed may be considered some evidence, but not conclusive evidence that a victim with high self-esteem will not be observed in the future.[9]

Deductive arguments are considered "truth preservers," while inductive arguments can be a source of new information.[2,9] Scientific generalizations about instances not observed in the present or projections about the future are examples. Although this form of reasoning is useful in advancing science, the very nature of induction may introduce error into the scientific process.[3] Even if we could be sure the premises were accurate, we could not be absolutely certain of the accuracy of the conclusion. In Giere's view, if we assume the premises are true:

> The difference between a *good inductive argument* and a *valid deductive argument* is that the deductive argument guarantees the *truth* of its conclusion while the inductive argument guarantees only an *appropriately high probability* of its conclusion.[2:37-38]

RETRODUCTION*

Whereas deduction and induction may explicate and evaluate ideas, retroduction originates ideas.[13] The retroductive form of reasoning is an approach to inquiry using analogy as a method for devising theory. In 1878 Pierce described three kinds of reasoning as comprising the major steps of inquiry: retroduction, deduction and induction.[14] Pierce viewed retroductive reasoning as the first stage in the search for understanding some "surprising phenomenon" in which a viewpoint offering a possible explanation is identified. Pierce stated that once a viewpoint was identified that held the promise of explanation for the observed phenomenon, deductive reasoning was used to develop the explanation. Pierce considered the final stage of inquiry in terms of induction with the focus on checking out the devised hypotheses in experience.[14] The theory models approach using retroductive inference was further developed by Steiner* as a method for devising theory. The form of the retroductive inference follows:

*References 3, 4, 11, 12. Elizabeth Steiner-Maccia's earlier published work on theory models was under her married name of Maccia.

Table 4-1. Deduction, induction, and retroduction summary table

Type	Question	Techniques
Deduction	Given the premises are true, what other propositions may be inferred as necessary conclusions from the premises?[12:67]	Logical and conceptual analysis
Induction	Given the premises are true, what is the strength of the link between them and the conclusion?[12:87]	Logical and conceptual analysis based on statistical analysis[11,15]
Retroduction	Given a surprising observation, what explanation would result in the expectation that the observation would be a matter of course?[12]	Logical and conceptual analysis[11]

1. The surprising fact C, is observed.
2. But if A were true, C would be a matter of course.
3. Hence, there is reason to suspect that A is true.[14:9]

An analysis of the above form reveals that the theory models (or retroductive) approach does not establish truth. Its function is to originate ideas about selected phenomena that can be developed further and tested. The theory models approach is most useful as a strategy for devising theory in a field in which there are few available theories and innovation is indicated to advance knowledge in describing and understanding selected observations.[14,16]

The retroductive theorist approaches the development of a wanted theory by identifying a source theory in another field that may have potential for developing the wanted theory. The theory models approach is based on the use of analogy and metaphor between two sets of phenomena, which requires considerable creativity on the part of the theorist and an intuitive knowledge of the phenomena of interest. The theory models approach is represented as:[13,14]

$$\text{THEORY}_1 \dashrightarrow \text{THEORY MODEL} \dashrightarrow \text{THEORY}_2$$

(Source theory)

(Wanted theory)

Definition	Example	Function
1. If A were true, then B would be true. 2. A is true. 3. Hence, B is true.[14:9]	*Premises* All victims of abuse have low self-esteem. Marty & Tom are victims of abuse. *Conclusion* Marty & Tom have low self-esteem.	*Explicates and derives further truths* If premises are true, establishes truth of something else by derivation[11:9]
1. A is true of $b_1, b_2 \ldots b_n$. 2. $b_2, b_2 \ldots b_n$ are members of some class B. 3. Hence, A is true of all members of class B.[14:9]	*Premise* $b_1, b_2 \ldots b_n$ victims of abuse that have been observed have low self-esteem. *Conclusion* All victims of abuse have low self-esteem.	*Evaluates and expands information* Based on probability of observed cases. Does not establish truth. Establishes probability of certainty. New data may change conclusion[2,8,11]
1. The surprising fact C is observed. 2. But if A were true, C would be a matter of course. 3. Hence, there is reason to suspect that A is true.[14:9]	*Proposition 1* The role of expecting *reward* determines a relation between *student* and *teacher* that establishes a path for influence of the *teacher* on the *student*.[4:121] *Proposition 2* The role of expecting *care and comfort* determines a relation between *patient* and *nurse* that establishes a path for influence of *nurse* on the *patient*.	*Originates ideas* Does not establish truth. Suggests lines of thought worthy of exploration and testing.[11:9]

Thus theory models are not "models-of," but are "models-for" devising representations of selected phenomena.[12] The theory model is essentially a meta-model which serves as a model to develop theory.[13]

To devise theory using retroductive inference, the theorist seeks out a source theory to form a theory model from which the wanted theory will be devised. The source theory is selected on the basis of a "suspected similarity in the structure of form or pattern of relations" between the two sets of phenomena.[14] The selected source theory is perceived to present ideas that may be useful for developing a theory about the observations of interest. These ideas are selected from $theory_1$ and formed into a point of view or theory model that will serve as the framework for developing $theory_2$. This approach is based on the assumption that new conjectures, or ideas, in a given field may be devised from other conjectures in theories in other fields.[3,4,14] The ideas selected from $theory_1$ for the theory model may involve any combination of concepts, hypothesized relationships or theory structures. The viewpoint presented by the theory model is used to develop $theory_2$ by adding content to the theory model and by altering concepts and relationships to fit with the phenomenon of interest for $theory_2$. It should be clear that this process of theory building is not simply borrowing a theory from one field and applying it unchanged to another. The deliberate selection of aspects of $theory_1$ to form the theory model, the addition of new information, and the alteration of concepts and relationships for congruence with different phenomena in a new context, result in a new theory. Of course a theory devised by this method must meet the criteria for adequacy of a theory (see Chapter 1). As Steiner[4,13,14] argued, the theory models approach cannot be considered reductive since $theory_1$ is not equivalent to $theory_2$. To be reductive, the theorist would simply borrow concepts and hypotheses and use them as formu-

lated in a new context. Neither can this approach be considered deductive, since $theory_2$ was not developed by deduction from $theory_1$. The hypotheses in $theory_2$ cannot be derived from $theory_1$.[13,14]

The use of analogy to develop theory has been a common occurrence in the development of a number of scientific fields. In Sigmund Freud's day, the machine model was a popular advanced model of the times. Freud used the notion of machine operations to develop his theoretical assertions about psychological tension-reduction relationships in his theory of psychosexual development. Three or more decades ago basic texts in human anatomy and physiology used the telephone switchboard as an analogy for explaining the functioning of the brain. Currently, the computer is often used as a model for thinking about the brain and in developing theories of human information processing.[5,10] In nursing, General Systems Theory has been used as a model for developing nursing theory.[6] Steiner's development of the theory models approach provides guidelines for using this strategy in theory building.

Stevens[15] has argued that one of the reasons much of nursing research has so little impact on nursing practice is nursing research is often based on the "categories and characteristics" of borrowed theories. A borrowed theory tends to be used unchanged in the new context. Although theories in other fields may suggest a possible framework for addressing phenomena in the field of nursing, this framework may need to be contextualized within nursing. That is, aspects of the "borrowed theory" may need to be altered to reflect the appropriate categories and characteristics within nursing. Walker and Avant's "derivation strategy" for theory construction[16] draws from the theory models approach developed by Steiner. Walker and Avant[16] present a number of examples of using the derivation strategy to "shift and reformulate" concepts, theoretical statements, and theories from other fields to nursing. The theory models approach permits the translation and expansion of ideas within the milieu of nursing and may result in the development of a new nursing theory. A nursing theory devised by this method can be further developed through the use of deductive and inductive strategies.

A summary of deductive, inductive, and retroductive forms of reasoning is presented in Table 4-1.

REFERENCES

1. Geach, P.T. (1979). *Reason and argument*. Los Angeles: University of California Press.
2. Giere, R.N. (1979). *Understanding scientific reasoning*. New York: Holt, Rinehart & Winston.
3. Maccia, E.S., & Maccia, G. (1966). *Construction of educational theory derived from three educational theory models* (Project No. 5-0638). Washington, D.C.: U.S. Department of Health, Education, and Welfare.
4. Maccia, E.S., Maccia, G., & Jewett, R. (1963). *Construction of educational theory models* (Cooperative Research Project No. 1632). Washington, D.C.: Office of Education, U.S. Department of Health, Education, and Welfare.
5. Norman, D.A. (1976). *Memory and attention: An introduction to human information processing*. New York: John Wiley & Sons.
6. Nursing Theories Conference Group (1980). *Nursing theories: The base for professional nursing practice*. Englewood Cliffs, N.J.: Prentice-Hall.
7. Pospesel, H. (1974). *Propositional logic*. Englewood Cliffs, N.J.: Prentice-Hall.
8. Salmon, W.C. (1967). *The foundations of scientific inference*. Pittsburgh: University of Pittsburgh Press.
9. Salmon, W.C. (1973). Logic. Englewood Cliffs, N.J.: Prentice-Hall.
10. Shepherd, G.M. (1974). *The synaptic organization of the brain*. New York: Oxford University Press.
11. Steiner, E. (1976). *Logical and conceptual analytic techniques for educational researchers*. Paper presented at the American Educational Research Association, San Francisco. © Copyright Elizabeth Steiner. All rights reserved.
12. Steiner, E. (1976). *The complete act of educational inquiry*. © Copyright Elizabeth Steiner. All rights reserved.
13. Steiner, E. (1977). *Criteria for theory of art education*. Paper presented at the Seminar for Research in Art Education, Philadelphia. © Copyright Elizabeth Steiner. All rights reserved.
14. Steiner, E. (1978). *Logical and conceptual analytic techniques for educational researchers*. Washington, D.C.: University Press.
15. Stevens, B. (1979). *Nursing theory: Analysis, application, evaluation*. Boston: Little, Brown.
16. Walker, L., & Avant, K. (1983). *Strategies for theory construction in nursing*. Norwalk, Conn.: Appleton-Century-Crofts.
17. Weiner, P. (1958). *Values in a universe of chance*. New York: Doubleday.

Theory Development Process

Sue Marquis Bishop

5

Nursing theory development is not a mysterious, magical activity. Many nurses have been developing their own private ideas of nursing since their first day in nursing (or perhaps before) and have continued to develop private assumptions based on their readings and experiences. These private notions may include such generalizations as "A clean, smooth bed allows greater rest and less need for pain medication for a patient," or "Encouraging the patient to have some say in his or her care leads to greater cooperation with treatment procedures." Nurses usually don't talk explicitly about their private theories, although these theories may influence the nursing activities they choose to implement and the manner in which they practice nursing.

If, in fact, all nurses are evolving private theories of nursing, why all the fuss about studying published theories? The major reason is that nurses' private conceptions of nursing may be "incomplete, inconsistent, or muddled."* This leads to considerable problems in using the private theory as a sound basis for practice. Further, an incomplete, inconsistent, or muddled theory may be difficult to use in studying clini-

cal nursing situations to advance our knowledge of nursing. If we agree that the availability of more systematic theories would provide a clearer understanding and enable us to explore whether this understanding corresponds with activities in the nursing environment, then we also must agree with Hardy[7] and others that rigorous development of nursing theory is a priority. The systematic development of nursing theory has a better chance of advancing nursing and may lead to the basis for nursing science.

It is important to grasp the concept of *systematic development*. Approaches to the construction of theory differ. But one aspect they have in common is the agreement among scientists to approach this task in a systematic fashion and to make the stages in development explicit so others can review the logical processes and test the hypotheses presented. The nurse who devises a theory of nursing and presents it for public review by the nursing community is engaging in the process essential to advancing theory development.

THEORY COMPONENTS

Hage[6] identified six components of a complete theory and specified the contribution each makes to the whole theory (Table 5-1). He ar-

---

*I wish to acknowledge my indebtedness to Nicholas Mullins, one of my former teachers, for his discussion of private and public theories, and for communicating both the complexity and creative playfulness in theoretical work.

Table 5-1. Theory components and their contributions to the theory

Theory Components	Contributions
Concepts	Description and classification
Theoretical state-ments	Analysis
Definitions	
Theoretical	Meaning
Operational	Measurement
Linkages	
Theoretical	Plausability
Operational	Testability
Ordering of concepts and definitions into primitive and derived terms	Elimination of overlap (tautology)
Ordering of state-ments and linkages into premises and equations	Elimination of inconsistency

Modified from Hage, J. (1972). *Techniques and problems in theory construction in sociology.* New York: John Wiley & Sons.

gued that the failure to include one or more of the components resulted in the elimination of that particular contribution to the total theory. These six aspects of a theory are discussed as a basis for understanding the function of each element in the theory building process.

Concepts

Concepts, the building blocks of theories, classify the phenomena with which we are concerned.[8] It is crucial in any separate discussion of concepts to recognize that concepts must not be considered separately from the theoretical system in which they are embedded and from which they derive their meaning.[2] Concepts may have completely different meanings in different theoretical systems. Because scientific progress is based on the critical review and testing of a researcher's work by others in the scientific community, consensus regarding the meaning of scientific concepts is important.[2,6]

Concepts may be abstract or concrete. Abstract concepts are independent of a specific time or place, while concrete concepts relate to a particular time and place.[6,13]

Abstract concepts	Concrete concepts
Social System	The Vaughn Family
	Indiana University
	School of Nursing
Debate	Reagan-Mondale Debate

In the above example, the Vaughn family is an instance of the more general abstract concept of social system.

Concepts may label discrete categories (or classes) of phenomena (such as patient, nurse, or environment), or dimensions of phenomena (the amount of self-care or degree of marital conflict, for example).[3,6,11,13] Theories may be developed by using nonvariable discrete concepts to build typologies.[6,13,16]

The nonvariable concept is devised to capture a number of different aspects.[6] Phenomena are then identified as belonging or *not* belonging to a given class. The sorting of phenomena into nonvariable, discrete categories carries the assumption that the reality associated with the given phenomena is captured by the classification.[6] The nonvariable concept of bureaucracy was devised by Max Weber as an ideal type to characterize organizations.[9] Organizations can thus be classified as bureaucratic or nonbureaucratic.

On the other hand, the use of variable concepts based on a range or continuum tend to be focused on one dimension without the assumption that a single dimension "captures all the reality" connected with the phenomenon.[6] Additional dimensions may be devised to measure further aspects of the phenomenon. In contrast to the nonvariable term *bureaucracy,* variable concepts such as rate of conflict, ratio of professional to nonprofessional staff, and communication flow may be used to characterize organizations. Although nonvariable concepts are useful in classifying phenomena in theory development, it has been argued that major breakthroughs occurred in several fields when the focus shifted from nonvariable to variable concepts.[6] Variable concepts permit scoring the full range of the phenomenon on a continuum.

The development of theoretical concepts permits the *description* and *classification* of phenomena.[6] The labeled concept suggests boundaries for selecting phenomena to observe and for reasoning about the phenomena of interest. New concepts may focus attention on new phenomena or may facilitate thinking about and classifying phenomena in a different way.[6]

Theoretical Statements

Although concepts are considered the building blocks of theory, they must be connected in some way with a set of theoretical statements to devise theory.* The development of theoretical statements asserting a connection between two or more concepts introduces the possibility of *analysis*.[6]

Statements in a theory can be classified into three general categories: existence statements, definitions, and relational statements.[13,18] Existence statements and definitions relate to specific concepts. Whereas definitions provide descriptions of the concept, existence statements simply assert that a given concept exists and is labeled with the concept name. Relational statements assert relationships between the properties of two or more concepts (or variables). Various types of relational statements have been described in the literature.[11,13,18] Discussion in this chapter is limited to an introduction to probabilistic statements and necessary and sufficient conditional statements. These types of statements are important in understanding scientific reasoning.[5]

In the connections between variables, one variable may be assumed to influence a second variable. In this instance, the first variable may be labeled a determinant (or antecedent) and the second variable a resultant (or consequent).[5,16,20] The first variable may be viewed as the independent variable and the second as the dependent variable.[5] Because of its complexity, nursing presents a situation in which multiple antecedents and consequents may be involved in studying a selected phenomenon. Zetterberg[20] concluded, however, that the development of two-variate theoretical statements may be an important intermediate step in the development of a theory. These statements later can be reformulated as the theory evolves or new information is known.

An example of a relational statement expressed as a sufficient condition is, "If nurses react with approval of patients' independent behaviors, patients increase their efforts in self-care activities." This is a type of compound statement linking antecedent and consequent. The statement does not assert the truth of the antecedent. Rather, the assertion is made that *if* the antecedent is true, then the consequent also is true.[5] In addition, there is no assertion in the statement explaining *why* the antecedent is related to the consequent.[6] In symbolic notation form, the above statements can be expressed as:

$$NA \dashrightarrow PSC$$

$$
\begin{array}{ll}
\text{(Nurse} & \text{(Patient} \\
\text{Approval)} & \text{Self-Care)}
\end{array}
$$

This statement asserts that nurse approval of a patient's independent behaviors is sufficient for the occurrence of the patient's self-care activities. However, patient assumption of self-care activities resulting from other factors such as the patient's health status and personality variables is not ruled out. In other words, there could be other antecedents that are sufficient conditions for the patient's assumption of self-care activities.

A statement in the form of a necessary condition asserts that one variable is required for the occurrence of another variable.[5,12,15] For example:

> Without the motivation to get well (MGW), patients will not assume strict adherence to following their prescribed treatment regimen (PTR).

$$MGW \dashrightarrow PTR$$

---

*References 2, 3, 6, 13, 20.

This means PTR never occurs when MGW does not occur.[5,12] No assertion is made that patients' strict adherence to the prescribed treatment regimen follows from their motivation to get well. It is asserted, however, that if motivation to get well is absent, patients will not assume strict adherence to their treatment regimen. The motivation to get well is thus a necessary, but not a sufficient, condition for the occurrence of this consequent.

The term *if* is most generally used to introduce a sufficient condition, whereas, *only if* and *if . . . then* are used to introduce necessary conditions.[5] In most instances conditional statements are not both necessary and sufficient.[5] It is possible, however, for a statement to express both conditions. In such instances the term, *if and only if* is used to imply the conditions are both necessary and sufficient for one another.[5] In this case: (1) the consequent never occurs in the absence of the antecedent, and (2) the consequent always occurs when the antecedent occurs.[5,12]

Although causal statements (one variable causes another) may be expressed as a conditional statement, not all conditional statements are causal.[5] For example, the statement "If this month is March, then the next month is April," does not assert that March causes April to occur. Rather the sequence of months suggests that April follows March.[5] (For an extensive discussion of conditional and unconditional causal statements see Nowak.[12])

Probabilistic statements are generally derived from statistical data and express connections that do not always occur but are likely to occur based on some estimate of probability.[18] Walker and Avant[18] used as an example the statement "Cigarette smoking will most likely lead to cancer of the lung." It is clear that cigarette smoking does not always lead to lung cancer since some persons who smoke do not develop this disease. However, the probability of developing cancer of the lung is enhanced for cigarette smokers. In symbolic notation:[18]

$$\text{If CS} \text{ ------} \rightarrow \text{P } \text{LC.}$$

The development of relational statements asserting connections between variables provides for *analysis* and establishes the basis for explanation and prediction.[6]

Definition

The development of science is a collaborative endeavor in which the community of scientists critique, test, and build upon one another's work.[2] It is therefore crucial that concepts be as clearly defined as possible to reduce ambiguity in understanding a given concept or a set of concepts. While it is not possible to entirely eliminate perceived differences in meaning, these differences can be minimized by setting forth explicit definitions. In the development of a complete theory, both theoretical and operational definitions provide meaning for the concept and a basis for searching for empirical indicators.[6] *Theoretical definitions* also permit consideration of the relationships of a given concept to other theoretical ideas.

But a clear meaning for concepts is not sufficient. If theories are to be tested against reality, concepts also must be measurable.[6] *Operational definitions* relate the concepts to observable phenomena by specifying empirical indicators.[6] Hage[6] asserted that the concept name and the theoretical and operational definitions establish reference points for "locating the concept," that is, viewing the concept as related to both theoretical systems and the observable environment.

Linkages

The specification of linkages is an important part of the development of theory.[6] Although the theoretical statements assert connections between concepts, the rationale for the stated connections need .to be developed. The development of *theoretical linkages* offers a reasoned explanation of why the variables may be connected in some manner, that is, the theoretical reasons for asserting particular interrelation-ships.[6] This rationale contributes *plausability* to the theory.[6]

Operational linkages, on the other hand, con-tribute the element of *testability* to the theory by specifying how variables are connected.[6] Whereas operational definitions provide for measurability of the concepts, operational link-ages provide for testability of the assertions. The operational linkage contributes a perspec-tive for understanding the nature of the rela-tionship between concepts, such as whether the relationship between concepts is negative or positive and linear or curvilinear.[6]

Ordering

Finally, Hage,[6] concluded that a theory may be considered to be "fairly complete" if it presents the elements of *concepts, definitions, statements,* and *linkages*. Complete development of the theory, however, requires the organization of concepts and definitions into primitive and de-rived terms and the organization of statements and linkages into premises and equations.[6] As the theory evolves, concepts and theoretical statements multiply, and the need arises to es-tablish some logical arrangement or ordering of the theoretical components and bring concep-tual order to the theory.[6] Hage stated the con-cepts should be ordered if the theory contains more than ten variables. He also recommended the concepts and definitions be ordered into primitive and derived terms. Primitive terms are terms not defined within the theory. Derived terms are defined with primitive terms or other terms already defined. Derived terms are thus defined within the theory. This process of or-dering may point up any existing overlap be-tween concepts and definitions.[6] The concep-tual arrangement of statements and linkages into premises and equations may reveal areas of inconsistency.[6] Premises (or axioms) are re-garded as the more general assertions from which the hypotheses are derived in the form of equations. Hage suggested that the ordering of

statements and linkages is indicated when the theory contains a large number of theoretical statements.

FORMS OF THEORY ORGANIZATION*

A formal theory is a systematically developed conceptual system that addresses a given set of phenomena. There are different ideas of how this conceptual system should be organized so as to constitute a theory. Three forms for or-ganizing theory include: set-of-laws, axiomatic, and causal process.

Set-of-laws Form

The set-of-laws approach attempts to organize findings from empirical research.[13] The theorist first reviews the research literature in an area of particular interest. Empirical findings from available research are identified and selected from the literature for evaluation. Findings are evaluated and sorted into categories based on the degree of empirical evidence supporting each assertion.[13] The available categories are *laws, empirical generalizations* and *hypotheses.*[13]

Since construction of the set-of-laws theory requires the selection and evaluation of re-search findings in terms of degree of empiri-cal support, several limitations emerge as a re-sult of this approach to constructing theory. Reynolds[13] discussed these limitations as disad-vantages to the set-of-laws approach to theory building. First, the nature of research requires focusing on relationships between a limited set of variables, often two variables. Therefore at-tempts to develop a set-of-laws theory from statements of findings may result in a lengthy number of statements that assert relationships between two or more variables. This lengthy set of generalizations may be difficult to organize and interrelate. Second, in order for research to

---

*The section on forms of theory organization is largely based on Reynolds' discussion[13] of these forms.

CLASSIFICATION OF EMPIRICAL FINDINGS

Laws (Overwhelming empirical support)
1.
2.
3.
Empirical Generalizations (Some empirical support)
1.
2.
3.
4.
Hypotheses (No empirical support)
1.
2.
3.
4.
5.

From Reynolds, P. (1971). *A primer in theory construction.* Indianapolis: Bobbs-Merrill.

---

be conducted, concepts must be operationally defined so as to be measurable. Concepts in the statements of empirical findings are therefore most likely to be measurable and operational concepts. This procedure eliminates other more highly abstract or theoretical concepts that might be useful in developing an understanding of the phenomenon of interest. Reynolds[13] concluded that although the set-of-laws forms may provide for classification of phenomena or predictions of relationships between selected variables, it does not permit a "sense of understanding" crucial for the advancement of science. Finally, Reynolds[13] noted that each statement in the set-of-laws form is considered to be independent in that the various statements have not been interrelated into a system of description and explanation (see box above). Therefore each statement must be tested. Because the statements are not interrelated, research support for one statement does not provide support for any other statement. Research efforts must therefore be more extensive.

The set-of-laws approach to theory building is consistent with the view that scientific knowledge consists of the body of empirical findings and that science is advanced by conducting research and then looking for patterns in the data.[13] This strategy is clearly an inductive one and may be based on the positivist belief that knowledge exists independent of theories and is waiting for discovery.[2,13] Patterns do not, of their own accord, arise from empirical data.[16] The theorist must bring "ideas to experience" to conceptualize and order theoretical relationships.[16] Reynolds[13] stated this may be difficult to do with a "lengthy catalogue" of empirical findings in the set-of-laws form.

Axiomatic Form

In contrast to the set-of-laws form, the axiomatic form of theory organization is an interrelated logical system. Specifically, an axiomatic theory consists of a set of concepts, explicit definitions, a set of existence statements, and a set of relationship statements arranged in hierarchical order.[13,17,20] The concepts include highly abstract concepts, intermediate concepts, and more concrete concepts. The set of existence statements describes situations in which the theory is applicable.[13,17,18] Statements helping delineate the boundaries of the theory are referred to as describing the scope conditions of the theory.[3,6,13] The relational statements consist of axioms and propositions. The highly abstract theoretical statements, called axioms, are organized at the top of the hierarchy.[17] All other propositions are developed through logical deduction from the axioms or from other more abstract propositions[17] (see box p. 46).

The axiomatic theory is determined to be integrated when there are no propositions in Set B that cannot be logically derived from Set A.[19] This results in a highly interrelated explanatory system. An essential criterion for the axiomatic form is that the theoretical statements may not

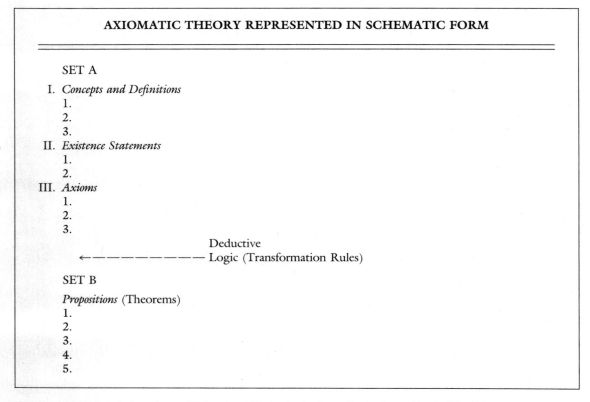

SET A

I. *Concepts and Definitions*
  1.
  2.
  3.
II. *Existence Statements*
  1.
  2.
III. *Axioms*
  1.
  2.
  3.

Deductive
←————————— Logic (Transformation Rules)

SET B

Propositions (Theorems)
  1.
  2.
  3.
  4.
  5.

This schemata on axiomatic theory is a modified version of Werkmeister's schemata[19] using Reynolds' terms[13] for the theory comments.

be contradictory.[19] A basic principle of logic asserts that when two statements are contradictory, one or both of the statements must be false.[15,19] Thus, axiomatic theorists seek to avoid this problem by developing a conceptual system with a few broad axioms from which a set of propositions can be derived.[19] As science progresses and new empirical data become known, the general axioms may be modified or extended. If, however, these additions to the logical system produce contradictions in the theory, the theory must be rejected for one without contradictions.[19] New theories often subsume portions of previous theories as special cases.[2,19] For example, Einstein's theory of relativity incorporated Newton's law of gravitation as a special case within the theory.

Axiomatic theories are not common in the social and behavioral sciences, but are clearly evident in the fields of physics and mathematics. For example, Euclidean geometry is an axiomatic theory.[19,20]

Developing theories in axiomatic form has several advantages.[13,20] First, since theory is a highly interrelated set of statements, some of which are derived from others, all concepts do not need to be operationally defined.[13] This allows the theorist to incorporate some highly abstract concepts that may be unmeasurable but provide for explanation. The interrelated axiomatic system may also be more efficient for explanation than the lengthy number of theoretical statements in the set-of-laws form. In addition, empirical support for one theoretical

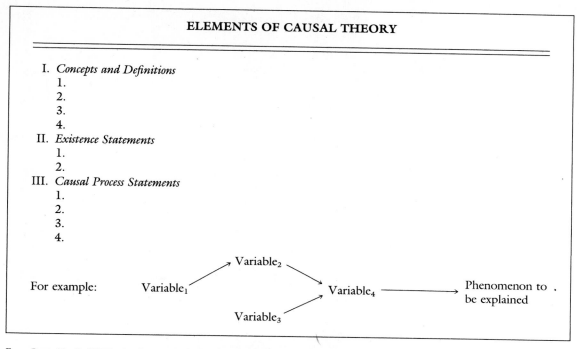

ELEMENTS OF CAUSAL THEORY

 I. *Concepts and Definitions*
    1.
    2.
    3.
    4.
 II. *Existence Statements*
    1.
    2.
III. *Causal Process Statements*
    1.
    2.
    3.
    4.

For example: Variable$_1$ → Variable$_2$ → Variable$_4$ → Phenomenon to be explained; Variable$_3$ → Variable$_4$

From Reynolds, P. (1971). *A primer in theory construction*. Indianapolis: Bobbs-Merrill Educational Publishing; and Turner, J. (1978). *The structure of sociological theory*. Homewood, Ill.: The Dorsey Press.

statement may be judged to provide support for the theory, thus permitting less extensive research than the requirement to test each statement in the set-of-laws form. Finally, Reynolds[13] concluded that in certain instances the axiomatic theory may be organized in a causal process form to increase a sense of understanding.

Causal Process Form

The distinguishing feature of the causal process form of theory is the development of theoretical statements specifying causal mechanisms between independent and dependent variables.[12,13] This form of theory organization consists of a set of concepts, a set of definitions, a set of existence statements, and a set of theoretical statements specifying causal process.[13] Concepts include abstract as well as concrete concepts. Existence statements function as in axiomatic

theories to describe the scope conditions of the theory—the situations to which the theory applies.[3,6,13] In contrast to the hierarchical arrangement in the axiomatic theory, causal process theories contain a set of statements describing the causal mechanisms or effects of one variable on one or more other variables.[11,13] Causal process theories may be limited to a few variables or may be quite complex with several variables (see box above).

The causal statements specify the hypothesized effects of one variable on one or more variables. In complex causal process theories, feedback loops and paths of influence through several variables may be hypothesized in the set of interrelated causal statements.[11,12] Reynolds concluded that the causal process form of theory provides for an explanation of "how something happens." He identified several advantages of the causal process form of organization. First, it provides for highly abstract theoretical concepts, as does axiomatic theory. Second, also like axiomatic theory, this form with its interrelated theoretical statements permits more efficient research testing. Finally, the causal process statements provide a sense of understanding about the phenomenon of interest not possible with other forms. However Turner[17] observed that causal process theories may not necessarily include highly abstract concepts, since a number of available theories contain simply "descriptions of causal connections among events." This approach does permit the development of a causal explanation of the sequence of events that may effect the phenomenon of interest.[17]

CREATIVITY IN THEORY BUILDING

Although a number of strategies for developing theory have been presented in the literature, the theorist who attempts to approach theory construction in a mechanical way by applying structured procedures may have limited success. Theory building involves discovery and creativity. A scientific theory is clearly "a creation of the human mind."[1] Bronowski[1] has written about the similarities in the processes of constructing theories and works of art, with each requiring a high level of imagination. In his view, "There is no difference in the use of such words as 'beauty' and 'truth' in the poem, and such symbols as 'energy' and 'mass' in the equation."[1:21]

While it is possible to teach specific techniques and content, we don't really know how to facilitate creativity and originality in students. In Rosenberg's words,[14:2] "You can teach someone how to look, but not how to see; how to search, but not how to find." Bronowski[1] suggests a sense of imagination, playfulness, and participation is essential not only for the theorist but for the reader who seeks to understand theories:

If science is a form of imagination, if all experiment is a form of play, then science cannot be dry-as-dust. . . . Science, or art, every creative activity is fun. . . . If a theorem in science seems dull to you, that is because you are not reading it with the same active sense of participation (and imagination) which you bring to the reading of a poem.[1:22-23]

In addition to imagination, developing and presenting theories requires personal discipline. Novel ideas tend to occur in a vague, disconnected, and tenuous form.[10] Self-discipline is required to work with the idea, develop it, and express it in written form for others to review. Rosenberg[14] stated that although "critical acumen" and creativity cannot be taught, they can be "nourished, enhanced, and matured." The individual's role is to attain familiarity with the phenomenon of interest and "practice, practice, practice."[14]

DO WE HAVE NURSING THEORIES?

It has been argued that there has been a preoccupation in nursing with the question of whether current nursing formulations are really theories. Flaskerud and Halloran[4] noted that although nurses identify formulations in nursing as "simply models or conceptual frameworks," they are not reluctant to label frameworks from other fields, such as psychology and sociology, as "theories." They argued that this has resulted in a depreciation of available efforts to systematize nursing. I recently encountered a nursing colleague who informed me she had returned to graduate school for doctoral work and had just completed a graduate course on nursing theories. When I inquired about what she had learned from the course, she responded, "Well, I didn't learn anything. You know there *really* aren't any nursing theories anyway." The application of rigorous criteria for a scientific theory will surely result in nursing theories being found deficient since theory construction in nursing is currently in the early stages of development. However, is the conclusion of negation of theory work in nursing (that there are no theories) the desired outcome from the study of nursing formulations?

The debate about whether nursing formulations are theories is often based on the conceptual sorting of theories into two categories: theories (T) and not-theories (T).

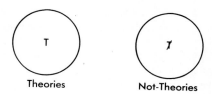

In using these conceptual classes for analysis, there are two categories for placing nursing formulations. If the T category (theory) is defined on the basis of rigorous criteria for a scientific theory, most and perhaps all nursing formulations would fall into the T category. The result may be that all nursing formulations would occupy only one category. What has been gained, in terms of advancing knowledge of nursing, by the time spent on the analysis of whether nursing formulations are or are not *theories,* especially if analysis ends at this point? Turner[17] labeled this approach the "game" of "criticize-the-discipline."

Suppose, hypothetically, we have two distinct sets of nursing formulations, X and Y. Let's assume we determine X meets the rigorous criteria for the theory class, while Y is incompletely developed and does not. However, let's further suppose that the formulations in X do not address the phenomenon we are interested in describing, understanding, or predicting. It is also possible that X does not even address anything we find particularly interesting. On the other hand, Y, which is now labeled *not-theory,* addresses a domain of interest that fits our particular concerns in our practice area. What do we do? Develop Y further!

In our efforts to prepare a new generation of nurse scholars to advance theory building in nursing, it may be more fruitful to give less attention to whether a given nursing formulation is a theory or not, and concentrate on analyzing how much of a theory it is.[6] In this perspective the category of theory is defined so a range of theoretical formulations can be considered (see Mullins[11]; Hage[6]). We have therefore expanded the conceptual categories from two, in which all nursing formulations tend to fall into the T category, to the notion of a continuum in the theory category. In this sorting system, sets of nursing formulations can be evaluated in terms of their relative completeness, according to where they fall in the following schematic:

T			T
Complete theories	Incomplete theories High Medium Low		Not-theory

Once a set of nursing formulations that fit our area of interest has been identified, several questions arise: How complete is it? What components or relationships are missing? Is it internally consistent? What is its correspondence with available empirical findings? Is it operationally defined for testing? Analyses of this nature logically lead to the question: What are the next steps in the further development of this theory? In Turner's view[17:12-13]:

> As soon as the question becomes one of *potential* for theory building, critical analysis must move beyond the mechanical comparisons of a particular theoretical perspective with the canons of scientific theory. While such comparisons . . . are an important and appropriate concern . . . , their polemic intent often gets in the way of the productive analysis of a particular conceptual perspective.

Turner recommended for his own discipline of sociology that any analysis of theory should begin with the "blunt admission" that theory construction in sociology "has a long way to go" and progress to the more important questions of beginning to identify and address current inadequacies in available theories. Hage's similar conclusions about sociological knowledge are quoted below, substituting nursing for sociology to illustrate relevance for states of affairs in nursing.

> The major difficulty in discussing whether there is any [nursing] knowledge is that many individuals think about this issue in either-or terms. . . . We do not want an either-or conception of knowledge. Because we are used to reasoning in this way, we are prevented from perceiving that perhaps there is some knowledge in [nursing], albeit it is incomplete.[6:182]

I recommend that at this point in the development of nursing, we acknowledge the following:

1. Widespread interest in the development of nursing theory is only a recent phenomenon in the history of the discipline.
2. The systematic development of nursing theories is currently in its infancy.
3. The application of rigorous criteria for a scientific theory to nursing formulations will most likely result in nursing theories being found to be far from the ideal scientific theory.
4. There is an increasing priority in nursing for the development of nursing science.

If we can accept there is a reasonable consensus in the community of nurse scholars on these assertions, perhaps we can direct our attention and energies to the critical analysis of existing incomplete theories in terms of their potential for further development.

REFERENCES

1. Bronowski, J. (1979). *The visionary age: Essays with arts, literature, and science.* Cambridge, Mass.: The MIT Press.
2. Brown, H. (1977). *Perception, theory and commitment: The new philosophy of science.* Chicago: The University of Chicago Press.
3. Dubin, R. (1978). *Theory building.* New York: The Free Press.
4. Flaskerud, J., & Halloran, E. (1980). Area of agreement in nursing theory development. *Advances in Nursing Science, 3:*1-7.
5. Giere, R.N. (1979). *Understanding scientific reasoning.* New York: Holt, Rinehart, & Winston.
6. Hage, J. (1972). *Techniques and problems in theory construction in sociology.* New York: John Wiley & Sons.
7. Hardy, N. (1983). Metaparadigms and theory development. In N. Chaska (Ed.), *The nursing profession: A time to speak.* New York: McGraw-Hill.
8. Kaplan, A. (1964). *The conduct of inquiry: Methodology for behavioral science.* New York: Chandler.
9. Merton, R., et al. (Eds.). (1952). *Reader in Bureaucracy.* New York: The Free Press.
10. Mills, C.W. (1959). On intellectual craftmanship. In L. Gross (Ed.), *Symposium on sociological theory.* Evanston, Ill.: Row, Peterson, & Co.
11. Mullins, N. (1971). *The art of theory: Construction and use.* New York: Harper & Row.
12. Nowak, S. (1975). Causal interpretations of statistical relationships in social research. In Blalock, H., et al. (Eds.), *Quantitative sociology: International perspectives on mathematical and statistical modeling.* New York: Academic Press.
13. Reynolds, P. (1971). *A primer in theory construction.* Indianapolis: Bobbs-Merrill.
14. Rosenberg, J. (1978). *The practice of philosophy.* Englewood Cliffs, N.J.: Prentice-Hall.
15. Salmon, W.D. (1973). *Logic.* Englewood Cliffs, N.J.: Prentice-Hall.
16. Steiner, E. (1978). *Logical and conceptual analytic techniques for educational researchers.* Washington, D.C.: University Press.
17. Turner, J. (1978). *The structure of sociological theory.* Homewood, Ill.: The Dorsey Press.
18. Walker, L., & Avant, K. (1983). *Strategies for theory construction in nursing,* Norwalk, Conn.: Appleton-Century-Crofts.
19. Werkmeister, W. (1959). Theory construction and the problem of objectivity. In L. Gross (Ed.), *Symposium on sociological theory.* Evanston, Ill.: Row, Peterson, & Co.
20. Zetterberg, H.L. (1966). *On theory and verification in sociology.* New York: John Wiley & Sons.

Evolution of Nursing Theory Development

Elizabeth Chong Choi

6

Nursing as a profession has been practiced for more than a century, but theory development in nursing has evolved most rapidly in the past three decades. In the mid 1800s, Nightingale[37] expressed her firm conviction that nursing required knowledge distinct from medical knowledge. She described what she believed was a nurse's proper function—to put the patient in the best condition for nature to act upon him. However, as Chinn and Jacobs noted,[5] not until the 1950s did members of the profession begin serious efforts to develop, articulate, and test nursing theory. Until the emergence of nursing as a science in the 1950s, nursing practice was based on rules, principles, and traditions passed on through an apprenticeship form of education and common wisdom that came from years of experience. Meleis[32] states that progress in nursing theory is a most significant aspect of scholarly evolution and the cornerstone of the nursing discipline.

Today there are many debates about theory in nursing that characterize the preparadigm period.[26] It is marked by frequent and deep debates over legitimate methods, problems, and standards of solutions, though these serve to define schools of thought rather than to produce agreement.[26] Kuhn[26] states that science progresses only when groups that now doubt

their own status achieve consensus about their past and present accomplishments.

Kim[22] identified that interest in nursing theory development emerged for two reasons. First, nursing leaders saw theory development as a means of clearly establishing nursing as a profession. Theory development was inherent in the long-standing interest in defining nursing's unique body of knowledge. Second, the theorists were motivated by the intrinsic value of theory for nursing and the importance of the growth and enrichment of theory for nursing in itself. "Today's theories represent the individual and collective efforts of nurses to define and direct the profession and, as such, provide the basis for continued theoretical development."[5:5]

Furthermore, two kinds of efforts are formed in the works of nursing scientists, both dealing with the definitional ambiguities in nursing. The first type is the grand theorist in nursing. Related models are used to describe the aspects of human conditions the discipline is concerned with and what the members of the discipline do as practitioners in a scientific field. On the other hand, middle range theorists have focused on developing elementary theoretical statements that deal with a few selected concepts relative to nursing.[22] This chapter examines both the grand theorists and middle range theorists in their theory development and traces the origin of their influence and their orientation to paradigms such as philosophy, interpersonal relationship, energy field, and system, that have influenced nursing.

FLORENCE NIGHTINGALE

The first author to be examined is Florence Nightingale. Her theory of nursing is closely related to her philosophical orientation of the client-environment interaction, and the principles and rules on which nursing practice was founded. Nightingale's emphasis on environment reflected a predominant concern of the late 1800s when sanitation was a major health problem.[58] Nightingale believed that disease was a reparative process. The manipulation of the external environment such as ventilation, warmth, light, diet, cleanliness, and noise would contribute to the reparative process and the patient's well being. She did not believe in the germ theory that was being postulated during her lifetime.[41] Nightingale's beliefs about nursing, what it is and what it is not, form the foundation upon which her notes on nursing were written. Her contribution to theory development is in explicating nursing's domain as the patient environment relationship and in pioneering statistical analysis for health and professional nursing. Nightingale's writings represent philosophy of nursing.[60]

HILDEGARD PEPLAU

Hildegard Peplau[43] referred to a partial theory for the practice of nursing. Her work was heavily influenced by Sullivan's interpersonal relationship model and reflects the view of the contemporaneous psychoanalytic model. Peplau is the first author to borrow from other scientific fields and relate this to nursing theory. Her influence in nursing through her theory development is praised as the second order of change in nursing.[55] Blake[4] calls Peplau's model developmental. However, it has strong emphasis on

interaction too. Thus it can be categorized as an interpersonal relationship.

IDA JEAN ORLANDO

Ida Jean Orlando[39,40] uses the interpersonal relationship as the basis for her work. She focuses on the patient's verbal and nonverbal expressions of needs. The nurse reacts to the patient's behavior by discerning both the meaning of the distress and what would alleviate the distress. Three elements—patient behavior, nurse reaction, and nursing actions—comprise a nursing situation. Orlando delineated automatic actions and deliberate actions. The deliberate actions are those that may yield solutions to problems and also prevent problems. She used the nursing process to meet the patient's need and thus alleviate distress. Her contribution as a theorist has advanced nursing, from personal and automatic responses to disciplined and professional practice responses.[54] Orlando's model can be categorized as interpersonal relationship.

JOYCE TRAVELBEE

Joyce Travelbee's model[59] is an extension of Peplau and Orlando's Interpersonal Relationship Model, but her unique synthesis of their ideas has strengthened her model in terms of the therapeutic relationship between nurse and patient. Her emphasis on caring, which stresses empathy, sympathy, and rapport, focuses on the emotional aspect and can be used as a philosophy for nursing. The model is categorized an interpersonal relationship.

ERNESTINE WIEDENBACH

Ernestine Wiedenbach[64] concentrated on the art or practice aspect of nursing. She focused on the need of the patient. Wiedenbach's model grew from 40 years of experience, primarily in maternity nursing, and her definition of nursing reflects that background. She said, "People may differ in their concept of nursing, but few would disagree that nursing is nurturing or caring for someone in a motherly fashion."[64:1] Wiedenbach's orientation[64] is a philosophy of nursing. It tells the nurse what to do or is a prescriptive level of theory.[6] According to Wiedenbach, clinical nursing has four elements: (1) philosophy, (2) purpose, (3) practice, and (4) art. Clinical nursing is directed toward the fulfillment of a specific purpose. The nurse's goal is to meet the perceived need-for-help the patient is experiencing.[64:15] Wiedenbach's theory of practice is influenced by her conception of nursing as an art. Her vision of nursing reflects the period of nursing theory development during which emphasis was on the art of nursing. She also follows Orlando's tradition of automatic versus deliberate nursing and incorporates the steps of the nursing process. Wiedenbach's model can be called philosophy of nursing.

LYDIA HALL

Lydia Hall[15] stressed the autonomous function of nursing. She identified three overlapping parts that comprise nursing: (1) the therapeutic use of self (the core aspect), (2) treatment within the health team (the cure aspect), and (3) the nurturing component (the care aspect). Her model is a philosophy of nursing influenced by Carl Rogers and other psychologists.[48,49] Her conceptualization encompasses adult patients who have passed the acute stage of illness. The goal for the client is rehabilitation and feelings of success in self-actualization and self-love. Her contribution to theory development is the actual implementation of her philosophy of care in Loeb Center and encouragement of professional nursing's contribution to client outcome. Hall's model is philosophy of nursing.

VIRGINIA HENDERSON

Virgina Henderson[16] views the patient as an individual who requires help toward indepen-

dence. She envisions the practice of nursing as independent from physicians. Henderson acknowledges her interpretation of the nurse's function as a synthesis of many influences. Her conceptual model is based on Thorndike's work, her experience in rehabilitation nursing, and Orlando's work regarding the continuation of deliberate nursing action.[2] Henderson emphasizes the art of nursing. She has identified fourteen problems. Her contributions include delineating autonomous nursing functions, stressing goals of interdependence for the patient, and creating self-help concepts that influenced Abdellah and Adam. Henderson's model is philosophy of nursing.

FAYE ABDELLAH

Faye Abdellah's model is based on the problem solving method, which had a great impact on nursing curriculum development.[1,56:165] Problem solving is the vehicle for delineating the nursing problems as the client is moved toward a healthy outcome. According to Abdellah[1], nursing is both an art and a science that mold the attitude, intellectual competencies, and technical skills of the individual nurse into the desire and ability to help people, whether ill or not, cope with their health needs. She believes nursing actions are carried out under general or specific medical direction. Abdellah has formulated twenty-one nursing problems based on research studies. Her work seems to be based somewhat on Henderson's fourteen principles and on research studies to establish the classification of nursing problems.[10] Abdellah may have been influenced by Maslow's hierarchy of needs, which encompasses both physical and psychological needs of a client.[10] The major difference between Henderson and Abdellah is that Abdellah's problems are formulated in terms of nursing-centered services, which can be incorporated to determine the client's needs. Abdellah's contribution to nursing theory development is the systematic use of research data in formulating and validating twenty-one nursing problems. Abdellah's model is philosophy of nursing.

DOROTHY JOHNSON

Dorothy Johnson[18,21] developed the behavioral system and labeled it a model for nursing practice, education, and research. Her model is influenced by ethological theorist and general systems theory. Johnson[21:212] considered attachment, or the affiliative subsystem, the corner stone and critical for all social organizations. Her behavioral system also includes the dependency, achievement, aggressive, ingestive, eliminative, and sexual subsystems. "Nursing problems arise because there are disturbances in the structure or function of the subsystems or the system, or because the level of behavioral functioning is at less than a desirable optimal level."[21:214] Johnson's contributions to nursing theory development are her actual model development, her writings related to philosophical issues on theory development, and her influence on students, such as Roy and Adams, who have subsequently contributed to nursing theory development.[19,20] Her model employs the system theory orientation.

MYRA LEVINE

Myra Levine borrowed from sciences such as psychology, sociology, and physiology, used this knowledge to analyze varied nursing practice suggestions, and described detailed nursing skills and activities.[29,30,44] Levine's Nursing Activity Analysis resulted in the formulation of four conservation principles in helping clients adapt to environment. She presented the person in a holistic manner and as the center of nursing activities. Her emphasis on the ill person in the health care setting is also reflective of the history of health care in the 1960s and the fact that she was writing a textbook to teach medical-surgical nursing to beginning students. Levine's model building has been influenced by the use of borrowed theory as well as nursing practice theory development.[44] She, in turn, influenced Roy. Levine's model can be categorized as energy field.

MARTHA ROGERS

Martha Rogers was influenced by general systems theory as well as electromagnetic theory. She clearly emphasizes the science of nursing versus the art of nursing in her delineation of the unitary human being as central to the discipline of nursing. Quillen and Runk have stated that Rogers' model had a significant influence on current scientific inquiry and professional nursing practice.[45] In addition, the model has served as a basis for the explication of other nursing conceptualizations, including those of Newman, Parse, and Fitzpatrick. It has also promoted research that has influenced the scientific community of nursing scholars who are investigating this model. Rogers' model can be categorized as energy field.

DOROTHEA OREM

Dorothea Orem[38] explicated self-care as a human need. Orem defines nursing as a human service and indicates that nursing's special concern is a person's need for the provision and management of self-care actions on a continuous basis in order to sustain life and health or to recover from disease or injury.[38] Fawcett[11] stated that the components of Orem's model, which focuses primarily on the individual, are capable of generating theories. Orem's contribution to theory development is further delineating nursing function in self-care needs and continuing to work for empirical support through research and previous work. Orem's model is philosophy of nursing.

IMOGENE KING

Imogene King[24,25] believes the patient is a personal system within an environment, coexisting with other personal systems. The nurse and the patient perceive one another and the situation, act and react, interact, and transact. King[25:144] defined nursing as a process of human interactions between nurse and clients, who communicate to set goals, explore means for achieving the goals, and then agree on the means to be used. King speaks of nursing as a discipline and an applied science, with emphasis on the derivation of nursing knowledge from other disciplines. King's model can be categorized as an interpersonal relationship. Fawcett[11] commented that King's conceptual framework is capable of generating a theory. Her contribution in theory development can be characterized as specifying outcome for nurse-client interactions, which are the end state of transaction for mutual satisfaction.

SISTER CALLISTA ROY

Sister Callista Roy[53] has based her work on Helson's adaptation model. Her model is a good example of how borrowed knowledge becomes unique in nursing.[53] It combines divergent thinking, such as systems, stress, and adaptation, into convergent views for explication of a person interacting with the environment. According to Roy, humans are biopsychosocial beings who exist within an environment. Environment and self provide three classes of stimuli: focal, residual, and contextual. Stimuli impact on humans and create needs in one or more interrelated adaptation modes, that is, physiological needs, self-concept, role function, and interdependence. Through two adaptive mechanisms, a regulator and a cognator, an individual can demonstrate adaptive responses (some successful, some not) or ineffective responses that require nursing intervention. The strength of Roy's model[52] is continued work related to the model, linking it to education, practice, and research and continued changes in the model to fit the growing empirical evidences. Roy's model is a system.

BETTY NEUMAN

Betty Neuman's model[34,35] is influenced by Gestalt theory, stress, and levels of prevention and can be characterized a system's model. Her conceptualization of the total person approach to client care is to help individuals, families, and groups attain and maintain a maximum level of total wellness by purposeful interventions.[35:119] Nursing intervention is aimed at the reduction of stress factors and adverse conditions that potentially or actually impact on optimal client functions. Her model represents the grand level theory focusing on the problem of summative concepts that are difficult at best to delineate for empirical testing.[8] At present, these are highly abstract and lack consistent operational definitions.[61] Her contribution to theory development is differentiating the level of prevention in nursing intervention as it relates to stress reduction. Neuman's model can be called a system.

MADELEINE LEININGER

Madeleine Leininger[27,28] espouses caring as the central theme in nursing care, nursing knowledge, and practice. Caring includes assistive, supportive, or facilitative acts toward an individual or a group with evident or anticipated needs. Caring serves to ameliorate or improve human conditions and life ways. Her methodology is borrowed from anthropology, but the concept of caring is an essential characteristic of nursing practice. She is credited with the foundation of transcultural nursing, and the resultant nursing research, education, and practice in this subfield of nursing. Leininger's model is philosophy of nursing.

JEAN WATSON

Jean Watson's theory[63] could be an extension of the Leininger model and borrows from an existential phenomenologist's view of psychology, and humanities. Nursing concerns itself with promoting health, preventing illness, caring for the sick, and restoring health. Clients require holistic care that promotes humanism, health, and quality living. Caring is a universal social phenomena that is only effectively practiced interpersonally. The ten caring factors represent both feelings and actions pertaining to the nurse, the patient, and the professional and include things to be felt, experienced, communicated, expressed, and promoted by every nurse.

Her theory contribution is in sensitizing individual practitioners to humanistic aspects and caring. Further work is needed for testability, but her work may currently be classified as a philosophy of nursing.

MARGARET NEWMAN

Margaret Newman's model[36] of health is a direct expansion of Rogers' theory. The goal of nursing is not to make well or to prevent illness, but to help people use the power within them as they evolve toward a higher level of consciousness.[36:37] Her contribution to theory development is the replication of earlier works and further expansion on the interaction of time, movement, space, and consciousness in maintaining life processes. She had also defined health differently, as a fusion of disease and nondisease. Further research and testing are needed to clarify relationships among variables. Newman's model, like Rogers', is highly abstract in its present form and further linking of concept to operational definition is needed for validation or refutation. The model can be categorized as an energy field.

JOAN RIEHL SISCA

Joan Riehl Sisca's interaction model[47] is a synthesis of works by Mead, Rose, and Erickson and uses symbolic interaction as the focus of nurse-client interaction. Her symbolic interaction was developed primarily to explain a philosophy of meaning. Communication is a major ingredient of symbolic interaction. Her work is borrowed from sociology and is categorized as interpersonal relationship.

ROSEMARIE RIZZO PARSE

Rosemarie Rizzo Parse[42] derives her theory from Rogers' principles and concepts, and synthesizes this with the existential-phenomenological views, such as those of Heidegger, Ponty, and Sartre. Parse's view of nursing is based on humanism as opposed to positivism.[31] Even though Parse developed her model largely from Rogers, whose model is highly abstract and lacking in testability, further work is needed in explicating each concept to form an operational definition and in linking existentialist relevancy to nursing phenomena. The strength of Parse's model may be a more humanistic approach as a philosophy of nursing. In addition, more emphasis on the relationship of man, environment, and health is addressed. Parse's model can be categorized as a philosophy of nursing.

HELEN ERICKSON, EVELYN TOMLIN, MARY ANN SWAIN

Helen Erickson, Evelyn Tomlin, and Mary Ann Swain's conceptual model is a synthesis of the works of Erickson, Maslow, Selye, Engel, and Piaget. They view nursing as interventions based on the client's perception of the world and adaptations related to stressors, and incorporate a self-care model. The model's contribution to nursing theory may be the interrelationships among disparate theories, such as motivation, stress development, and adaptation; but its major weakness may also originate from combining all of highly abstract theories into major summative concepts.[8] Erickson, Tomlin, and Swain's model can be categorized as interpersonal relationship.

JOYCE FITZPATRICK

Joyce Fitzpatrick's rhythm model[12] is based on research, which extends and refines Rogers' theory. Fitzpatrick uses Rogers' conceptualization of unitary man as a building block for her life perspective rhythm model.[50,51] She proposes that human development occurs within the context of continuous person-environment interaction.[12:300] Fitzpatrick's major concept relates to the development of persons as indices of temporal patterns, motion patterns, and consciousness patterns. She believes the meaning attached to life as the basic understanding of human existence is a central concern of nursing science and the nursing profession.[12:301] The model's contribution to theory development is that one of the indices—the temporal pattern—was developed by previous researchers. Other indices are largely untested, and research is needed to explicate the interrelation of indices in the future. Fitzpatrick's model can be called energy field.

KATHERINE BARNARD

Katherine Barnard's middle range theory[3] borrows from psychology and human development and focuses on the mother-infant interaction with the environment. Her model is based on empirical evidence accumulated through scales developed to measure feeding, teaching, and environment. Barnard's theory is at a descriptive level that follows traditional science. Her contribution to theory development is the limitation of her concepts to mother-infant interaction and environment during the first 3 years of life, allowing the development of conceptual and operational definitions. Continuous research refined the model by providing a closer link between the available data and the model. Barnard further extended scientific knowledge across disciplines, since knowledge is not unique to nursing. She has provided a role model for future scholars who would engage in theory development for furthering the science

of nursing. Barnard's model is interpersonal relationship.

EVELYN ADAM

Evelyn Adam[2] is a Canadian nurse who uses Johnson's model to show how Henderson's fourteen basic needs can be focused in terms of the nursing process and gives implications for research, practice, and education. Adam's model is a good example of using a unique basis of nursing for further expansion or addition. Adam has contributed to theory development by clarification of the earlier theorists' models. Adam's model is philosophy of nursing.

Through this overview, one can sense complete evolution of theory development in nursing (see box p. 58). First evolving a philosophy for nursing (Nightingale), then an emphasis on interpersonal relationships (Peplau, Orlando, Travelbee), the art of nursing (Henderson, Wiedenbach, Hall), and the beginning emphasis on the scientific aspects of nursing (Abdellah). These are followed by the systems approach and the emphasis of science (Johnson, Neuman, Roger, King, Orem, Roy, Barnard), with the philosophy for a humanistic nursing approach resurfacing (Watson, Leininger, Parse). Finally, there is further elaboration of earlier models (Parse, Newman, Fitzpatrick, Adam).

Before we look to the future, a prospective critical reexamination of where we are may help clarify our goals for the future of theory development. After reading all the theorists, it seems as if we are in the midst of a coined word explosion. Every theorist has defined nursing, environment, health, and person differently along with other terms such as adaptation, system, and stress. This profusion of definitions only creates further confusion.

A think tank should be created where all the theorists could work together to eliminate the redundancies and inconsistencies among the theories when defining identical phenomena,

THE EVOLUTION OF NURSING THEORY DEVELOPMENT

PHILOSOPHY

Nightingale (1860)
Abdellah (1960s-70s)
Wiedenbach (1960s)
Hall (1960s)
Henderson (1960s)
Leininger (1970s-80s)
Orem (1950s-80s)
Watson (1979-80s)
Adam (1980s)
Parse (1980s)

INTERPERSONAL RELATIONSHIP

Peplau (1950s)
Orlando (1960s)
Travelbee (1970s)
King (1970s-80s)
Barnard (1970s-80s)
Riehl (1980s)
Erickson, Swain, Tomlin (1980s)

ENERGY FIELD

Levine (1960s-70s)
Fitzpatrick (1970s-80s)
Rogers (1970s-80s)
Newman (1979-80s)

SYSTEMS

Neuman (1970s-80s)
Roy (1970s-80s)
Johnson (1980s)

such as Roy and Riehl attempted in suggesting a unified nursing model.[52] In this regard, Wortofsky[62:5] may have referred to the present status of nursing theory development by noting:

> Philosophy is nothing if not a dedicated search for coherence, for the synthesis of what we know in one field with what we know in others. Sometimes this enthusiasm for synthesis leads to excess, to fanciful systems and wishful unities of every-

thing-all-at-once which evaporate under critical examination, and are often no more than expressions of scientifically illiterate goodwill and pious hopes for coherence.

As Naisbitt[33] said in *Megatrends,* we are living in the time of the parenthesis, the time between eras. "It is as though we have bracketed off the present from both the past and the future, for we are neither here nor there."[33:279] This is a period of change, when anything can take place, and perhaps the rapid changes in nursing that are resulting from the theory development occurring now reflect the time.

The future of nursing is bright and full of hope. The theorists' different conceptualizations of nursing will enrich the discipline and its search for truth about persons, health, environment, and nursing. Our task for the future is to use further testing and collaboration to refute or support the truth about the nature of human beings from conceptual models. Kuhn[26:42] eloquently stated that a "paradigm can guide research in the absence of rules"; however, normal science cannot progress without the paradigm. These contributions represent the status of nursing as a discipline, and further development needs to occur for the explication of nursing phenomena. A great debate has occurred over what is nursing phenomena, whether nursing is an applied or a basic science, and whether it has a borrowed or unique body of knowledge.* What is more important is that models can predict or account for the phenomena of nursing, and are becoming more and more accepted by the nursing community of scholars. The debate should not be what each model represents, but rather how does it represent the truth we are seeking. The future direction should be toward the further clarification of each testable conceptual model so that each theorist's efforts should be replicating and refining her original model. Some theorists such as Roy,

*References 7, 11, 17, 18, 60.

Orem, Rogers, King, Leininger, and Barnard, have already been working in this regard. The development of nursing theory has come a long way, but there is still much to be done, for the future of nursing as a discipline depends on theory development.

The ultimate goal in theory development for nursing could be a multiple model, or a paradigm, that could guide scientists, and those who learn from them, closer and closer to the truth.[26] In addition, we should not insist on including all four concepts of person, health, environment, and nursing within a conceptual framework. Working at micro or middle range theory development would facilitate testability and establish further a scientific knowledge base. A philosophy of nursing should address the issues related to nursing practice or nursing as a discipline. Theory development should be directed toward explicating person, health, and environment interactions (although not simultaneously) by learning more about each relationship through theory and through research strategy.[46]

REFERENCES

1. Abdellah, F., et al. (1973). *New direction in patient-centered nursing.* New York: MacMillan.

2. Adam, E. (1980). *To be a nurse.* Toronto: W.B. Saunders.

3. Barnard, K.E., et al. (1977). *The nursing child assessment satellite training study guide.* Unpublished program learning manual. Seattle: University of Washington.

4. Blake, M. (1980). The Peplau development model. In J. Riehl & C. Roy (Eds.), *Conceptual models for nursing practice* (2nd ed.). New York: Appleton-Century-Crofts.

5. Chinn, P., & Jacobs, M. (1983). *Theory and nursing.* St. Louis: C.V. Mosby.

6. Dickoff, J., & James, P. (1968). A theory of theories: A position paper. *Nursing Research, 17*:197-203.

7. Donaldson, S.K., & Crowley, D.M. (1978). The discipline of nursing. *Nursing Outlook, 26*:113-120.

8. Dubin, R. (1978). *Theory building.* New York: The Free Press.

9. Erickson, H., Tomlin, E., & Swain, M. (1983). *Modeling and role-modeling: A theory and paradigm for nursing.* Englewood Cliffs, N.J.; Prentice-Hall.

10. Falco, S.M. (1980). Faye G. Abdellah. In Nursing Theories Conference Group, J.B. George (Ed.), *Nursing Theories: The base for professional practice.* Englewood Cliffs, N.J.: Prentice Hall.

11. Fawcett, J. (1983). Hallmarks of success in nursing theory development. In P. Chinn (Ed.), *Advances in nursing theory development.* Rockville, Md.: Aspen Systems.

12. Fitzpatrick, J. (1983). A life perspective rhythm model. In J. Fitzpatrick & A. Whall (Eds.), *Conceptual models of nursing: Analysis and application.* Bowie, Md.: Robert J. Brady.

13. Gale, G. (1979). *Theory of science: An introduction to the history, logic and philosophy of science.* New York: McGraw-Hill.

14. Giere, R.N. (1979). *Understanding scientific reasoning.* New York: Holt, Rinehart & Winston.

15. Hall, L. (1969). The Loeb Center for Nursing and Rehabilitation. *International Journal of Nursing Studies, 6*:81-95.

16. Henderson, V. (1966). *The nature of nursing: A definition and its implications, practice, research, and education.* New York: Macmillan.

17. Jacox, A. (1974). Theory construction in nursing: An overview. *Nursing Research, 23*:4-13.

18. Johnson, D.E. (1968). State of the art of theory development in nursing. In *Theory development: What, why, how?* New York: National League for Nursing.

19. Johnson, D.E. (1968). *One conceptual model of nursing.* Unpublished paper presented April 25 at Vanderbilt University, Nashville, Tenn.

20. Johnson, D.E. (1974). Development of a theory: A requisite for nursing at a primary health profession. *Nursing Research, 23*(5):372-377.

21. Johnson, D.E. (1980). The behavioral system model for nursing. In J.P. Riehl & S.C. Roy (Eds.), *Conceptual models for nursing practice* (2nd ed.). New York: Appleton-Century-Crofts.

22. Kim, H.S. (1983). *The nature of theoretical thinking in nursing.* Norwalk, Conn.: Appleton-Century-Crofts.

23. King, I. (1968). A conceptual frame of references for nursing. *Nursing Research, 17*:27-31.

24. King, I. (1971). *Towards a theory of nursing.* New York: John Wiley & Sons.
25. King, I. (1981). *A theory of nursing: systems, concepts, process.* New York: John Wiley & Sons.
26. Kuhn, T.S. (1970). *The structure of scientific revolutions.* Chicago: University of Chicago Press.
27. Leininger, M. (1981). *Caring: An essential human need. Proceedings of the Three National Caring Conferences.* Thorofare, N.J.: Charles B. Slack.
28. Leininger, M. (1978). *Transcultural nursing concepts, theories, and practice.* New York: John Wiley & Sons.
29. Levine, M.E. (1967). The four conservation principles of nursing. *Nursing Forum, 6:*45-59.
30. Levine, M.E. (1973). *Introduction to clinical nursing.* Philadelphia: F.A. Davis.
31. Limandri, B. (1982). Review of *Man-living-health: A theory of nursing* by Rosemarie Rizzo Parse. *Western Journal of Nursing Research, 4*(1):105.
32. Meleis, A. (1983). The evolving nursing scholars. In P. Chinn (Ed.), *Advances in nursing theory development.* Rockville, Md.: Aspen Systems.
33. Naisbitt, J.C. (1984). *Megatrends: Ten new directions transforming our lives.* New York: Warner.
34. Neuman, B. (1980). The Betty Neuman healthcare systems model: A total person approach to patient problems. In J. Riehl & C. Roy (Eds.), *Conceptual models for nursing practice* (2nd ed.). New York: Appleton-Century-Crofts.
35. Neuman, B. (Ed.) (1982). *The Neuman systems model.* New York: Appleton-Century-Crofts.
36. Newman, M. (1979). *Theory development in nursing.* Philadelphia: F.A. Davis.
37. Nightingale, F. (1969). *Notes on nursing: What it is and what it is not.* New York: Dover. (Originally published, 1859.)
38. Orem, D.E. (1985). *Nursing: Concepts of practice.* (3rd ed). New York: McGraw-Hill.
39. Orlando, I.J. (1961). *The dynamic nurse-patient relationship.* New York: G.P. Putnam's Sons.
40. Orlando, I.J. (1972). *The discipline and teaching of nursing process.* New York: G.P. Putnam's Sons.
41. Palmer, I.S. (1977). Florence Nightingale: Reformer, reactionary, researcher. *Nursing Research, 26*(2):84-89.
42. Parse, R.R. (1981). *Man-living-health: A theory of nursing.* New York: John Wiley & Sons.
43. Peplau, H.E. (1952). *Interpersonal relations in nursing.* New York: G.P. Putnam's Sons.
44. Pieper, B.C. (1983). Levine's nursing model. In J. Fitzpatrick, & A. Whall (Eds.), *Conceptual models of nursing: Analysis and application.* Bowie, Md.: Robert J. Brady.
45. Quillen, S., & Runk, J. (1983). Martha Rogers' model. In J. Fitzpatrick, & A. Whall (Eds.), *Conceptual models of nursing: Analysis and application.* Bowie, Md.: Robert J. Brady.
46. Reynolds, P. (1971). *A primer in theory construction.* Indianapolis: Bobbs-Merrill.
47. Riehl, J. (1980). The Riehl interaction model. In J. Riehl & C. Roy (Eds.), *Conceptual models for nursing practice* (2nd ed.). New York: Appleton-Century-Crofts.
48. Rogers, C. (1951). *Client-centered therapy.* Boston: Houghton Mifflin.
49. Rogers, C. (1961). *On becoming a person.* Boston: Houghton Mifflin.
50. Rogers, M.E. (1970) *The theoretical basis of nursing.* Philadelphia: F.A. Davis.
51. Rogers, M.E. (1980). A science of unitary man. In J.P. Riehl & C. Roy (Eds.). *Conceptual models for nursing practice* (2nd ed.). New York: Appleton-Century-Crofts.
52. Roy, C. (1984). *An introduction to nursing: An adaptation model* (2nd ed.). Englewood Cliffs, N.J.: Prentice-Hall.
53. Roy, C.S. (1976). *Introduction to nursing: An adaptation model.* Englewood Cliffs, N.J.: Prentice-Hall.
54. Schmieding, N.C. (1983). An analysis of Orlando's nursing theory based on Kuhn's Theory of science. In P. Chinn (Ed.), *Advances in nursing theory development.* Rockville, Md.: Aspen Systems.
55. Sills, G. (1978). Leader, practitioner, academician, scholar, theorist. *Perspectives in Psychiatric Care, 16*(3):122-128.
56. Stevens, B.J. (1984). *Nursing Theory: Analysis, Application, Evaluation* (2nd ed.). Boston: Little, Brown.
57. Sullivan, H.S. (1952). *The interpersonal theory of psychiatry.* New York: W.W. Norton.
58. Torres, G. (1980). Florence Nightingale. In Nursing Theories Conference Group, J.B. George, Chairperson, *Nursing theories: The base for professional nursing practice.* Englewood Cliffs, N.J.: Prentice-Hall.

59. Travelbee, J. (1971). *Interpersonal aspects of nursing*. Philadelphia: F.A. Davis.
60. Walker, L.O. (1971). Toward a clearer understanding of the concept of nursing theory. *Nursing Research, 20:*428-435.
61. Walker, L.O., & Avant, K.C. (1983). *Strategies for theory construction in nursing*. Norwalk, Conn.: Appleton-Century-Crofts.
62. Wartofsky, M. (1968). *Conceptual foundations of scientific thought*. New York: Macmillan.
63. Watson, J. (1979). *Nursing: The philosophy and science of caring*. Boston: Little, Brown.
64. Wiedenbach, E. (1964). *Clinical nursing: A helping art*. New York: Springer.

UNIT II

Art and Science of Humanistic Nursing

Florence Nightingale

7

Modern Nursing

Karen R. deGraaf, Cynthia L. Mossman, Maribeth Slebodnik

CREDENTIALS AND BACKGROUND OF THE THEORIST

Florence Nightingale, the matriarch of modern nursing, was born May 12, 1820, while her British parents were on an extended European tour. Her parents, Edward and Frances Nightingale, named their daughter for her birthplace, Florence, Italy.

The Nightingales were affluent and well-educated members of a Victorian family. So as Nightingale grew older her father tutored her in mathematics, languages, religion, and philosophy. In her teens Nightingale was active in aristocratic society, but she felt her life should be more useful. In 1837 she confided in her diary that "God spoke to me and called me to his service."[6:8;7:41]

In 1851, Nightingale went to Kaiserswerth, Germany, for her early nursing training. After leaving Kaiserswerth, she continued to examine the facilities at hospitals, reformatories, and charitable institutions. In 1853 she became Superintendent of the Hospital for Invalid Gentlewomen in London.

During the Crimean War Nightingale volunteered to go to Scutari, Turkey. There she organized a nursing department and devoted her efforts to eliminating sanitation problems in the wards. At that time women working in hospitals were not respectable, reliable, or educated. There were no trained nurses and no British Red Cross. Consequently, Nightingale solicited and received help from the Sisters of Mercy.

Conditions in the army wards were poor. In addition to their wounds, the soldiers suffered from exposure, frostbite, lice infestations, and disease. There were few chamber pots; latrines were blocked; cess pools overflowed; and the water was contaminated. Patients who couldn't feed themselves starved. There were no surgery tables or anesthesia.

Nightingale's work made her popular with the men. They called her "the Lady of the Lamp" in recognition of her Turkish candle lantern she carried through the corridors packed with wounded soldiers. While at Scutari Nightingale became critically ill with Crimean fever, which might have been typhus.

Nightingale returned to England following the war and established a teaching institution for nurses at St. Thomas Hospital and at King's College Hospital in London. These were established from funds received in recognition of her war service. Nightingale kept close contact with her graduates through encouraging letters. Within a few years after its foundation, the Nightingale School began receiving requests for nurses to found new schools at hospitals worldwide and Florence Nightingale's reputation as the founder of modern nursing was assured.

During her carreer Nightingale concentrated on army sanitation reform, army hospitals, and sanitaiton in India and among the poorer classes in England. She wrote *Notes on Matters Affecting the Health, Efficiency, and Hospital Administration of the British Army* (1858), *Notes on Hospitals* (1858), *Notes on the Sanitary State of the Army in India* (1871), and *Life or Death in India* (1874). For her efforts, Nightingale received numerous awards, including the Order of Merit from King Edward VII, Germany's Cross of Merit, and France's Secours aux Blesses Militaires.

Nightingale wrote between 15,000 and 20,000 letters to friends and distinguished acquaintances. These often displayed her beliefs, observations, and desire for change in health care. She worked into her eighties gathering data and writing about nursing and health care. She enjoyed a robust old age before suffering a gradual loss of vision, which made reading and writing difficult. She was widely recognized for her knowledge, drive, and compassion.

Nightingale died in her sleep at the age of 90 on August 13, 1910, in London. But many of her revolutionary ideas continue to inspire contemporary nursing.

THEORETICAL SOURCES FOR THEORY DEVELOPMENT

Many factors influenced the development of Nightingale's theory for nursing. Individual, societal, and professional values were all integral in the development of her work. She combined her individual resources with societal and professional resources to produce change.

Nightingale, who considered nursing a religious calling to be answered only by women, believed she should strive to change the things she saw as unacceptable. Chinn and Jacobs[2:46] note that "When individual or professional values are in conflict with and challenge societal values, there is potential for creating change in society." Nightingale lived up to that potential. The health care system of her era used the uneducated and incompetent to care for the ill. But Nightingale transformed it into the system of professional nursing practices we value today.

Nightingale knew that contact with the professionals of her time was important. She expanded her philosophy of nursing through association with numerous prominent physicians and other influential members of society.

The strongest influences on the development of her practice were her education, experience, and observation. She gained these through years of charitable and hospital work and military nursing. They established the logical base for her nursing philosophy.

USE OF EMPIRICAL EVIDENCE

Nightingale was a devoted statistician. She used her carefully collected information to prove the efficacy of her system of hospital nursing and organization during the Crimean War. The report of her data and experiences, entitled *Notes on Matters Affecting the Health, Efficiency, and Hospital Administration of the British Army,* was given to the British Royal Sanitary Commission, which had been organized in response to Nightingale's charges of poor sanitary conditions. "It showed that for every man killed in battle in the Crimea, seven died from disease. Even in peacetime the mortality rate in the barracks was twice that of the general population."[3:396]

Palmer[12:88] identified Nightingale's research skills as recording, communicating, ordering, coding, conceptualizing, inferring, analyzing, and synthesizing. Nightingale viewed observation and practice as concurrent activities.

MAJOR CONCEPTS AND DEFINITIONS

Nightingale's grand theory focused on the environment. Murray and Zentner[8:149] state that the environment, which is capable of preventing, suppressing or contributing to disease, accidents, or death, is all the external conditions and influences affecting the life and development of an organism. While the term environment does not itself appear in Miss Nightingale's writings, her major concepts of ventilation, warmth, light, diet, cleanliness, and noise comprise the components of environment as defined above.

Although Nightingale usually defined concepts precisely, she did not clearly separate the patient's environment into physical, emotional, or social aspects. She assumed these aspects were encompassed by the environment, but made no clear distinction of how to differentiate them. "Although she tends to emphasize the physical more than the psychological or social environment, this needs to be viewed in the context of her time and her activities as a nurse leader in a war-torn environment."[11:28]

Nightingale emphasized several aspects of the environment in her work. She believed healthy surroundings were necessary for proper nursing care. Although she specifically addressed the issue of health in homes with this passage, it may be assumed she was referring to hospitals as well when she said:

> There are five essential points in securing the health of houses: (1) pure air, (2) pure water, (3) efficient drainage, (4) cleanliness, [and] (5) light. Without these, no house can be healthy. And it will be unhealthy just in proportion as they (sic) are deficient.[10:24]

Nightingale felt the public needed to believe and practice these procedures in order to have healthy homes. She wanted people to use common sense, but only after they were educated to essential facts regarding health.

The aspect of the environment that concerned Nightingale most was providing proper ventilation for a patient. This meant the nurse was "to keep the air he breathes as pure as the external air, without chilling him."[10:12] Nightingale believed a steady supply of fresh air was the most important principle in nursing. She said pure air was "the very first canon of nursing, the first and the last thing upon which a nurse's attention must be fixed, the first essential to a patient, without which all the rest you can do for him is nothing."[10:12]

Light was another element of nursing care that Nightingale believed could not be ignored.

> It is the unqualified result of all my experience with the sick, that second only to their need of fresh air is their need of light. . . . And that it is not only light, but direct sun-light they want. . . . Without going into any scientific exposition we must admit that light has quite as real and tangible effects upon the human body. . . . Who has not observed the purifying effect of light, and especially of direct sunlight, upon the air of a room?[10:84-85]

Nightingale firmly believed in the beneficial aspects of direct sunlight. She even suggested that a nurse might have to carry the patient "about after the sun, according to the aspects of the rooms, if circumstances permit."[10:84]

The need for cleanliness extended to the patient, the nurse, and the environment, Nightingale believed. She stated that dirty carpets and walls contained large quantities of organic matter and provided a ready source of infection, just as dirty sheets and beds did. A well-ventilated dirty room and a clean unventilated room were both deemed dirty areas. Nightingale also believed that unwashed skin interfered with the healing process and that washing removed noxious matter from the system quickly. Therefore nurses should wash their hands frequently and keep their patients very clean.[10:94]

In addition to her five main points of emphasis, Nightingale also believed a nurse should attend to a patient's warmth, quiet, and diet.[10:8] She advised nurses to constantly monitor patients' body temperatures by palpatating the extremities to prevent the effects of vital heat loss.[10:17] Nightingale delineated specific instructions for providing fresh air while avoiding a chilly climate. She castigated medical and nursing personnel who neglected ventilation for the sake of warmth and thereby exposed their patients to the dangers of foul, infected air.[10:15] "The safest atmosphere of all for a patient is a good fire and open window, excepting in extremes of temperature."[10:19]

Noise was another environmental element Nightingale believed the nurse should manipulate. "Unnecessary noise, or noise that creates an expectation in the mind, is that which hurts a patient. . . . Any sacrifice to secure silence . . . is worthwhile, because no air, however good, no attendance however careful, will do anything . . . without quiet."[10:45,47] By maintaining that noise could impede the progress of the patient's recovery, even if there were fresh air and good attendance by nurses, she clarified the interrelatedness of her major concepts.

Nightingale was also concerned with a patient's diet. She believed a nurse should not only assess the dietary intake, but also assess the timeliness of the food and its effect on the patient. Observation, ingenuity, and perserverance were the qualities Nightingale felt should distinguish a good nurse so that patients were not starved to death because of chronic illnesses.[10:65] She said "If the nurse is an intelligent being, and not a mere carrier of diets to and from the patient, let her exercise her intelligence in these things."[10:67]

MAJOR ASSUMPTIONS

Nightingale believed that every woman, at one time or another, would be a nurse in the sense that nursing was to have the responsibility for someone's health. Thus, she provided women with guidelines for nursing care and advice on how to "think how to nurse."[10:3-4]

Nightingale refers to the person as a patient in most of her writings. However, the patient is regarded as being acted upon by the nurse or affected by the environment. The patient is passive and does not seem to influence the nurse or the environment.

Nightingale defined health as being well and using to the fullest extent every power we have.[10:334-5] Additionally, she saw disease as a reparative process nature instituted because of some want of attention.[10:7] Nightingale envisioned health as being maintained through the prevention of disease via environmental health factors. She called this health nursing and distinguished it from nursing proper, which was nursing of the diseased patient so he could survive or at least live better until his death.[10:199]

The environment, Nightingale asserted, was one of the chief sources of infection. Fitzpatrick and Whall[4:16-7] state that Nightingale's concept of the environment was "those elements external to and which affect the health of the sick and healthy person" and included "everything from the patient's food and flowers to the nurse's verbal and nonverbal interactions with the patient."

THEORETICAL ASSERTIONS

Nightingale believed disease was a reparative process. Disease, she felt, was nature's effort to remedy a process of poisoning or decay, or a reaction against the conditions in which a person was placed. Nightingale directed that nursing's role was to prevent the reparative process from being interrupted and to provide optimal conditions for its enhancement. Nurses encouraged this process by providing proper environmental conditions such as fresh air, light, pure water, efficient drainage, cleanliness, warmth, quiet, and appropriate diet. Nightingale also felt nurses had to use common sense to achieve these conditions, but that it had to be coupled with perserverance, observation, and ingenuity. Nightingale assumed the person was desirous of health, so that the nurse, nature, and the person would cooperate to allow the reparative process to occur.

LOGICAL FORM

Nightingale used inductive reasoning to extract laws of health and nursing from her observations and experiences. For example, she noticed that disease flourished in confined, dark, damp areas and concluded it was generated in such environments. She also derived from this observation her belief that disease could be prevented, or its cure hastened, by providing an environment antithetical to the one in which disease originated. Many of these observations and derived principles originated during her wartime experiences.

ACCEPTANCE BY NURSING COMMUNITY
Practice

Nightingale's nursing principles remain applicable to nursing practice today. Ventilation, warmth, quiet, diet, and cleanliness are integral parts of nursing care. Pure water and efficient drainage are controlled by public health regulations. In her book, *Notes on Nursing,* Nightingale suggested concepts that are relatively simple to apply in practice, yet many of them are overlooked in the highly technical areas of nursing. Contemporary practitioners would find value in examination and use of her concepts.

Much of Nightingale's rationale has been modified or disproved because of advances in medicine and nursing. However, it is important to remember Nightingale's background and the advances she made in her era. Her inclusion of both health teaching and sick nursing within nursing's domain was a then-revolutionary concept that still defines nursing practice, and her insistence upon proper education and social support systems for nursing remains pertinent today. The numerous articles and books written regarding Nightingale's attitudes and contributions demonstrate her continued acceptance by nursing in the area of practice.

Education

The Nightingale system was the basis for the origination of many early nurse training schools, including St. Thomas Hospital and King's College Hospital in London. This system is no longer in general use, but its influence lingers on in the combination of practical and didactic training found in today's nursing programs. Nightingale advocated the nursing school's independence from hospitals so that students were not involved in the hospital's labor pool as part of their training. Nightingale felt the "art of nursing" could not be standardized and therefore licensing examinations were inappropriate, but her opinion was overridden shortly after her death. Scholarships and grants in her honor continue to allow students to pursue advanced studies in nursing.

Research

Nightingale's interest in statistics and their importance to nursing continues to influence nursing research. She was exceptionally efficient and resourceful in her ability to gather and analyze data. Much of these data may be found in her numerous letters. She was one of the first to use graphic illustrations in statistics.[1:665] Many of these illustrations continue to be used by statisticians today. Nightingale recognized the importance of data collection in nursing care. While her methods have had a continued effect on research in nursing, her theory lacks complexity and testability.[4:23] Therefore, it has not generated nursing research.

FURTHER DEVELOPMENT

Nightingale's theory for nursing is stated clearly and concisely. *Notes on Nursing* was Nightingale's most widely known work and one that seems most amenable to theory analysis. The organization of chapters treating various aspects of nursing care suggests that perhaps the main goal is definition and elaboration of concepts rather than organization of a theory. Fitzpatrick and Whall[4:18] state that this theory can be described as a "set of laws" theory. Laws are theoretical statements with overwhelming empirical support.

It might also be proposed that Nightingale formulated a grand theory, as described by Margaret Hardy:[5:42]

A theory in the early stage of development is characterized by discursive presentation and descriptive accounts of anecdotal reports to illustrate and support its claims. The theoretical terms are usually vague and ill defined, and their meaning may be close to everyday language. A paradigm at this embryonic stage is very readable and provides a perspective rather than a set of interrelated theoretical statments. . . . This type of formulation, the "grand theory" or "general orientation," is aimed at explaining the totality of behavior. Grand theories tend to use vague terminology, leave the relationships between terms unclear and provide formulations that cannot be tested.

Nightingale's intention to provide a first step for the formalization and development of nursing seems to have been accomplished. Her achievements spawned the beginning of nursing as we know it today. Nightingale's theory

was a lower level theory, but it sets the stage for further work in the development of nursing theories.

CRITIQUE
Simplicity

Nightingale's theory contains three major relationships: environment to patient, nurse to environment, and nurse to patient. She viewed environment as the main factor acting upon the patient to produce an illness state, and regarded disease as "the reactions of kindly nature against the conditions in which we have placed ourselves."[10:32] The nurse as manipulator of environment and actor on the patient is described when Nightingale said nursing "ought to signify the proper use of fresh air, light, warmth, cleanliness, quiet, and the proper selection and administration of diet—all at the least expense of vital power to the patient."[10:8] These relationships are expanded on in the text of *Notes on Nursing*. The book is organized into chapters dealing with the components of environment, such as ventilation, warmth, light, noise, and cleanliness. Relationships between these environmental components are also described, as when Nightingale states, "Without cleanliness, within and without your house, ventilation is comparatively useless."[10:27]

The concepts and their relationships cannot be combined in order to increase simplicity; they are in economical form as Nightingale stated them. Various diagrams for the theory have been proposed, suggesting that it is simple and logical enough to allow such visual representation. This theory tends toward description and explanation rather than prediction. Nightingale did not intend to develop theory, but to define nursing and set forth general rules for its practice and development. Simplicity of the theory was therefore necessary and is present.

Generality

Nightingale's theory attempts to provide general guidelines for all nurses in all times. Although many of her specific directives are no longer applicable, the general concepts, such as the relationships between nurse, patient, and environment, are still pertinent. The theory is specifically directed toward the nurse, defined as a woman who at some time has charge of somebody's health, and is thus not restricted to the professional nurse. In order to address her audience, the proposed theory is of necessity very broad. Generality is a criterion met by Nightingale's theory.

Empirical Precision

Concepts and relationships within Florence Nightingale's theory are frequently stated implicitly and are presented as established truths rather than tentative, testable statements. Little or no provision is made for empirical examination. Indeed, Nightingale suggested that the practice of nursing should be built upon individual observation rather than systematic research when she advised, "Let experience, not theory, decide upon this as upon all other things."[10:76]

The generality implicit in Nightingale's theory and hence its lack of specificity make empirical generalization of the theory difficult.

Derivable Consequences

Nightingale's writings, to an extraordinary degree, direct the nurse to action in the behalf of her patient and herself. These directives encompass the areas of practice, research, and education. Most specific are her principles attempting to shape nursing practice. She urges nurses to provide doctors with "not your opinion, however respectfully given, but your facts."[10:113] She goes on to say, "If you cannot get the habit of observation one way or other, you had better give up the being a nurse, for it is not your calling, however kind and anxious you may be."[10:122] Her encouragement of a measure of independence and precision previously unknown in nursing may still guide and motivate us today as nursing continues to evolve.

Nightingale's view of humanity was consistent with her theories of nursing. She believed in creative, universal humanity with the poten-

tial and ability for growth and change.[12:85] Deeply religious, she viewed nursing as a means of doing the will of her God. Perhaps it is because of this concept of nursing as a divine calling that she relegated the patient to a passive role, essentially infantile, with every want and need provided by the nurse. The excessive zeal and self-rightousness of a religious reformer might partially account for this behavior. Although the lack of patient involvement in health seems to be a gap in Nightingale's views, it may be accounted for by the historical period in which she lived and wrote.

Basic principles of environmental manipulation and psychological care of the patient can be applied with modification in many contemporary nursing settings. Of course, many technological and societal changes have occurred since Nightingale's day, which reduce some of her fondest assertions to the ludicrous. Her unshakable disdain for the germ theory of disease and adherence to the belief that dirt and dampness are pathogenic now seems less than progressive.[12:87] Likewise, her emphasis on personal observation rather than formation of a unified body of nursing knowledge has fallen into disuse.

Lack of specificity has hindered use of Nightingale's ideas for the generation of nursing research. However, her writings continue to stimulate productive thinking for the individual nurse and the nursing profession. Nightingale was brilliant and creative. She gave nursing much food for thought—food that continues to nourish us 120 years later.

REFERENCES

1. Agnew, L.R. (1958, May). Florence Nightingale, statistician. *American Journal of Nursing, 58:*644.
2. Chinn, P., & Jacobs, M. (1983). *Theory and nursing: A systematic approach.* St. Louis: C.V. Mosby.
3. Cruse, P. (1980, Sept.). Florence Nightingale. *Surgery 88*(3):394-9.
4. Fitzpatrick, J., & Whall, A. (1983). *Conceptual models of nursing.* Bowie, Md.: Prentice-Hall.

5. Hardy, M. (1978). Perspectives on nursing theory. *Advances In Nursing Science, 1*:37-48.

6. Isler, C. (1970). *Florence Nightingale: Rebel with a cause*. Oradell, N.Y.: Medical Economics.

7. Isler, C. (1970, May). Florence Nightingale: Rebel with a cause, *RN, 33*:39-55.

8. Murray, R., & Zenter, J. (1975). *Nursing concepts in health promotion*. Englewood Cliffs, N.J.: Prentice Hall.

9. Nightingale, F. (1954). *Selected writings*. Compiled by Lucy R. Seymer. New York: Macmillan.

10. Nightingale, F. (1969). *Notes on nursing: What it is and what it is not*. New York: Dover.

11. Nursing Theories Conference Group, J.B. George, Chairperson. (1980). *Nursing theories: The base for professional practice*. Englewood Cliffs, N.J.: Prentice-Hall.

12. Palmer, I.S. (1977, March-April). Florence Nightingale: Reformer, reactionary, researcher. *Nursing Research*, 26:84-9.

13. *World Who's Who in Science*. (1968). Florence Nightingale. Chicago: A.N. Marquis.

BIBLIOGRAPHY
Primary Sources
Books

Nightingale, F. (1911). *Letters from Miss Florence Nightingale on health visiting in rural districts*. London: King.

Nightingale, F. (1954). *Selected writings*. Compiled by Lucy R. Seymer. New York: Macmillan.

Nightingale, F. (1956). *The institution of Kaiserswerth on the Rhine, Dusseldorf, Germany*. Anna Sticker.

Nightingale, F. (1957). *Notes on nursing*. Philadelphia: Lippincott. (Originally published, 1859).

Nightingale, F. (1969). *Notes on nursing: What it is and what it is not*. New York: Dover.

Nightingale, F. (1974). *Letters of Florence Nightingale in the history of nursing archive*. Boston: Boston University.

Nightingale, F. (1976). *Notes on hospitals*. New York: Gordon.

Nightingale, F. (1978). Notes on nursing. London: Duckworth.

Nightingale, F. (1979). *Cassandra, an essay*. Old Westbury, N.Y.: Feminist Press.

Journal Articles

Nightingale, F. (1930, July). Trained nursing for the sick poor, *International Nursing Review, 5*:426-433.

Nightingale, F. (1954, May 7). Maternity hospital and midwifery school. *Nursing Mirror, 99*:ix-xi, 369.

Nightingale, F. (1954). The training of nurses, *Nursing Mirror, 99*:iv-xi.

Secondary Sources
Book Reviews

Nightingale, F. (1954). Selected writings. *Nursing Mirror 100*:846, Dec. 24, 1954. Roy San Inst. J. *75*:275-276, April 1955. *American Journal of Nursing, 55*:162, May 1955. *Nursing Times, 51*:502-503, 507, May 6, 1955.

Nightingale, F. (1969). *Notes on Nursing: What it is and what it is not*. *Nursing Times, 66*:828, June 25, 1970. *Nursing Mirror, 131*:47, Oct. 9, 1970.

Nightingale, F.: *Notes on nursing: What it is and what it is not, the science and art*. *Nursing Times, 76*:187, Oct. 23, 1980. *Nursing Mirror, 151*:41, Dec. 11, 1980. *Australian Nurses Journal, 10*:29, Feb. 1981.

Nightingale, F. (1979). *Cassandra, an essay. American Journal of Nursing, 81*:1059–1061, May 1981.

Seymer, L.R.: *Florence Nightingale*. (1950). *Nursing Mirror, 92*:31, Nov. 17, 1950. *Nursing Times, 46*:1285, Dec. 16, 1950. *Journal of the American Medical Association, 146*:605, June 9, 1951. *Public Health Nursing, 43*: 459, Aug. 1951.

Books

Aiken, C.A. (1915). *Lessons from the life of Florence Nightingale*. New York: Lakeside.

Aldis, M. (1914). *Florence Nightingale*. New York: NOPHN.

Andrews, M.R. (1929). *A lost commander*. Garden City, N.J.: Doubleday.

Barth, R.J. (1945). *Fiery angel: The story of Florence Nightingale*. Coral Gables, Fla.: Glade House.

Bishop, W.J. (1962). *A bio-bibliography of Florence Nightingale*. London: Dawson's of Pall Mall.

Boyd, N. (1982). *Three Victorian women who changed their world*. New York: Oxford.

Columbia University Faculty of Medicine and Department of Nursing. (1937). *Catalogue of the Florence Nightingale collection* New York: the Department.

Cook, E.T. (1913). *The life of Florence Nightingale.* London: Macmillan.

Cook, E.T. (1941). *A short life of Florence Nightingale,* New York: Macmillan.

Cope, Z. (1958). *Florence Nightingale and the doctors.* Philadelphia: Lippincott.

Cope, Z. (1961). *Six disciples of Florence Nightingale.* New York: Pitman.

Editors of *RN.* (1970). *Florence Nightingale: Rebel with a cause.* Oradell, N.J.: Medical Economics.

French, Y. (1953). *Six great Englishwomen.* London: H. Hamilton.

Goldsmith, M.L. (1937). Florence Nightingale: The woman and the legend. London: Hodder and Stoughtons.

Goldwater, S.S. (1947). *On hospitals.* New York: Macmillan.

Gordon, R. (1979). *The private life of Florence Nightingale.* New York: Atheneum.

Haldale, E. (1931). *Mrs. Gaskell and her friends.* New York: Appleton.

Hall, E.F. (1920). *Florence Nightingale.* New York: Macmillan.

Hallock, G.T., & Turner, C.E. (1928). *Florence Nightingale.* New York: Metropolitan Life Insurance Co.

Herbert, R.G. (1980). *Florence Nightingale: Saint, reformer, or rebel? Melbourne, Fla.: Krieger.*

Holmes, M. (n.d.) *Florence Nightingale—A cameo life-sketch.* London: Woman's Freedom League.

Huxley, E.J. (1975). *Florence Nightingale.* London: Putnam.

Hyndman, J.A. (1969). *Florence Nightingale: Nurse to the world.* Cleveland, Ohio: World Publishing.

Keele, J. (Ed.). (1981). *Florence Nightingale in Rome.* Philadelphia, Pa.: American Philosophical Society.

Lammond, D. (1935). *Florence Nightingale.* London: Duckworth.

Miller, B.W. (1947). *Florence Nightingale: The lady with the lamp.* Grand Rapids, Mich.: Zondervan.

Mosby, C.V. (1938). Little journey to the home of Florence Nightingale. New York: C.V. Mosby.

Muir, D.E. (1946). *Florence Nightingale.* Glasgow: Blackie and Son.

Nash, R. (1937). *A sketch for the life of Florence Nightingale.* London: Society for Promoting Christian Knowledge.

Newton, M.E. (1949). *Florence Nightingale's philosophy of life and education.* Ed.D. dissertation. Stanford, Calif.: Stanford University.

O'Malley, I.B. (1931). *Life of Florence Nightingale, 1820-1856.* London: Butterworth.

Pollard, E. (1902). *Florence Nightingale: The wounded soldiers' friend.* London: Partridge.

Presbyterian Hospital, School of Nursing. (1937). *Catalogue of the Florence Nightingale collection.* New York: the School.

Quiller-Couch, A.T. (1927) *Victors of peace.* New York: Nelson.

Rappe, E.C. (1977). *God bless you, my dear Miss Nightingale.* Stockholm: Almqvist and Wiksell.

Sabatini, R. (1934). *Heroic lives.* Boston: Houghton.

St. Thomas's Hospital. (1960). *The Nightingale Training School: St. Thomas's Hospital, 1860-1960.* London: St. Thomas's Hospital.

Saleeby, C.W. (1912). *Surgery and society: A tribute to Listerism.* New York: Moffat, Yard & Co.

Schmidt, M.M. (1933). *400 outstanding women of the world and costumology of their time.* Chicago: the author.

Seymer, L.R. (1951). *Florence Nightingale.* New York: Macmillan.

Smith, F.B. (1982). *Florence Nightingale: Reputation and power.* New York: St. Martin.

Stephenson, G.E. (comp.) (1924). *Some pioneers in the medical and nursing world.* Shanghai.: Nurse's Association of China.

Strachey, L. (1918). *Eminent Victorians.* London: Chatto & Windus.

Tabor, M.E. (1925). *Pioneer Women.* London: Sheldon.

Todey, S.A. (1905). *The life of Florence Nightingale.* New York: Macmillan.

Wilson, W.G. (1940). *Soldier's heroine.* Edinburgh: Missionary Education Movement.

Woodham-Smith, C.B. (1951). *Florence Nightingale, 1820-1910.* New York: McGraw-Hill.

Woodham-Smith, C.B. (1951). *Lonely crusader: The life of Florence Nightingale, 1820-1910.* New York: Whittlesey House.

Woodham-Smith, C.B. (1956). *Lady-in-chief.* London: Methven.

Woodham-Smith, C.B. (1977). *Florence Nightingale, 1820-1910.* London: Collins.

Woodsey, A.H. (1950). *A century of nursing.* New York: Putnam.

World Who's Who in Science: Florence Nightingale (entry). (1968). Chicago: A.N. Marquis.

Wren, D. (1949). *They enriched humanity: Adventurers of the 19th century.* London: Skilton.

Book Chapters

Reed, P.G., & Zurakowski, T.L. (1983). Nightingale: A visionary model for nursing. In J. Fitzpatric, & A. Whall, *Conceptual models of nursing: Analysis and application.* Bowie, Md.: Robert J. Brady.

Torres, G.C. (1980). Florence Nightingale. In Nursing Theories Conference Group, J.B. George, Chairperson, *Nursing theories: The base for professional nursing practice.* Englewood Cliffs, N.J.: Prentice-Hall.

Journal Articles

Abbott, M.E. (1916, Sept. 14). Portraits of Florence Nightingale. *Boston Medical and Surgical Journal 1975:*361-367.

Abbott, M.E. (1916, Sept. 21), Portraits of Florence Nightingale. *Boston Medical Surgery Journal, 175:*413-422.

Abbott, M.E. (1916, Sept. 28). Portraits of Florence Nightingale, *Boston Medical Surgery, 175:*453-457.

Address by the Archbishop of York. (1970, May 21). Florence Nightingale *Nursing Times, 66:*670,

Address given at fiftieth anniversary of founding by Florence Nightingale of first training school for nurses at St. Thomas's Hospital, London, England. (1911, Feb.). *American Journal of Nursing 11:*331–361.

Agnew, L.R.C. (1958, May). Florence Nightingale: Statistician. *American Journal of Nursing, 58:*644+.

At Embley Park and East Wellow. (1937, July 24). *Nursing Times, 33:*730-731.

Ball, O.F. (1952, May). Florence Nightingale. *Modern Hospital, 78:*88-90, 144.

Baly, M.E.: (1969, Jan. 2). Florence Nightingale's influence on nursing today. *Nursing Times, 65(suppl.):*1-4.

Barber E.M. (1935, July). A culinary compaign. *Journal of the American Dietetic Association, 11:*89-98.

Barritt, E.R. (1973). Florence Nightingale's values and modern nursing education. *Nursing Forum, 12:*7-47.

Boylen, J.O. (1974, April). The Florence Nightingale—Mary Stanley controversy: Some unpublished letters. *Medical History, 18(2):*186-193.

Berentson, L. (1982, April-May), Florence Nightingale: Change agent. *RN, Idaho, 6(2):*3, 7.

Berman J.K. (1974, Aug.). Florentia and the Clarabellas—a tribute to nurses. *Journal of the Indiana State Medical Association, 67:*717-719.

Bishop, W.J. (1957, January). Florence Nightingale bibliography. *International Nursing Review, 4:*64+.

Bishop W.J. (1957, May). Florence Nightingale's letters. *American Journal of Nursing, 57:*607+.

Bishop, W.J. (1960, May). Florence Nightingale's message for today. *Nursing Outlook, 8:*246+.

Black, B.W. (1939, July). A tribute to Florence Nightingale. *Pacific Coast Journal of Nursing, 35:*408-409.

Blanc, E. (1980, May). Nightingale remembered: Reflections on times past. *California Nurse, 75(10):*7.

Blanchard, J.R. (1939, June). Florence Nightingale: A study in vocation. *New Zealand Nursing Journal, 32:*193-197.

Book reviews and digests. (1920, May). *Public Health Nursing, 12:*442-448.

Bridges, D.C. (1954, April). Florence Nightingale centenary. *International Nurses Review 1:*3.

Brow, E.J. (1954, April). Florence Nightingale and her international influence. *International Nursing Review, (ns) 1:*17-19.

The call to war. (1970, May). *RN, 33:*42+.

Cartwright, F.F. (1976, March). President's address: Miss Nightingale's dearest friend. *Proceedings of the Royal Society of Medicine, 69(3):*169-175.

Centenary celebrations [Florence Nightingale]. (1954, Nov.). *Nursing Times, 50:*1213-1214.

Centenary (ed.). (1960, May). *Nursing Times, 56:*587.

Cherescavich, G.: (1971, June). *Nursing clinics of North America, 6:*217-223.

Choa, G.H. (1971, May). Speech by Dr. the Hon. G.H. Choa at the Florence Nightingale Day Celebration on Wednesday, 12th May, 1971, at City Hall, Hong Kong. *Nursing Journal, 10:*33-34.

Clayton, R.E. (1974, April). How men may live and not die in India: Florence Nightingale. *Australasian Nurses Journal, 2:*10-11 passim.

Collins, W.J. (1945, May 12). Florence Nightingale and district nursing. *Nursing Mirror 81:*74.

Cope, Z. (1960, May 13). Florence Nightingale and her nurses. *Nursing Times, 56:*597.

Coxhead, E. (1973, May 10). Miss Nightingale's country hospital. *Nursing Times, 65:*615-617.

A criticism of Miss Florence Nightingale. (1907, Feb. 2). *Nursing Times, 3:*89.

Crowder, E.L.: (1978, May). Florence Nightingale. *Texas Nursing, 52(5):*6-7.

Cruse, P. (1980, Sept.). Florence Nightingale. *Surgery, 88(3):*394-399.

Davidson, C. (1937, March). Jeanne Mance and Florence Nightingale. *Hospital Progress, 18:*83-85.

de Guzman, G. (1935, July). [Florence Nightingale]. *Filipino Nurse, 10:*10-14.

Dennis, K.E. & Prescott, P.A. (1985, Jan.). Florence Nightingale: Yesterday, today, and tomorrow. *Advances in Nursing Science, 7(2):*66-81.

de Tornayay, R. (1976, Nov.-Dec.). Past is Proloque: Florence Nightingale. *Pulse, 12(6):*9-11.

The death of Florence Nightingale. (1910, Sept.). *American Journal of Nursing, 10:*919-920. (Editorial).

Draper, J.M. (1907, Jan.). A brief sketch of the life of Florence Nightingale. *Trained Nurse, 38:*1-4.

Duggan, R. (1981, June). Florence Nightingale memorial service. *Australasian Nurses Journal 10(6):*30.

Dunbar, V.M. (1954, Oct.). Florence Nightingale's influence on nursing education. *International Nursing, Review, (ns) 1:*17-23.

Dwyer, B.A. (1937, Jan.). The mother of our modern nursing system. *Filipino Nurse, 12:*8-10.

Echoes of the past. (1907, Nov. 16). *British Journal of Nursing, 39:*396-397.

Echoes of the past. (1907, Dec. 21). *British Journal of Nursing, 39:*497-498.

Ellett, E.C. (1904, May). Florence Nightingale. *Trained Nurse, 32:*305-310.

Extracts from letters from the Crimea. (1932, May). *American Journal of Nursing, 32:*537-538.

Fink, L.G. (1934, Dec.). Catholic influences in the life of Florence Nightingale. *Hospital Progress, 15:*482-489.

Florence Nightingale. (1903, July). *Medical Dial, 5:*122-124. (Editorial).

Florence Nightingale. (1964, May 15.). *Nursing Mirror, 118:*131. (Editorial).

Florence Nightingale as a leader in the religious and civic thought of her time. (1936, July). *Hospitals, 10:*78-84.

The Florence Nightingale bibliography. (1956, April). *South African Nursing Journal, 22:*16.

Florence Nightingale bibliography. (1956, Oct.). *Nursing Research, 5:*87.

Florence Nightingale bibliography is compiled. (1931, May). *Modern Hospital, 36:*126.

Florence Nightingale: Looking back. . .notes on hospitals. (1979, Sept.). *Lamp, 36:*39-43.

Florence Nightingale O.M. (1910, Aug. 20). *British Journal of Nursing, 45:*141-147.

Florence Nightingale: The original geriatric nurse. (1980, May). *Oklahoma Nurse, 25(4):*6.

Florence Nightingale: Rebel with a cause. (1970, May). *RN, 33:*39-55.

Florence Nightingale's influence on nursing today. (1969, Jan. 3). *Nursing Times, 65:*1+.

Florence Nightingale's letter. (1932, July 2). *Nursing Times, 28:*699.

Florence Nightingale's letter of advice to Bellevue. (1911, Feb.). *American Journal of Nursing 11:* 361-364.

Florence Nightingale's tomb. (1957, June). *Canadian Nurse, 53:*529.

Florence Nightingale's work for public health. (1914, June). *American Journal of Public Health 4:*510-511. (Editorial).

Food for thought. (1958, Aug.). *Nursing Outlook, 6:*437. (Editorial).

Footnote to a dedicated life. (1958, Aug.). *RN, 21:*53+.

Fraga, M., & Tanenbaum, L. (1980, May). Florence Nightingale: Model for today's nurse. *Florida Nurse, 29(5):*11.

Frankenstein, L. The lady with a lamp. *Red Cross Courier, 16:*15-17.

Gordon, J.E. (1972, Oct.). Nurses and nursing in Britain. 21. The work of Florence Nightingale. I. For the health of the army, *Midwife Health Visitor and Community Nurse, 8:*351-359.

Gordon, J.E. (1972, Nov.). Nurses and nursing in Britain. 22. The work of Florence Nightingale. II. The establishment of nurse training in Britain, *Midwife Health Visitor and Community Nurse, 8:*391-396.

Gordon, J.E. (1973, Jan.). Nurses and nursing in Britain. 23. The work of Florence Nightingale. III. Her influence throughout the world. *Midwife Health Visitor and Community Nurse, 9:*17-22.

Gottstein, W.K. (1956, May). Miss Nightingale's personality. *RN, 19:*58-60, 80, 82.

Gould, M.E. (1970, May 7). A woman of parts. *Nursing Times, 66:*606+.

Graham, S. (1980, Oct. 23). Notes on nursing, 1860-1980: Angels of plain speech. *Nursing Times, 76(43):*1874.

Greatness in little things. (1954, May 8). *Nursing Times, 50:*508-510.

Grier, B., & Grier, M. (1978, Oct.). Contributions of the passionate statistician (Florence Nightingale). *Research in Nursing and Health, 1(3)*:103-109.

Grier, M.R.: Florence Nightingale: Saint or scientist? (1978, Oct.). *Research in Nursing and Health, 1(3)*:91. (Editorial).

Hallowes, R. (1957, Sept. 27). Florence Nightingale. In Distinguished British nurses. *Nursing Mirror, 105*:viii-x.

Hamash Dash, D.M. (1971, June). Florence Nightingale's writings. *Nursing Journal of India, 62*:179.

Headberry, J. (1966, Feb.). Florence Nightingale and modern nursing. *Australian Nurses Journal, 64*:32-36.

Headberry, J.E. (1966, Jan.). Florence Nightingale and modern nursing. *Journal of the West Australian Nurses, 32*:7-16.

Headberry, J.E. (1966, March-April). Florence Nightingale and modern nursing. *UNA Nursing Journal, 64*:80-87.

Headberry, J.E. (1966, Sept. 2). Florence Nightingale and modern nursing. *Nursing Mirror, 122*:xiii.

Health as a personal and community asset. (1926, Dec. 13). *Journal of Education 104*:566.

Hearn, M.J. (1920, April). Florence Nightingale. *Quart. J. Chinese Nurses, 1*:12-14.

Her letters [Florence Nightingale]. (1955, June). *Nursing Journal of India, 46*:210.

Her letters [Florence Nightingale]. (1955, July). *Nursing Journal of India, 46*:236.

Her letters [Florence Nightingale]. (1955, Aug.). *Nursing Journal of India, 46*:268.

Her letters [Florence Nightingale]. (1955, Oct.). *Nursing Journal of India, 46*:326.

Holly, H. (1967, Winter). Wanted: A day's work for a day's pay. *Nevada Nurses Association Newsletter.* 1 passim.

Hurd, H.M. (1910, June). Florence Nightingale: A force in medicine. *Johns Hopkins Nurses Alumnae Magazine, 9*:68-81.

Ifemesia, C.C. (1976, July-Sept.). Florence Nightingale (1820-1910). *Nigerian Nurse, 8(3)*:26-34.

In her memory. (1957, May). *RN, 20*:53.

Isler, C. (1970, May). Florence Nightingale. *RN, 33*:35-55.

Iu, S. (1971, May). President's address at Florence Nightingale Day Celebration 12th May 1971, City Hall Theatre. *Hong Kong Nursing Journal, 10*:27-32.

Iveson-Iveson, J. (1983, May 11). Nurses in society: A legend in the breaking (Florence Nightingale). *Nursing Mirror 156(19)*:26-27.

Jake, D.G. (1975, Nov.). Florence Nightingale: Mission impossible. *Arizona Medicine 32(11)*:894-895.

Jamme, A.C. (1920, May). Florence Nightingale, the great teacher of nurses. *Pacific Coast Journal of Nursing, 16*:282-285.

Jones, H.W. (1940, Nov.). Some unpublished letters of Florence Nightingale. *Bulletin of the History of Medicine, 8*:1389-1396.

Jones, O.C. (1972, Aug.). A useful memorial (Florence Nightingale). *Canadian Nurse, 68*:38-39.

Journey among women: Responsibility at the top. Part 2. (1970, June 4). *Nursing Times, 66*:77+.

Kalisch, B.J., & Kalisch, P.A. (1983, April). Heroine out of focus: Media images of Florence Nightingale. *Nursing and Health Care, 4*:181-187.

Kalisch, B.J. & Kalisch, P.A. (1983, May). Heroine out of focus: Media images of Florence Nightingale. *Nursing and Health Care, 4*:270-278.

Kelly, L.Y. (1976, Oct.). Our nursing heritage: Have we renounced it? (Florence Nightingale). *Image* (NY) 8(3):43-48.

Kerling, N.J. (1976, July 1). Letters from Florence Nightingale. *Nursing Mirror, 143(1)*:68.

Kiereini, E.M. (1981, June). The way ahead: On the occasion of Florence Nightingale oration at the Perth Concert Hall, Australia, 24th October, 1979. *Kenya Nursing Journal, 10(1)*:5-8.

King, A.G. (1964, June). The changing role of the nurse. *Hospital Topics 42*:89+.

King, F.A. (1954, Oct. 22). Miss Nightingale and her ladies in the Crimea. *Nursing Mirror, 100*:xi-xii.

King, F.A. (1954, Oct. 29). Miss Nightingale and her ladies in the Crimea. *Nursing Mirror, 100*:viii-ix.

King, F.A. (1954, Nov. 5). Miss Nightingale and her ladies in the Crimea. *Nursing Mirror, 100*:v-vi.

King, F.A. (1954, Nov. 12). Miss Nightingale and her ladies in the Crimea. *Nursing Mirror, 100*:x-xi.

Konderska, Z. (1971, Oct.). [The birthday of nursing, (Florence Nightingale)]. *Pielig Polozna, 8*:12-13.

Konstantinova, M. (1923, Oct.). In the cradle of nursing. *American Journal of Nursing, 24*:47-49.

Kopf, E.W. (1978, Oct.). Florence Nightingale as statistician. *Research in Nursing & Health, 1(3)*:93-102.

Kovacs, A.F. (1973, May-June). The personality of

Florence Nightingale. *International Nursing Review, 20*:78-79 + .

The lady with a lamp. (1929, Feb. 9). *Nursing Times, 25*:154.

Levine, M.E. (1963, April). Florence Nightingale: The legend that lives. *Nursing Forum, 2*:24 + .

Literature of Florence Nightingale. (1931, April). *Hospital Progress, 12*:188.

Loane, S.F. (1911, Feb.). Florence Nightingale and district nursing. *American Journal of Nursing, 11*:383-384.

McKee, E.S. (1909, Sept.). Florence Nightingale and her followers. *Nashville Journal of Medicine and Surgery, 103*:385-392.

Mackie, T.T. (1942, Jan.). Florence Nightingale and tropical and military medicine. *American Journal of Tropical Medicine, 22*:1-8.

Materials for the study of Florence Nightingale. (1931, May). *Trained Nurse and Hospital Review* 86:656-657.

The meaning of the lamp. (1956, May). *RN, 19*:61 + .

Menon, M. (1980, Aug.). The lamp she lit (Florence Nightingale). *Nursing Journal of India, 81(8)*:214-215.

Miss Nightingale's book of the Crimea. (1954, May 7). *Nursing Journal of India, 99*:ii-iii.

Monteiro, L. (1972, Nov.-Dec.). Research into things past: Tracking down one of Miss Nightingale's correspondents. *Nursing Research, 21*:526-529.

Monteiro. L. (1973, Nov. 8). Letters to a friend. *Nursing Times, 69*:1474-1476.

The most beautiful old lady. (1951, May 11). *Nursing Journal of India, 93*:101.

Nelson, J. (1976, May 13). Florence: The legend (Florence Nightingale). *Nursing Mirror, 142(20)*: 40-41.

Newton, M.E. (1952, May). Florence Nightingale's concept of clinical teaching. *Nursing World, 126*:220-221.

Newton, M.E. (1951, Sept.). The power of statistics. *Public Health Nursing, 43*:502-502.

Nightingale bibliography. (1957, May). *American Journal of Nursing, 57*:585.

Nightingale letter to Alice Fisher in Philadelphia. (1976, Jan.). *American Nurse, 8(2)*:2.

The Nightingale Saga (Vol. 1). (1962, Aug. 13). *Nursing Mirror 114*:425.

Ninan, R. (1982, June). The lady with the lamp: A profile. *Nursing Journal of India, 73(6)*:154-155.

No other earth. (1962, Nov.). *Today's Health, 40*:63.

Noguchi, M. (1969, Oct.). [Nightingale's philosophy and its limitations: My theory on Nightingale]. *Japanese Journal of Nursing, Art 10*:65-75.

Noyes, C.D. (1931, Jan.). Florence Nightingale: sanitarian and hygienist. *Red Cross Courier, 10*:41-42.

Notting, M.A. (1927, May). Florence Nightingale as a statistician. *Public Health Nursing, 19*:207-209.

O'Malley, I.B. (1935, May). Florence Nightingale after the Crimean War (1856-1861). *Trained Nurse, 94*:401-407.

Oman C. (1950, Nov. 17). Florence Nightingale as seen by two biographers, *Nursing Mirror, 92*:30-31.

The other side of the coin. (1967, May). *New Zealand Nursing Journal, 60*:40. (Editorial).

Palmer I.S. (1976, Sept.-Oct.). Florence Nightingale and the Salisbury incident. *Nursing Research 25(5)*:370-377.

Palmer, I.S. (1977, March-April). Florence Nightingale: Reformer, reactionary, researcher. *Nursing Research, 26*:84-89.

Palmer, I.S. (1981, June). Florence Nightingale and international origins of modern nursing. *Image, 13*:28-31.

Palmer, I.S. (1983, July-Aug.). Nightingale revisited. *Nursing Outlook, 31(4)*:229-233.

Palmer, I.S. (1983, Aug. 3). Florence Nightingale: The myth and the reality. *Nursing Times, 79*:40-42.

Parker, P. (1977, March). Florence Nightingale: First lady of administrative nursing. *Supervisor Nurse, 8*:24-25.

The passing of Florence Nightingale. (1910, Nov.). *Pacific Coast Journal of Nursing, 6*:481-519.

A passionate statistician. (1931, May). *American Journal of Nursing, 31*:566.

Pearce, E.C. (1954, April). The influence of Florence Nightingale on the spirit of nursing. *International Nursing Review, (ns)1*:20-22.

Peter, M. (1936, May). A personal interview with Florence Nightingale. *Pacific Coast Journal of Nursing, 32*:270-271.

Phillips, E.C. (1920, May). Florence Nightingale: A study. *Pacific Coast Journal of Nursing, 16*:272-274.

Pickering, G. (1974, Dec. 14). Florence Nightingale's illness. *British Medical Journal, 4(5945)*:656. (Letter).

Public health nursing: Florence Nightingale as a consultant. (1920, May). *Pacific Coast Journal of Nursing, 16*:299-300.

Rains, A.J. (1982, Feb.). Mitchiner memorial lecture: 'The Nightingale touch.' *Journal of the Royal Army Medical Corps, 128(1)*:4-17.

Rao, G.A. (1971, June). Florence Nightingale's writings. *Nursing Journal of India, 62*:179.

The real Florence Nightingale. (1912, April 6). *British Journal of Nursing, 48*:267.

Remembering Florence Nightingale. (1979, Sept.). *Nursing Focus, 1(1)*:34.

The revolting revisionist historian perspective. (1979, Jan.). *Arizona Medicine, 36(1)*:65-66.

Rhynas, M. (1931, May). Intimate sketch of the life of Florence Nightingale. *Canadian Nurse 27*:229-233.

Richards, L. (1920, May). Recollections of Florence Nightingale. *American Journal of Nursing, 20*:649.

Richards, L. (Ed.).(1934). Letters of Florence Nightingale, *Yale Review, 24*:326-347.

Roberts, M.M. (1937, July). Florence Nightingale as a nurse educator. *American Journal of Nursing, 37*:773-778.

Rogers, P. (1982, July). Florence Nightingale: The myth and the reality. *Nursing Focus, 3(11)*:10.

The romantic Florence Nightingale. (1968, May). *Canadian Nurse, 64*:57+.

Ross, M. (1954, May). Miss Nightingale's letters. *American Journal of Nursing, 53*:593-594.

Scovil, E.R. (1911, Feb.). Personal recollections of Florence Nightingale. *American Journal of Nursing, 11*:365-368.

Scovil, E.R. (1913, Oct.). Florence Nightingale. *American Journal of Nursing, 14*:28-33.

Scovil, E.R. (1914, Oct.). Florence Nightingale and her nurses. *American Journal of Nursing, 15*:13-18.

Scovil, E.R. (1916, Dec.). The love story of Florence Nightingale. *American Journal of Nursing, 17*:209-212.

Scovil, E.R. (1920, May). The later activities of Florence Nightingale. *American Journal of Nursing, 20*:609-612.

Scovil, E.R. (1927, May). Florence Nightingale's notes on nursing. *American Journal of Nursing, 27*:355-357.

Seden, F. (1947, July). Florence Nightingale and Turkish education. *Public Health Nursing, 39*:349.

Seymer, L.R. (1947, Sept.). Florence Nightingale oration. *International Nursing Bulletin, 3*:12-17.

Seymer, L.R. (1951, July). Florence Nightingale at Kaiserswerth. *American Journal of Nursing, 51*:424-426.

Seymer, L.R. (1954, April 2). Florence Nightingale. *Nursing Mirror, 99*:34-36.

Seymer, L.R. (1960, May). Nightingale Nursing School: 100 years ago. *American Journal of Nursing, 60*:658+.

Seymer, S. (1979, May). The writings of Florence Nightingale. *Nursing Journal of India, 70(5)*:121-128.

Skeet, M. (1980, Oct. 23). Nightingale's notes on nursing, 1860-1980 [interview by Alison Dunn]. *Nursing Times, 76(43)*:1871-1873.

Smith, F.T. (1981, May). Florence Nightingale: Early feminist. *American Journal of Nursing, 81*:1059-1061.

Some letters from Florence Nightingale. (1935, Feb.). *Hospital (London), 31*:50.

Sotejo, J.V. (1970, April-June). Florence Nightingale: Nurse for all seasons. *ANPHI Papers, 5*:4.

Stewart, I.M. (1939, Dec.). Florence Nightingale: Educator. *Teacher's College Record, 41*: 208-223.

Swain V. (1983, March 16-22). No plaster saint! *Nursing Times, 79(11)*:62-63.

That lamp. (1966, May 13). *Nursing Times, 62*:631.

Thompson, J.D. (1980, May). The passionate humanist: From Nightingale to the new nurse. *Nursing Outlook, 28(5)*:290-295.

Tinkler, L.F. (1973, Aug. 2). The barracks at Scutari: Start of a nursing legend. *Nursing Times, 69*:1006-1007.

Tobin, J. (1969, March). Observations on Florence Nightingale. *Tar Heel Nurse, 31*:52-55 passim.

Tracy, M.A. (1940, July). Florence Nightingale and her influence on hospitals. *Pacific Coast Journal of Nursing, 36*:406-407.

Trautman, M. J. (1971, April). Nurses as poets. *American Journal of Nursing, 71*:725-728.

Two unpublished letters. (1937, May). *Public Health Nursing, 29*:307.

Verney, H. (1980, Spring). The perfect aunt: FN 1820-1910. *News Letter of the Florence Nightingale International Nurses Association, 70*:13-16.

Walton, P. (1972, Jan.-March). The lady with the lamp: Florence Nightingale. *Phillipine Journal of Nursing, 41*:11-12.

Watkin, B. (1976, May 6). Notes on Nightingale. *Nursing Mirror, 142(19)*:42.

Westminster Abbey Florence Nightingale Commemoration Service, May 12th, 1970: The 150th anniversary of her birth. (1970, Autumn). *News Letter of the Florence Nightingale Internation Nurses Association, pp. 21-4.*

White, F.S. *(1923, June). At the gate of the temple. Public Health Nursing, 15:279-283.*

Whittaker, E. & Olesen, V.L. (1967, Nov.). Why Florence Nightingale? *American Journal of Nursing, 67:*2338 + .

The wider education of the nurse. (1951, Sept. 14). *Nursing Journal of India, 93:*438.

Williams, C.B. (1961, May). Stories from Scutari. *American Journal of Nursing, 61:*88.

Winchester, J.H. (1967, May). Tough angel of the battlefield. *Today's Health, 45:*30 + .

Winslow, C.E.A. (1946, July). Florence Nightingale and public health nursing, *Public Health Nursing, 38:*330-332.

Wolstenholme, G.E. (1980, Dec.). Florence Nightingale: New lamps for old. *Proceedings of the Royal Society of Medicine, 63:*1282-1288.

Woodham-Smith, Mrs. C. (1947, May 10). Florence Nightingale as a child. *Nursing Mirror, 85:*91-92.

Woodham-Smith, Mrs. C. (1952, May). Florence Nightingale revealed. *American Journal of Nursing, 52:*570-572.

Woodham-Smith, Mrs. C. (1954, July 10). The greatest Victorian. *Nursing Times, 50:*737, 738-741.

The works of mercy window (1956, May). *American Journal of Nursing, 56:*574.

Yeates, E.L. (1962, May 11). The prince consort and Florence Nightingale. *Nursing Mirror, 114:*iii-iv.

Virginia Henderson

Definition of Nursing

Deborah Wertman DeMeester, Tamara Lauer, Susan E. Neal

CREDENTIALS AND BACKGROUND OF THE THEORIST

Virginia Henderson was born in 1897, the fifth of eight children in her family. A native of Kansas City, Mo., Henderson spent her developmental years in Virginia because her father practiced law in Washington, D.C.

During World War I Henderson developed an interest in nursing. So in 1918 she entered the Army School of Nursing in Washington, D.C. Henderson graduated in 1921 and accepted a position as a staff nurse with the Henry Street Visiting Nurse Service in New York. In 1922 Henderson began teaching nurs-

ing in the Norfolk Protestant Hospital in Virginia. Five years later she entered Teacher's College at Columbia University, where she subsequently earned her B.S. and M.A. degrees in nursing education. In 1929 Henderson served as a teaching supervisor in the clinics of Strong Memorial Hospital in Rochester, New York. She returned to Teacher's College in 1930 as a faculty member, teaching courses in the nursing analytical process and clinical practice until 1948.*

Henderson has enjoyed a long career as an

The authors wish to express appreciation to Virginia Henderson for critiquing the chapter.
*References 3:49; 20:87; 21:116-117.

author and researcher. While on the Teacher's College faculty she rewrote the fourth edition of Bertha Harmer's *Textbook of the Principles and Practice of Nursing* following the author's death. This edition was published in 1939. The fifth edition of the textbook was published in 1955 and contained Henderson's own definition of nursing. Henderson has been associated with Yale University since the early 1950s, and has done much to further nursing research through this association. From 1959 to 1971 Henderson directed the Nursing Studies Index Project sponsored by Yale. The *Nursing Studies Index* was developed into a four-volume annotated index to nursing's biographical, analytical, and historical literature from 1900 to 1959. Concurrently, Henderson authored or coauthored several other important works. Her pamphlet, *Basic Principles of Nursing Care,* was published for the International Council of Nurses in 1960 and translated into more than 20 languages. Henderson's 5-year collaboration with Leo Simmons produced a national survey of nursing research that was published in 1964. Her book, *The Nature of Nursing,* was published in 1966 and described her concept of nursing's primary, unique function. The sixth edition of *The Principles and Practice of Nursing,* published in 1978, was coauthored by Henderson and Gladys Nite and edited by Henderson. This textbook has been widely used in the curriculums of various nursing schools. In the 1980s, Henderson remains active as a Research Associate Emeritus at Yale. Henderson's achievements and influence in the nursing profession have brought her more than seven honorary doctoral degrees and the first Christiane Reimann Award.*

THEORETICAL SOURCES FOR THEORY DEVELOPMENT

Henderson first published her definition of nursing in the 1955 revision of Harmer and Henderson's, *The Principles and Practice of Nurs-*

ing. There were three major influences upon Henderson's decision to synthesize her own definition of nursing. First, she revised the *Textbook of Principles and Practice of Nursing* in 1939. Henderson identifies her work for this text as the source that made her realize "the necessity of being clear about the function of nurses."[21:119] A second source was her involvement as a committee member in a regional conference of the National Nursing Council in 1946. Her committee work was incorporated into Ester Lucile Brown's 1948 report, *Nursing for the Future.* Henderson[7:62] says this report represented "my point of view modified by the thinking of others in the group." Finally, the American Nurses' Association's 5-year investigation of the function of the nurse interested Henderson, who was not fully satisfied with the definition adopted by the ANA in 1955.

Henderson labels her work a definition rather than a theory because theory was not in vogue at that time. She describes her interpretation as the "synthesis of many influences, some positive and some negative."[7:64] In *The Nature of Nursing* she identifies sources of influence during her early years of nursing. These include the following.

ANNIE W. GOODRICH. Goodrich was the Dean of the Army School of Nursing, where Henderson achieved her basic nursing education, and served as an inspiration to Henderson. Henderson[8:7] recalls, "Whenever she visited our unit, she lifted our sights above techniques and routine." She also attributes Goodrich with "my early discontent with the regimentalized patient care in which I participated and the concept of nursing as merely ancillary to medicine."[8:7]

CAROLINE STACKPOLE. Stackpole was a physiology professor at Teacher's College, Columbia University when Henderson was a graduate student. She impressed upon Henderson the importance of maintaining physiological balance.[8:10-11]

*References 20:87; 21:117-130; 22:58.

JEAN BROADHURST. Broadhurst was a microbiology professor at Teacher's College. The importance of hygiene and asepsis made an impact on Henderson.[8:10-11]

DR. EDWARD THORNDIKE. Thorndike worked in psychology at Teacher's College. He conducted investigational studies on the fundamental needs of humans. Henderson[8:11] realized that illness is "more than a state of disease" and that most fundamental needs are not met in hospitals.

DR. GEORGE DEAVER. Deaver was a physicist at the Institute for the Crippled and Disabled and, later, at Bellevue Hospital. Henderson observed that the goal of the rehabilitative efforts at the Institute was rebuilding the patient's independence.[8:12]

BERTHA HARMER. Harmer, a Canadian nurse, was the original author of *Textbook of the Principles and Practice of Nursing,* which Henderson revised. Henderson never met Harmer, but similarities of their respective definitions of nursing are obvious. Harmer's 1922 definition begins, "Nursing is rooted in the needs of the humanity."[3:54]

IDA ORLANDO. Henderson identifies Orlando as an influence upon her concept of the nurse-patient relationship. She says, "Ida Orlando (Pelletier), [has] made me realize how easily the nurse can act on misconceptions of the patient's needs if she does not check her interpretation of them with him."[8:14]

USE OF EMPIRICAL EVIDENCE

Henderson incorporated physiological and psychological principles into her personal concept of nursing. Her background in these areas stems from her association with Stackpole and Thorndike during her graduate studies at Teacher's College.

Stackpole based her physiology course on Claude Bernard's dictum that health depends on keeping lymph constant around the cell.[8:10] From this, Henderson surmised that "A definition of nursing should imply an appreciation of the principle of physiological balance."[8:11] From Bernard's theory, she also gained an appreciation for psychosomatic medicine and its implications for nursing. She states, "It was obvious that emotional balance is inseparable from physiological balance once I realized that an emotion is actually our interpretation of cellular response to fluctuations in the chemical composition of the intercellular fluids."[8:11]

Henderson does not identify the precise theories supported by Thorndike, only that they involved the fundamental needs of man. A correlation with Abraham Maslow's Hierarchy of Needs is seen in Henderson's 14 components of nursing care, which begin with physical needs and progress to the psychosocial components. Although she doesn't cite Maslow as an influence, she describes his theory of human motivation in the sixth edition of *Principles and Practice of Nursing Care* in 1978.

MAJOR CONCEPTS AND DEFINITIONS

NURSING. Henderson[8:15] defines nursing in functional terms:

> The unique function of the nurse is to assist the individual, sick or well, in the performance of those activities contributing to health or its recovery (or to peaceful death) that he would perform unaided if he had the necessary strength, will, or knowledge. And to do this in such a way as to help him gain independence as rapidly as possible.

HEALTH. Henderson does not state her own definition of health. But in her writing she equates health with independence. In the sixth edition of *Textbook of Principles and Practice of Nursing* she cites several definitions of health from various sources, including the one from the charter of the World Health Organization.

She views health in terms of the patient's ability to perform the 14 components of nursing care unaided. She says it is "the quality of health rather than life itself, that margin of mental and physical vigor that allows a person to work most effectively and to reach his highest potential level of satisfaction in life."[15:122]

ENVIRONMENT. Again, Henderson does not give her own definition of environment. She uses *Webster's New Collegiate Dictionary,* 1961, which defines environment as "the aggregate of all the external conditions and influences affecting the life and development of an organism."[15:829]

PERSON (PATIENT). Henderson[7:65] views the patient as an individual who requires assistance to achieve health and independence or peaceful death. The mind and body are inseparable. The patient and his family are viewed as a unit.

NEEDS. No specific definition of need is found, but Henderson identifies 14 basic needs of the patient, which comprise the components of nursing care.* These include the need to:

1. Breathe normally.
2. Eat and drink adequately.
3. Eliminate body wastes.
4. Move and maintain desirable position.
5. Sleep and rest.
6. Select suitable clothes—dress and undress.
7. Maintain body temperature within normal range by adjusting clothing and modifying the environment.
8. Keep the body clean and well groomed and protect the integument.
9. Avoid dangers in the environment and avoid injuring others.
10. Communicate with others in expressing emotions, needs, fears, or opinions.
11. Worship according to one's faith.
12. Work in such a way that there is a sense of accomplishment.
13. Play or participate in various forms of recreation.
14. Learn, discover, or satisfy the curiosity that leads to normal development and health and use the available health facilities.

MAJOR ASSUMPTIONS

Virginia Henderson does not directly cite what she feels her underlying assumptions include. We have adapted the following assumptions from Henderson's publications.

Nursing

The nurse has a unique function to help well or sick individuals.

The nurse functions as a member of a medical team.

The nurse functions independently of the physician, but promotes his or her plan, if there is a physician in attendance. Henderson stressed that the nurse (for example, the nurse-midwife) can function independently and *must* if he or she is the best-prepared health worker in the situation. The nurse can and *must* diagnose and treat if the situation demands it. (Henderson is especially emphatic on this in the sixth edition of *Principles and Practice of Nursing*).

The nurse is knowledgeable in both biological and social sciences.

The nurse can assess basic human needs.

The 14 components of nursing care encompass all possible functions of nursing.*

Person (Patient)

The person must maintain physiological and emotional balance.

The mind and body of the person are inseparable.

---

*Reprinted with the permission of Macmillan Publishing Company *The Nature of Nursing* by Virginia Henderson. Copyright © 1966 by Virginia Henderson.

---

*References 7:63; 8:16-17; 15.

The patient requires help toward independence.

The patient and his family are a unit.

The patient's needs are encompassed by the 14 components of nursing.[8:11]

Health

Health is a quality of life.

Health is basic to human functioning.

Health requires independence and interdependence.

Promotion of health is more important than care of the sick.[11:33]

Individuals will achieve or maintain health if they have the necessary strength, will, or knowledge.[8:15]

Environment

Healthy individuals may be able to control their environment, but illness may interfere with that ability.

Nurses should have safety education.

Nurses should protect patients from mechanical injury.

Nurses should minimize the chances of injury through recommendations regarding construction of buildings, purchase of equipment, and maintenance.

Doctors use nurses' observations and judgments upon which to base prescriptions for protective devices.

Nurses must know about social customs and religious practices to assess dangers.[6:652]

THEORETICAL ASSERTIONS
The Nurse-Patient Relationship

Three levels comprising the nurse-patient relationship can be identified, ranging from a very dependent to a quite independent relationship: (1) the nurse as a *substitute* for the patient; (2) the nurse as a *helper* to the patient; and (3) the nurse as a *partner* with the patient. In times of grave illness, the nurse is seen as a "substitute for what the patient lacks to make him 'complete,' 'whole,' or 'independent,' by the lack of physical strength, will, or knowledge."[7:63] Henderson[8:16] portrays this view when she says the nurse "is temporarily the consciousness of the unconscious, the love life for the suicidal, the leg of the amputee, the eyes of the newly blind, a means of locomotion for the infant, knowledge and confidence for the young mother, the 'mouthpiece' for those too weak or withdrawn to speak, and so on."

During conditions of convalescence, the nurse helps the patient acquire or regain his independence. Henderson[21:120] states, "Independence is a relative term. None of us is independent of others, but we strive for a healthy interdependence, not a sick dependence."

As partners, the nurse and patient together formulate the care plan. Basic needs exist regardless of diagnosis but are modified by pathology and other conditions such as age, temperament, emotional state, social or cultural status, and physical and intellectual capacities.[6:415]

The nurse must be able not only to assess the patient's needs, but also those conditions and pathologic states that alter them. Henderson[7:63] says the nurse must "get 'inside the skin' of each of her patients in order to know what he needs." The needs must then be validated with the patient.

The nurse can alter the environment where she deems necessary. Henderson[15:831] believes, "In every situation nurses who know physiologic and psychologic reactions to temperature and humidity, light and color, gas pressures, odors, noise, chemical impurities, and microorganisms can organize and make the best use of the facilities available."

The nurse and patient are always working toward a goal, whether it be independence or peaceful death. One goal of the nurse must be to keep the patient's day as "normal as possible."[7:67] Promotion of health is another important goal of the nurse. Henderson[11:33] states, "There is more to be gained by helping every man learn how to be healthy than by preparing the most skilled therapists for service to those in crises."

The Nurse-Physician Relationship

Henderson insists the nurse has a unique function from that of physicians. The care plan, formulated by the nurse and patient together, must be implemented in such a way as to promote the physician's prescribed therapeutic plan. Henderson[11:34] stresses that nurses do *not* follow doctor's orders, for she "questions a philosophy that allows a physician to give orders to patients or other health workers." Recently she has extended this to emphasize that the nurse helps patients with health management when physicians are unavailable.[15:121] She also indicates that many nurse and physician's functions overlap.[19]

The Nurse as a Member of the Health Team

The nurse works in interdependence with other health professionals. The nurse and other team members help each other carry out the total program of care, but they should not do each others' jobs. Henderson[7:63] reminds us that "No one of the team should make such heavy demands on another member that anyone of them is unable to perform his or her unique function."

Henderson compares the entire medical team, including the patient and his family, to wedges on a pie graph (Figure 8-1). The size of each member's section depends on the patient's current needs, and therefore changes as the patient progresses toward independence. In some situations, certain team members are not included in the pie at all. The goal is for the patient to have the largest wedge possible or to take the whole pie.

Just as the patient's needs change, so may the definition of nursing. Henderson[21:121] admits, "This does not say that it is a definition that will stand for all time. I believe nursing is modified by the era in which it is practiced, and depends to a great extent on what other health workers do."

Henderson believes her sixth edition of *Principles and Practice of Nursing,* coauthored with Gladys Nite, expands her definition to include nurse practitioners. She says, "Nursing must not exist in a vacuum. Nursing must grow and learn to meet the new health needs of the public as we encounter them."[18]

LOGICAL FORM

Henderson appears to have used the deductive form of logical reasoning to develop her definition of nursing. She deduced her definition of nursing and 14 needs from physiological and psychological principles. One must study the assumptions of Henderson's definition to assess logical adequacy. Many of the assumptions have validity because of their high level of agreement with the literature and research conclusions of scientists in other fields. For example, her 14 basic needs correspond closely to Maslow's widely accepted human needs hierarchy, even though they were listed before she read Maslow's work.

In her book, *To be a Nurse,* Evelyn Adam analyzes Henderson's work using a framework she learned from Dorothy Johnson. Adam[1] identifies Henderson's assumptions, values, the goal of nursing, the client, the role of the nurse, the source of difficulty, the intervention, and the desired consequences.

ACCEPTANCE BY THE NURSING COMMUNITY
Practice

Henderson's definition of nursing as it relates to nursing practice points out that the nurse who sees her primary function as the direct care-giver to the patient will find an immediate

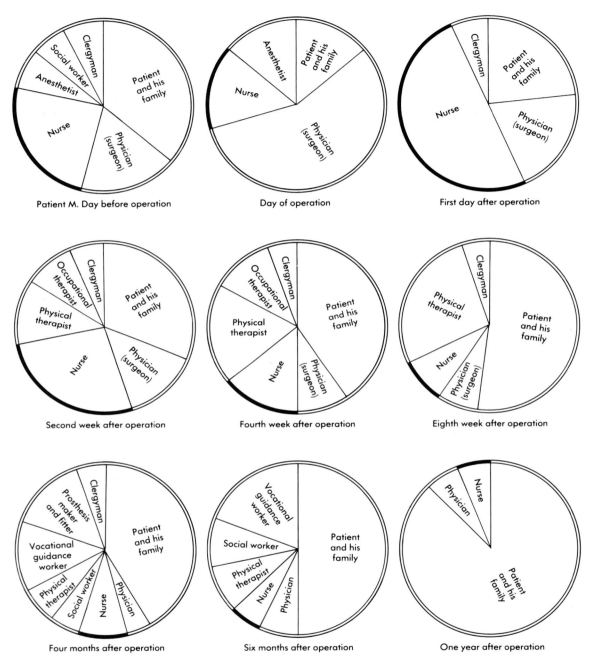

Figure 8-1. Showing how nurse's role diminishes as rehabilitation progresses in case of young man having leg amputated, for example.

Reprinted with permission of Macmillan Company from *The Nature of Nursing* by V. Henderson. Copyright © 1966 by Virginia Henderson.

reward in the patient's progress from dependence to independence. The nurse must make every effort to understand the patient when he lacks will, knowledge, or strength. As Henderson[8:24] states, the nurse will "get inside his skin." The nurse can help the patient move to an independent state by assessing, planning, implementing, and evaluating each of the 14 components of basic nursing care.

Henderson's approach to patient care is deliberative and involves decision-making. Although she does not specifically mention the steps in the nursing process, one can see how the concepts are interrelated. Henderson[17,18,19] believes the nursing process is the problem-solving process and is not peculiar to nursing.

In the assessment phase, the nurse would assess the patient in all 14 components of basic nursing care. After the first component was completely assessed, the nurse would move on to the next component until all 14 areas were assessed. In gathering data, the nurse uses observation, smell, feeling, and hearing. To complete the assessment phase, the nurse must analyze the data she has collected. This requires knowledge of what is normal in health and disease.

According to Henderson,[15:416] the planning phase involves making the plan fit the individual's needs, updating the plan as necessary based on the changes, using the plan as a record and ensuring it fits with the physician's prescribed plan. A good plan, in her opinion, integrates the work of all those on the health team.[18]

In the implementation phase, the nurse helps the patient perform activities to maintain health, to recover from illness, or to aid in peaceful death. Interventions are individualized, depending on physiological principles, age, cultural background, emotional balance, and physical and intellectual capacities. Henderson[8:24-31;12] would evaluate the patient according to the degree to which he performs independently. However, the infant cannot be independent, nor can the unconscious. In some phases of illness, we should accept the patient's desire to depend on others.

Education

Henderson[8:69] states, "In order for a nurse to practice as an expert in her own right and to use the scientific approach to the improvement of practice, the nurse needs the kind of education available only in colleges and universities." The nurse's education demands universal understanding of diverse human beings. The statement supports the position taken in 1965 by the American Nurses' Association.

In her book, *The Nature of Nursing: A Definition and Its Implications for Practice, Research, and Education,* Henderson has designed three phases of curriculum development students should progress through in their learning. The focus in all three phases remains the same—assisting the patient when he needs strength, will, or knowledge in performing his daily activities or in carrying out prescribed therapy with the ultimate goal of independence.

In the first phase, emphasis is placed on the fundamental needs of the patient, planning nursing care, and the unique function of the nurse in helping the patient carry out his activities of daily living. In this phase the curriculum plan does not emphasize pathological states or specific illnesses, but takes into account conditions always present that affect basic needs.[8:51] In the second phase, emphasis is placed on helping patients meet their needs during marked body disturbances or pathological states that demand modifications in the nurse's plan of care. The patient presents the student with problems of greater complexity. More medical science is involved, and the student begins to understand the rationale of symptomatic treatment.[8:51] In the third phase, instruction is patient- and family-centered. The student becomes involved in the complete study of the patient and all his needs.[8:55]

Henderson[16] has stressed the importance of having nursing students develop a habit of inquiry; take courses in biological, physical, and social sciences, and in the humanities; study with students in other fields; observe effective care; and give effective care in a variety of settings.

The textbook in which Henderson's definition of nursing is found, *Principles and Practices of Nursing,* is an excellent source that can be used by nursing students and by practicing nurses. It provides depth usually lacking in such texts. Kelly states, "If only one nursing book can be saved when the bomb falls, *PPN* is that book. In it are the breadth and depth of nursing, framed within the accumulated wisdom of law, medicine, and religion, documented from the world literature, fascinatingly footnoted—and eminently practical."[22:59]

Research

Henderson recommends library research and has done a vast amount of it herself. She has surveyed library resources and nursing research.[5] She supports developing nurses in a research atmosphere, introducing research at the baccalaureate level, and believes research is needed to evaluate and improve practice.[4] She recommends that nurses make greater use of library resources and hopes nurses will conduct research to improve practice rather than merely for academic respectability.*

In a survey and assessment of nursing research reported by Henderson and Leo W. Simmons in 1964 several reasons for lack of research in clinical nursing were identified. These reasons included:

1. Major energies of the profession have gone into improving the preparation for nursing.
2. Learning how to recruit and to hold sufficient numbers of nurses to meet the growing demand has taken considerable energy.
3. The need for administrators and educators has almost exhausted the supply of degree nurses.
4. A lack of support from administrators,

nursing service administrators, and physicians has discouraged researchers.[8:34]

Research questions arise from each of the 14 components for basic nursing care, and it is the nurse's function to assume responsibility for identifying problems, for continually validating her function, for improving the methods she uses, and for reassuring the effectiveness of nursing care.

Henderson[8:39] concludes, "No profession, occupation, or industry in this age can evaluate adequately or improve its practice without research." Research is the most reliable type of analysis.

FURTHER DEVELOPMENT

Henderson has no plans to further develop her definition of nursing.[18] Neither does she anticipate any further revisions of the text, *Principles and Practices of Nursing.* She stresses continued assessment of the patient's needs and continued revision of the patient's needs as his condition and goals change. Henderson[17] encourages the nurse to identify new needs beyond the 14 she enumerated.

CRITIQUE

Before one attempts to evaluate Virginia Henderson's theory of nursing with respect to the generally accepted criteria of simplicity, generality, empirical precision, and derivable consequences, one must understand that she did not intend to develop a definitive nursing *theory*. Instead, she developed a personal concept or definition in an attempt to clarify what she considers to be the unique function of nursing. She states, "My interpretation of the nurse's function is the synthesis of many influences, some positive and some negative. . . . I should first make clear that I do not expect everyone to agree with me. Rather, I would urge every nurse to develop her own concept."[7:64]

Henderson's definition can be considered a grand theory or philosophy within the preparadigm stage of theory development in nursing.

*References 9; 10; 13; 14:164.

Her concept is descriptive and easy to read. It is defined in common language terms. Her definitions of nursing and enumeration of the 14 basic nursing functions presents a perspective aimed at explaining a totality of nursing behavior. Because she had no intention of developing a theory, Henderson does not develop the interrelated theoretical statements or operational definitions necessary to provide the theory testability. However, that can be done.

Simplicity

Henderson's concept of nursing is complex rather than simplistic. It contains many variables and several different descriptive and explanatory relationships. It is not associated with structural organizations within a framework or model form to enhance simplicity, although some work has been done in this area. Diagrams of Henderson's and Orem's concepts of nursing from the Nursing Developmental Conference Group's book, *Concepts Formation in Nursing,* have been reproduced in the Henderson and Nite book.[15:23] In addition, the 14 basic needs appear simple as stated, but they become complex when an alteration of a need occurs and all the parameters relating to that need are considered. The sixth edition of *Principles and Practices of Nursing* is extremely comprehensive and well illustrated to add clarity.

Generality

Generality is present in Henderson's definition since it is broad in scope. It attempts to include the function of all nurses and all patients in their various interrelationships and interdependencies.

Derivable Consequences

Henderson's perspective has been useful in promoting new ideas and in furthering conceptual development of emerging theorists. In her many published works she has discussed the importance of nursing's independence from, and interdependence with, other branches of the health care field. She has also influenced curriculum development and made a great contribution in promoting the importance of research in the clinical practice of nursing. She has made extensive use of other theorist's research in her own work. Evans[2] states that *Principles and Practice of Nursing* has made "a revolutionary change in one's thinking about nursing research." He states that the revolutionary thesis of the book is:

> The habits of minds which inform the everyday tasks of a nurse are exactly the same as those which undergird the very finest published research; in this way, Everynurse ought not just to *do* simple research tasks as part of her work, but she ought also *always* to *be* a researcher, whether or not she writes or speaks a word in print or public.[2:338-339]

Since Henderson's definition of the unique function of nursing has been widely read, it has functioned as a major stepping-stone in the emergence of nursing as a professional scientific discipline.

REFERENCES

1. Adam, E. (1980). *To Be a Nurse.* New York: W.B. Saunders.
2. Evans, D.L. (1980). Everynurse as researcher: An argumentative critique of Principles and Practice of Nursing, *Nursing Forum, xix:*335-349.
3. Furukawa, C.Y., & Howe, J.K. (1980). Virginia Henderson. In Nursing Theories Practice Group, J.B. George, Chairperson, *Nursing theories: The base for professional nursing practice.* Englewood Cliffs, N.J. Prentice-Hall.
4. Henderson, V. (1956, Feb.). Research in nursing practice—when? *Nursing Research, 4:*99.
5. Henderson, V. (1957, Oct.). An overview of nursing research. *Nursing Research, 6:*61-71.
6. Henderson, V. (1958, May 9). The basic principles of nursing care. *Nursing Mirror, 107:*337-338, 415-416, 497-498, 583-584, 651-652, 733-734, 803-804.
7. Henderson, V. (1964, Aug.). The nature of nursing. *American Journal of Nursing, 64:*62-68.
8. Henderson, V. (1966). *The nature of nursing: A definition and its implications for practice, research, and education.* New York: Macmillan.
9. Henderson, V. (1968). Library resources in nursing: Their development and use. *Interna-*

*tional Nursing Review, 15:*164-174, 236-246.

10. Henderson, V. (1971, Jan.). Implications for nursing in the library activities of the regional medical programs. *Bulletin of the Medical Library Association, 59:*53-64.

11. Henderson, V. (1971, March). Health is everybody's business. *Canadian Nurse, 67:*31-34.

12. Henderson, V. (1973, June). On nursing care plans and their history. *Nursing Outlook, 21:*378-379.

13. Henderson, V. (1977). Awareness of library resources: A characteristic of professional workers; an essential in research and continuing education. *Reference resources for research and continuing education in nursing.* Kansas City, Mo.: American Nurses' Association.

14. Henderson, V. (1977, May-June). We've 'come a long way,' but what of the direction? *Nursing Research, 26:*163-164.

15. Henderson, V., & Nite, G.A. (1978). *The principles and practice of nursing.* New York: Macmillan.

16. Henderson, V. (1978, March). The concepts of nursing, *Journal of Advanced Nursing, 3:*13-30.

17. Henderson, V. (1982, March). The nursing process—is the title right? *Journal of Advanced Nursing, 7:*103-109.

18. Henderson, V. (1984-1985). Telephone interviews.

19. Henderson, V. (1985). Personal correspondence.

20. Runk, J.A., & Muth, Quillin, S.I. (1983). Henderson's definition of nursing. In J.J. Fitzpatrick, & A.L. Whall, *Conceptual models of nursing: An analysis and application.* Bowie, Md.: Robert J. Brady.

21. Safier, G. (1977). Virginia Henderson: Practitioner. In G. Safier, *Contemporary American leaders in nursing: An oral history.* New York: McGraw-Hill.

22. 70 Plus and going strong: Virginia Henderson, a nurse for all ages. (1983). *Geriatric Nursing, 4:*58-59.

BIBLIOGRAPHY
Primary Sources
Books

Harmer, B., & Henderson, V. (1939). *Textbook of the principles and practice of nursing* (4th ed.). New York: Macmillan.

Harmer, B., & Henderson, V. (1955). *Textbook of the principles and practice of nursing* (5th ed.). New York: Macmillan.

Henderson, V. (1966). *The nature of nursing: A definition and its implications for practice, research, and education.* New York: Macmillan.

Henderson, V. (1969). *ICN Basic principles of nursing care.* Geneva: International Council of Nursing.

Henderson, V. (1970). *Basic principles of nursing care.* Basel, N.Y.: Karger. (Pamphlet prepared for International Council of Nurses.)

Henderson, V., & Nite, G. (1978). *The principles and practice of nursing* (6th ed.). New York: Macmillan.

Henderson, V., & Simons, L.W. (1957). *The yearbook of modern nursing:1956.* New York: G.P. Putnam's Sons.

Simmons, L.W., & Henderson, V. (1964). *Nursing research: A survey and assessment.* New York: Appleton-Century-Crofts.

Yale University School of Nursing Index Staff under the direction of Virginia Henderson. (1963-1972). *Nursing Studies Index* (4 vols.). Philadelphia: J.B. Lippincott.

Book Chapters

Henderson, V. (1974). On nursing care plans and their history. In American Journal of Nursing, *The nursing process in practice.* Kansas City, Mo.: American Nurses' Association.

Henderson, V. (1977). Annie Warburton Goodrich. In *Dictionary of American Biography: Supplement Five, 1951-1955.* New York: Charles Scribners' Sons.

Henderson, V. (1977). Awareness of library resources: A characteristic of professional workers. In American Nurses' Association, *Reference resources for research and continuing education.* Kansas City, Mo.: American Nurses' Association.

Articles

Henderson, V. (1937, Jan.). Paper and other substitutes for woven fabric. *American Journal of Nursing, 37:*23-32.

Henderson, V., et al. (1938, Nov.). Oxygen therapy: A study of some aspects of the operation of an oxygen tent. *American Journal of Nursing, 38:*1203-1216.

Henderson, V. (1955, Dec.). Annie Warburton Goodrich. *American Journal of Nursing, 55:*1488-1492.

Henderson, V. (1956, Feb.). Research in nursing practice—when? *Nursing Research, 4:*99.

Henderson, V. (1957, Oct.). An overview of nursing research. *Nursing Research, 6:*61-71.

Henderson, V. (1958, May 2). The basic principles of nursing care. *Nursing Mirror, 107:*337-338.

Henderson, V. (1958, May 9). The basic principles of nursing care, *Nursing Mirror, 107:*415-416.

Henderson, V. (1958, May 16). The basic principles of nursing care. *Nursing Mirror, 107:*497-498.

Henderson, V. (1958, May 23). The basic principles of nursing care. *Nursing Mirror, 107:*583-584.

Henderson, V. (1958, May 30). The basic principles of nursing care. *Nursing Mirror, 107:*651-652.

Henderson, V. (1958, June 6). The basic principles of nursing care. *Nursing Mirror, 107:*733-734.

Henderson, V. (1958, June 13). The basic principles of nursing care. *Nursing Mirror, 107:*803-804.

Henderson, V. (1964, Aug.). The nature of nursing. *American Journal of Nursing, 64:*63-68.

Henderson, V. (1965, Jan.-Feb.). The nature of nursing. *International Nursing Review, 12(1):*23-30.

Henderson, V. (1968, Spring). Some comments for nurses today. *The Alumnae Magazine* (Columbia University-Presbyterian Hospital School of Nursing Alumnae Association), pp. 5-15.

Henderson, V. (1968, April). Library resources in nursing: Their development and use (Part I). *International Nursing Review, 15(2):*164-182.

Henderson, V. (1968, July). Library resources in nursing: Their development and use (Part II). *International Nursing Review, 15(3):*236-247.

Henderson, V. (1968, Oct.). Library resources in nursing: Their development and use (Part III). *International Nursing Review, 15(4):*348-358.

Henderson, V. (1968, Oct.). Is the role of the nurse changing? *Weather Vane,* pp. 12-43.

Henderson, V. (1969, Oct.). Excellence in nursing. *American Journal of Nursing, 69:*2133-2137.

Henderson, V. (1971, Jan.). Implications for nursing in the library activities in regional medical programs. *Bulletin of the Medical Library Association, 59(1):*53-61.

Henderson, V. (1971, March). Health is everybody's business. *Canadian Nurse, 67:*31-34.

Henderson, V. (1973, June). On nursing care plans and their history. *Nursing Outlook, 21:*378-379.

Henderson, V. (1977, Jan.-Feb.). We've come a long way, but what of the direction? *Nursing Research, 26:*163-164. (Guest editorial).

Henderson, V. (1977). The essence of nursing. *Virginia Nurse.*

Henderson, V. (1978, May 1). Professional writing. *Nursing Mirror and Midwives Journal,* pp. 5-18.

Henderson, V. (1978). The concept of nursing. *Journal of Advances in Nursing, 3:*113-130.

Henderson, V. (1979, Nov. 22-23). Preserving the essence of nursing in a technological age. *Nursing Times, 75:*2012.

Henderson, V. (1980, May). Preserving the essence of nursing in a technological age. *Journal of Advanced Nursing, 5:*245-260.

Henderson, V. (1980, May 22). Nursing—yesterday and tomorrow. *Nursing Times, 76:*905-907.

Henderson, V. (1982, March). The nursing process—in the title right? *Journal of Advanced Nursing, 7:*103-109.

Book Reviews

Henderson, V. (1969, January). Review of *Edith Cavell: Pioneer and patriot* by A.E. Clark-Kennedy. *Journal of the History of Medicine and Allied Sciences, 24(1):*100-101.

Henderson, V. (1973). Review of *Mary Adelaide Nutting: Pioneer of modern nursing* by Helen F. Marshall. *Journal of the History of Medicine and Allied Sciences.*

Henderson, V. (1976, Aug.). Review of *Equity in health services: Empirical analysis in social policy* by Ronald Anderson et al. *American Journal of Nursing, 76(1):*1339-1340.

Henderson, V. (1979, Aug.). Review of *The advance of American nursing* by Philip A. Kalish and Beatrice J. Kalish. *Nursing Outlook, 27(8):*554.

Henderson, V. (1969, March-April). Review of *A bibliography of nursing literature: 1859-1960* edited by Alice M.C. Thompson. *Nursing Research, 18(2):*174-176.

Thesis

Henderson, V. (1935, June). *Medical and surgical asepsis: The development of asepsis and a study of current practice with recommendations in relation to certain aseptic nursing methods in hospitals.* (Department of Nursing Education, Teacher's College, Columbia University).

Correspondence

Henderson, V. (1984-1985). Telephone interviews.

Henderson, V. (1985). Personal correspondence.

Interviews

Community Health Nursing Revisited: A conversation with Virginia Henderson. By S.L. Shamansky. *Public Health Nursing, 1(4)*.

70 plus and going strong: Virginia Henderson, a nurse for all ages. (1983). *Geriatric Nursing, 4:*58-59.

Virginia Henderson: A nursing's treasure. (1984). *Focus on Critical Care 11(3):*60-61.

Who's afraid of Virginia Henderson? (1977, May 11). By C. Darby. *Nursing Mirror and Midwives Journal, 146:*15-18.

Secondary Sources
Books

Adam, E. (1980). *To be a nurse.* New York: W.B. Saunders.

Chinn, P.L., & Jacobs, M.K. (1983). *Theory and nursing: A systematic approach.* St. Louis: C.V. Mosby.

Walker, L.O., & Avant, K.C. (1983). *Strategies for theory construction in nursing.* Norwalk, Conn.: Appleton-Century-Crofts.

Book Chapters

Furukawa, C.Y., & Howe, J.K. (1980). Virginia Henderson. In Nursing Theories Practice Group, J.B. George, Chairperson, *Nursing theories: The base for professional nursing practice.* Englewood Cliffs, N.J.: Prentice-Hall.

Runk, J.A., & Muth Quillin, S.I., (1983). Henderson's definition of nursing. In J.J. Fitzpatrick, & A.L. Whall, *Conceptual models of nursing: Analysis and application.* Bowie, Md.: Robert J. Brady.

Safier, G. (1977). Virginia Henderson: Practitioner. In G. Safier, *Contemporary American leaders in nursing: An oral history.* New York: McGraw-Hill.

Articles

Ellis, R. (1968, May-June). Characteristics of significant theories. *Nursing Research, 17:*217-222.

Hardy, M.E. (1978). Perspectives on nursing theory. *Advances in Nursing Science, 1:*37-48.

Faye Glenn Abdellah

Twenty-one Nursing Problems

Dorothy Kay Dycus, Donna N. Schmeiser, Roseanne Yancey

CREDENTIALS AND BACKGROUND OF THE THEORIST

Faye Glenn Abdellah was born in New York City. A 1942 Magna Cum Laude graduate of Fitkin Memorial Hospital School of Nursing, she received her B.S., M.A., and Ed.D. from Teacher's College at Columbia University. She completed her doctoral work in 1955.

Abdellah has practiced in many settings. She has been a staff nurse, a head nurse, a faculty member at Yale University and at Columbia

University, a public health nurse, a researcher, and an author of more than 132 articles and books. Since 1949, Abdellah has held various positions in the U.S. Public Health Service, including nurse consultant to the states, chief of the nurse education branch, senior consultant of nursing research, principle investigator in the progressive patient care project, chief of the research grants branch, director of nursing home affairs, and director of long-term care.

Abdellah was appointed Chief Nurse Officer of the USPHS in 1970. In 1982 she was selected as Deputy Surgeon General, the first nurse and first woman to hold the post. Her office makes her the focal point for nursing and a chief adviser on long-term care policy within

The authors wish to express their appreciation to Dr. Faye G. Abdellah for critiquing the chapter.

the Office of the Surgeon General. Abdellah represents the interests of health professionals in all categories in the PHS. She acts as advisor on matters related to nursing, long-term care policy, mental retardation, developmentally disabled, home health services, aging, and hospice. Because her efforts are directed toward improvement of the quality of health care for all Americans, she supervises the activities in both health and nonhealth agencies.

More than 36 academic awards and professional honors have been bestowed upon her. These include selection as a Charter Fellow of the American Academy of Nursing; six honorary degrees, including an honorary Doctor of Laws degree from Case Western Reserve University for pioneering nursing research and being responsible for the advent of the nurse-scientist scholar; the Federal Nursing Service Award for the advancement of professional nursing; and the Distinguished Service Honor Award of the U.S. Department of Health, Education, and Welfare for exceptional leadership and professional commitment.

Abdellah realized that for nursing to gain full professional status and autonomy, a strong knowledge base was imperative. Nursing also needed to move away from the control of medicine and toward a philosophy of comprehensive patient-centered care. Abdellah and her colleagues conceptualized 21 nursing problems to teach and evaluate students. The typology of 21 nursing problems first appeared in the 1960 edition of *Patient-centered Approaches to Nursing* and had a far-reaching impact on the profession.

THEORETICAL SOURCES

A critique of Abdellah's work cannot be isolated from the background in which her typology of nursing problems was developed. Nursing practice and education in the 1950s were facing major problems resulting from technological advancement and social change. Old methods of educational preparation and practice based on functions and medical services were inadequate to meet the demands of the rapid change. The definition of nursing was becoming clouded. In Abdellah's opinion, one of the greatest barriers keeping nursing from a professional status was lack of a scientific body of knowledge unique to nursing. The educational system was not providing students and practitioners a means to cope with changing technology. Evaluation of students' clinical experiences based on a services approach provided no measure of quality of that experience. The delivery of care to patients was organized around meeting the needs of the institution rather than those of the patient.

Abdellah formulated her model as a remedy to the problems facing nursing. The typology of 21 nursing problems and skills was developed to constitute the unique body of knowledge that is nursing (see box p. 95). Knowledge of the problem-solving approach to nursing problems would provide a method of change with advancing technology. A qualitative assessment of student experiences could be made based on the nursing problems encountered and alleviated, while providing patients with patient-centered nursing care.

USE OF EMPIRICAL EVIDENCE

The typology was developed from several studies conducted during the 1950s. In the study, *Appraising the Clinical Resources in Small Hospitals,* Abdellah and Levine[5] classified medical diagnoses of more than 1700 patients into 58 categories thought to represent common nursing problems. Abdellah's dissertation,[1] *Methods of Determining Covert Aspects of Nursing Problems as a Basis for Improved Clinical Teaching,* reported findings from her study designed to identify what interview technique provided the most complete list of patients' problems. The study revealed that a free-answer method was the most productive for identifying nursing

ABDELLAH'S TYPOLOGY OF 21 NURSING PROBLEMS

1. To maintain good hygiene and physical comfort.
2. To promote optimal activity: exercise, rest, and sleep.
3. To promote safety through prevention of accident, injury, or other trauma and through the prevention of the spread of infection.
4. To maintain good body mechanics and prevent and correct deformity.
5. To facilitate the maintenance of a supply of oxygen to all body cells.
6. To facilitate the maintenance of nutrition of all body cells.
7. To facilitate the maintenance of elimination.
8. To facilitate the maintenance of fluid and electrolyte balance.
9. To recognize the physiological responses of the body to disease conditions—pathological, physiological, and compensatory.
10. To facilitate the maintenance of regulatory mechanisms and functions.
11. To facilitate the maintenance of sensory function.
12. To identify and accept positive and negative expressions, feelings, and reactions.
13. To identify and accept interrelatedness of emotions and organic illness.
14. To facilitate the maintenance of effective verbal and nonverbal communication.
15. To promote the development of productive interpersonal relationships.
16. To facilitate awareness of self as an individual with varying physical, emotional, and developmental needs.
17. To create and/or maintain a therapeutic environment.
18. To facilitate awareness of self as an individual with varying physical, emotional, and developmental needs.
19. To accept the optimum possible goals in the light of limitations, physical, and emotional.
20. To use community resources as an aid in resolving problems arising from illness.
21. To understand the role of social problems as influencing factors in the cause of illness.

Reprinted with permission of Macmillan Publishing Co. from *Patient-centered approaches to nursing* by Faye G. Abdella, Irene L. Beland, Almeda Martin, and Ruth V. Matheney. Copyright © 1960 by Macmillan Publishing Co.

problems. When used with patients, this method elicited many more covert (emotional-social) problems than a pictorial interview technique or direct questioning approach.[2] Also in 1955, the National League for Nursing (NLN) Committee on Records formed a subcommittee to develop a meaningful clinical evaluation tool. The subcommittee members, with the assistance of faculties from 40 NLN-accredited collegiate schools of nursing, compressed the 58 patient categories into 21 common nursing problems, and reported their development and use in *Patient-centered Approaches to Nursing* in 1960.

MAJOR CONCEPTS AND DEFINITIONS

NURSING. In writing the typology of 21 nursing problems, Abdellah was creating a guide for nurses to use in identifying and solving patient problems. The concept of nursing was therefore a primary component of her writing. Abdellah[9:24] defined nursing as:

service to individuals and families; therefore, to society. It is based upon an art and science which mold the attitudes, intellectual competencies, and technical skills of the individual nurse into the desire and ability to help people sick or well cope with their health needs, and may be carried out under general or specific medical direction.

Abdellah was clearly promoting the image of the nurse who was not only kind and caring, but also intelligent, competent, and technically well prepared to provide service to the patient.

NURSING PROBLEM. A second major concept in Abdellah's work was the nursing problem. The "nursing problem presented by the patient is a condition faced by the patient or family which the nurse can assist him or them to meet through the performance of her professional functions."[9:7] The problem can be either an overt or covert nursing problem. An "overt nursing problem is an apparent condition faced by the patient or family which the nurse can assist him or them to meet through the performance of her professional functions."[2:4] The "covert nursing problem is a concealed or hidden condition faced by the patient or family which the nurse can assist him or them to meet through the performance of her professional functions."[2:4] Once again the focus of Abdellah's writing seems to be the nurse and nursing. Although Abdellah spoke of the patient-centered approaches, she wrote of nurses identifying and solving specific problems. This identification and classification of problems was called the typology of 21 nursing problems. Abdellah's typology[9:11] was divided into three areas: (1) the physical, sociological, and emotional needs of the patient; (2) the types of interpersonal relationships between the nurse and the patient; and (3) the common elements of patient care. Abdellah and her colleagues thought the typology would provide a method to evaluate a student's experiences and also a method to evaluate a nurses' competency.

PROBLEM SOLVING. "The process of identifying overt and covert nursing problems and interpreting, analyzing, and selecting appropriate courses of action to solve these problems" is problem solving, the final building block of Abdellah's writing.[9:26] Abdellah wrote that the nurse must be able to solve problems in order to give the best professional nursing care. This process, which closely resembles the steps of the nursing process, involves identifying the problem, selecting data, and formulating, testing, and revising hypotheses. According to Abdellah, the patient will not receive quality nursing care if the steps to problem solving are done incorrectly.

Abdellah identifies nursing diagnosis as a subconcept of the problem-solving process. It is defined as the "determination of the nature and extent of nursing problems presented by individual patients or families receiving care."[9:9]

MAJOR ASSUMPTIONS
Nursing

Nursing is a helping profession. In Abdellah's model, nursing care is doing something to or for the person or providing information to the person with the goal of meeting needs, increasing or restoring self-help ability, or alleviating an impairment.

Determination of nursing care strategies to be administered is based on the problem-solving approach. The nursing process is viewed as problem solving and the correct identification of nursing problems is a paramount concern. Direct observation of overt needs may be possible, but determination of covert needs requires mastery of communication skills and patient interaction. Deciding how patient needs can best be met is considered the responsibility of hospital and public health personnel.

"As long as self-help ability is developed and maintained at a level at which need satisfaction can take place without assistance, nursing care will not be required."[9:56] The role of the nurse in health promotion is limited to circumstances of anticipated impairment. In 1960 Abdellah[9:23] stated that physicians need more knowledge about prevention and rehabilitation than do nurses. But in correspondence with the authors in 1984, Abdellah indicated it is important that nurses also know about prevention and rehabilitation. No consideration is given to achievement of a higher level of wellness than is present when personal needs are met or when actual and anticipated impairments are absent.

Person

Abdellah describes people as having physical, emotional, and sociological needs. These needs may be overt, consisting of largely physical needs, or covert, such as emotional and social needs. The typology of nursing problems is said to evolve from the recognition of a need for patient-centered approaches to nursing. The patient is described as the only justification for the existence of nursing. But as previously discussed, the patient is not the central focus of Abdellah's work.

People are helped by the identification and alleviation of problems they are experiencing. The model implies that by resolving each problem the person returns to a healthy state or one with which he can cope; therefore, the idea of holism is absent in this model. The whole, which is the patient, is not greater than the sum of its parts, which are his problems.

In Abdellah's model all persons have self-help ability and the capacity to learn, both of which vary from one individual to another. Because identifying these qualities in a comatose patient or an infant without family resources may be difficult, omissions could result when organizing such patients' care with this model.

Environment

The environment is the least-discussed concept in Abdellah's model. Nursing problem number 17, from the typology, is "to create and/or maintain a therapeutic environment."[9:17] Abdellah also states that if the nurse's reaction to the patient is hostile or negative, the atmosphere in the room may be hostile or negative. This suggests that patients interact with and respond to their environment and that the nurse is part of that environment.

The environment is also the home and community from which the patient comes. Although fleetingly discussed, Abdellah urges that nurses not limit the identification of nursing problems to those existing only in the hospital. She predicts a future community center that will extend beyond the four walls of the hospital into the community.

Health

Health, as Abdellah discusses in *Patient-centered Approaches to Nursing,* is a state mutually exclusive of illness. Health is defined implicitly as a state when the individual has no unmet needs and no anticipated or actual impairments. Much of nursing practice in the 1950s focused on remedial or illness care, so it is not surprising that health was not clearly defined. But 30 years have passed since the book was published and Abdellah[4] now says she "would certainly place greater emphasis today on health status as an important part of the wellness-sickness continuum." She also fully supports the holistic approach to patient-centered care and the need for greater attention on environmental factors.

THEORETICAL ASSERTIONS

Several assertions were repeatedly stated by Abdellah although they were not labeled as such. These assertions are:

1. "The nursing problem and nursing treatment typologies are the principles of nursing practice and constitute the unique body of knowledge that is nursing."[9:12]
2. "Correct identification of the nursing problem influences the nurse's judgment in selecting steps in solving the patient's problem."[7:492]
3. The core of nursing is nursing problems that focus on the patient and his problems.[9:13]

According to Reynolds,[12:68] statements of assertion can be either existence or relational statements. Assertions 1 and 3 are of the existence type, while assertion 2 is rational.

Neither the major components of the nursing paradigm nor the central concepts are clearly linked with relational statements. Such structure cannot be diagrammed without imposing the critic's conclusions regarding the existence of relationships. Because the components of person, health, and environment were only implicitly defined, no attempt will be made to propose relationships between them. The major concepts that are more clearly defined by Abdellah are thought to be associated in this manner. Nursing, through the identification of nursing problems and usage of the problem-solving process, helps the client meet his needs. As late as 1972 Abdellah[3:234] stated, "The patient, his needs, and the nurse meeting his needs through nursing service is the only raison d'être for the nursing profession." Abdellah's statement exemplifies her major concerns and implied relationships.

LOGICAL FORM

The logical form can best be described as an inductive approach that generalizes from particulars. Abdellah used her multiple observations from the studies mentioned previously as the basis for her typology. Thus the typology developed from research toward theory.

ACCEPTANCE BY THE NURSING COMMUNITY

In discussing the acceptance by the nursing community, one must be aware of two distinct times within the history of nursing—the mid 1950s through early 1960s and the present. When *Patient-centered Approaches to Nursing* was published in 1960, the profession of nursing was striving to clarify its practice area and to identify rationale for its actions based on scientific knowledge. The introduction of the 21

nursing problems had profound effects on the areas of practice, education, and research.

Practice

Abdellah's typology of 21 nursing problems helps nurses practice in an organized, systematic way. The use of this scientific base enabled the nurse to understand the reasons for her actions. The clinical practitioner, using the 21 nursing problems, could assess the patient, make a nursing diagnosis, and plan interventions. Through the problem-solving process the nurse attempted to make the patient, rather than his medical condition, the central figure. By using the typology and the problem-solving process in the clinical setting, nurses gave their practice a scientific basis.

Education

Abdellah's 21 nursing problems had their most dramatic effect on the educational system within nursing. Nursing educators were aware that curricula changes were needed if nurses were to become autonomous. They recognized that the greatest weakness in the profession was the lack of a scientific body of knowledge unique to nursing. The typology provided such a body of knowledge and an opportunity to move away from the medical model of educating nurses. The typology of 21 nursing problems was widely accepted in the nursing community in all types of programs—2-, 3-, and 4-year.

Research

Because the typology of 21 nursing problems was created through research, it is not surprising that more research followed its introduction. Was this typology really necessary from an administrative point of view? Had not hospitals been doing well without it? The amount of time the nurse spent with the patient was examined in the form of function studies. How could the patient receive comprehensive patient care in 18 minutes per 8-hour shift? Does the hospital administration serve the patient or does it serve someone else? To answer these questions Abdellah and Strachan[8] extended the research and used the typology as the basis for developing the nursing care model used for planning staffing patterns in clinical settings. These staffing patterns were based on patients' identified needs and as Abdellah envisioned, consisted of intensive care, intermediate care, long-term care, self-care, and home-care units. By grouping patients with similar needs instead of diagnoses, nursing service could provide the best staffing patterns to meet patients' needs.

FURTHER DEVELOPMENT

According to Dickoff and James' categories,[11] Abdellah's typology may be recognized as a level one theory—categories or classifications. Currently, the nursing community's use of the 21 nursing problems has moved into a second generation of development, which includes patient problems and patient outcomes rather than nursing problems and outcomes.

Abdellah[4] is pleased with the shift of emphasis from nursing problems to patient outcomes. She believes that 30 years ago the concept of nursing problems was used to identify a strong nursing role in patient care. If the initial emphasis had been on patient problems instead, the concept would *not* have been accepted and the medical model would have been perpetuated.

The concepts of problem-solving and nursing diagnosis continue to be used in the settings of practice, education, and research. Critical thinking and validating of theory in the practice area is needed within the profession. More sophisticated research tools might be designed to thoroughly study problem solving and how nurses apply this concept. The nursing diagnosis classification system may be considered an outgrowth of the typology. Currently nursing diagnosis is a classification system de-

scribing patient signs and symptoms. Expanding this system to explain outcomes may be possible through additional research.

CRITIQUE
Simplicity

The typology is very simple and is descriptive of nursing problems thought to be common among patients. The concepts of nursing, nursing problems, and the problem-solving process, which are central to this work, are defined explicitly. The concepts of person, health, and environment, which are associated with the nursing paradigm today, are implied. There are no stated relationships between Abdellah's major concepts or those of the nursing paradigm in her writing. This model has a limited number of concepts, and its only structure is a list. A somewhat mixed approach to concept definition is present in this work. Nursing and nursing problems are connotatively defined, while the problem-solving process is defined denotatively. These approaches to definitions do not seem to detract from the clarity of definitions. The typology does not yet constitute a theory because it lacks sufficient relationship statements.

Generality

The 21 nursing problems are general and linked to neither time nor environment. Assuming that persons experience similar needs, the nursing goals stated in the list of 21 problems could be used by nurses in any time frame to meet patients' needs. However, according to this model, some persons do not need nursing.

Other service professions could use the typology of 21 nursing problems to focus on the psychosocial and emotional needs presented by patients. The goals of this model vary in generality. The broadest goal is to positively affect nursing education, while subgoals are to provide a scientific basis on which to practice and to provide a method of qualitative evaluation of educational experiences for students. The goals are appropriate for nursing.

Empirical Precision

The concepts are very specific with empirical referents easily identifiable. The concepts are within the domain of nursing. Ready linkage of the concepts and the typology to reality is secondary to an inductive approach to theory development. Validation of the typology was done by the faculty of 40 collegiate schools of nursing. Chapters 4, 5, and 6 of *Patient-centered Approaches to Nursing* describe different approaches to implementation and use of the typology in three programs of nursing.

Derivable Consequences

The typology provided a general framework in which to act, but continued neither specific nursing actions nor patient-centered outcomes, despite the title of the book. However, two subsequent publications did address outcome measures (effect variables) and suggested models for organizing curricula to emphasize patient-centered outcomes.[6,10] Except for stating the importance of nursing the whole patient, today's idea of holism is not apparent in this work. The skills list includes skills thought necessary for nurses to meet patients' needs but is not prescriptive. Abdellah suggests nursing research as a method for validating treatments toward resolution of patients' needs.

The emphasis on problem-solving is not limited by time or space and therefore provides a means for continued growth and change in the provision of nursing care. The problem-solving process and the typology of 21 nursing problems can be respectively considered precursors of the nursing care process and classification of nursing diagnoses in evidence today.

In *Patient-centered Approaches to Nursing Care*, Abdellah addressed nursing education problems linked to the use of the medical model. Her typology provided a new way to qualitatively evaluate experiences and emphasized a practice based on sound rationales rather than rote. Abdellah's work had a substantial impact on nursing education, practice, and research.

REFERENCES

1. Abdellah, F.G. (1955). *Methods of determining covert aspects of nursing problems as basis for improved clinical teaching*. Doctoral dissertation, New York Teacher's College, Columbia University.
2. Abdellah, F.G. (1957, June). Methods of identifying covert aspects of nursing problems. *Nursing Research, 6:4*.
3. Abdellah, F.G. (1972). Evolution of nursing as a profession: Perspective on manpower development. *International Nursing Review, 19:3*.
4. Abdellah, F.G. (1984, March 7). Personal Correspondence.
5. Abdellah, F.G., & Levine, E. (1954). *Appraising the clinical resources in small hospitals* (U.S. Public Health Service. Pub. No. 389). Washington, D.C.: U.S. Government Printing Office.
6. Abdellah, F.G. & Levine, E. (1958). Effect of nurse staffing on satisfactions with nursing care. In *Hospital Monograph Series No. 4*. Chicago: American Hospital Association.
7. Abdellah, F.G., & Levine, E. (1965). *Better patient care through nursing research*. New York: Macmillan.
8. Abdellah, F.G., & Strachan, E.J. (1959, May). Progressive patient care, *American Journal of Nursing, 59:5*.
9. Abdellah, F.G., et al. (1960). *Patient-centered approaches to nursing*. New York: Macmillan.
10. Abdellah, F.G., et al. (1973). *New directions in patient-centered nursing: Guidelines for systems of service, education, and research*. New York: Macmillan.
11. Dickoff, J., & James, P. (1968, March). A theory of theories: A position paper. *Nursing Research, 17:3*.
12. Reynolds, P.D. (1971). A primer in theory construction. Indianapolis: Bobbs-Merrill.

BIBLIOGRAPHY
Primary Sources
Books

Abdellah, F.G. (1968). *An overview of nurse-scientist programs in the country.* National League for Nursing No. 15-1342.

Abdellah, F.G. (1972). *A career in nursing.* B'nai B'rith Career and Counseling Services Occupational Brief Series. Washington, D.C.: B'na: B'rith.

Abdellah, F.G. (1972). *Extending the scope of nursing practice. National League for Nursing* Pub. No. 15-1473.

Abdellah, F.G., & Levine, E. (1954). *Appraising the clinical resources in small hospitals* (U.S. Public Health Service Pub. No. 389). Washington, D.C.: U.S. Government Printing Office.

Abdellah, F.G., & Levine, E. (1957). *Patients and personnel speak: A method of studying patient care in hospitals* (U.S. Public Health Service Pub. No. 527). Washington, D.C.: U.S. Government Printing Office.

Abdellah, F.G., & Levine, E. (1958). *Effect of nurse staffing on satisfactions with nursing care: A study of how omissions in nursing services, as perceived by patients and personnel, are influenced by the number of nursing hours available.* Chicago: American Hospital Association.

Abdellah, F.G., & Levine, E. (1965). *Better patient care through nursing research.* New York: Macmillan.

Abdellah, F.G., & Levine, E. (1979). *Better patient care through nursing research* (2nd ed). New York: Macmillan.

Abdellah, F.G., Meltzer, L.E., & Kitchell, J.R. (Eds.). (1969). *Concepts and practices of intensive care for nurse specialists.* Philadelphia: Charles Press.

Abdellah, F.G., Meltzer, L.E., & Kitchell, J.R. (Eds.). (1976). *Concepts and practices of intensive care for nurse specialists* (2nd ed). Bowie, Md.: Charles Press.

Abdellah, F.G., Schwartz, D.R., & Smoyak, S.A. (1975). *Models for health care delivery: Now and for the future* (American Nurses Association No. G 119). American Academy of Nursing.

Abdellah, F.G., Walsh, M.E., & Brown, E.L. (1979). *Health care in the 1980's: Who provides? Who plans? Who pays? National League for Nursing* Pub. No. 52-1755.

Abdellah, F.G., et al. (1960). *Patient-centered approaches to nursing.* New York: Macmillan.

Abdellah, F.G., et al. (1968). *Patient-centered approaches to nursing* (2nd ed.). New York: Macmillan.

Abdellah, F.G., et al. (1973). *New directions in patient-centered nursing.* New York: Macmillan.

Dissertation

Abdellah, F.G. (1955). *Methods of determining covert aspects of nursing problems as basis for improved clinical teaching.* New York Teacher's College, Columbia University.

Articles

Abdellah, F.G. (1952, June). State nursing surveys and community action. *Public Health Reports, 67:*554-560.

Abdellah, F.G. (1953, July) Some trends in nursing education. *American Journal of Nursing, 53:*841-843.

Abdellah, F.G. (1954, May). Surveys stimulate community action. *Nursing Outlook, 2:*268-270.

Abdellah, F.G. (1957, June). Methods of identifying covert aspects of nursing problems. *Nursing Research, 6:*4.

Abdellah, F.G. (1959, May). How we look at ourselves. *Nursing Outlook, 7:*273.

Abdellah, F.G. (1960, June). Progressive patient care: A challenge for nursing. *Hospital Management, 89:*102.

Abdellah, F.G. (1960, Aug.). Nursing patterns vary in progressive care. *Modern Hospital, 95:*85.

Abdellah, F.G. (1961, April). The decision is yours. *Nursing Outlook, 9:*223.

Abdellah, F.G. (1961, Winter). Criterion measures in nursing. *Nursing Research, 10:*21.

Abdellah, F.G. (1965, Oct.). Search or research? An experiment to stimulate research. *Nursing Outlook, 13:*65-67.

Abdellah, F.G. (1966). Frontiers in nursing research. *Nursing Forum, 5:*28-38.

Abdellah, F.G. (1967, Fall). Approaches to protecting the rights of human subjects. *Nursing Research, 16:*315-320.

Abdellah, F.G. (1969, Sept.-Oct.). The nature of nursing science. *Nursing Research, 18:*390-393.

Abdellah, F.G. (1969, Dec.). Nursing research in the health services, *Nursing Research Reports, 4:*2. (Editorial).

Abdellah, F.G. (1970, Jan.-Feb.). Overview of nursing research: 1955-1968 (Part I). *Nursing Research, 19:*6-17.

Abdellah, F.G. (1970, March-April). Overview of nursing research: 1955-1968 (Part II). *Nursing Research, 19:*151-162.

Abdellah, F.G. (1970, May-June). Overview of nursing research: 1955-1968 (Part III). *Nursing Research, 19:*239-252.

Abdellah, F.G. (1970, May). Training and development of the health care team. *AORN Journal, 11:*86-91.

Abdellah, F.G. (1970, Summer). Conference on the nature of science in nursing. The nature of nursing science. *Japanese Journal of Nursing Research, 3:*248-252.

Abdellah, F.G. (1971, May). Problems, issues, challenges of nursing research. *Canadian Nurse, 67:*44-46.

Abdellah, F.G. (1972, Oct.). No legal bars to expanded nursing practice. *Stat, 41:*4.

Abdellah, F.G. (1972, Sept.). The physician-nurse team approach to coronary care. *Nursing Clinics of North America, 7:*423-430.

Abdellah, F.G. (1972). Evolution of nursing as a profession: Perspective on manpower development. *International Nursing Review, 19:*219-238.

Abdellah, F.G. (1973, Jan.-Feb.). Criterios de avaliac as em enfermagen. *Revista Brasileira de Enfermagem, 26:*17-32. (Portugal).

Abdellah, F.G. (1973, May). Research on career development in the health professions: Nursing. *Occupational Health Nursing, 21:*12-16.

Abdellah, F.G. (1973, June). School nurse practitioner: An expanded role for nurses. *Journal of the American College Health Association, 21:*423-432.

Abdellah, F.G. (1973, Dec.). Nursing and health care in the USSR. *American Journal of Nursing, 73:*2096-2099.

Abdellah, F.G. (1974, Spring). Long-term care: A top health priority. *Journal of Long-Term Care Administration, 2(2):*1-3. (Guest editorial).

Abdellah, F.G. (1974, Fall). Health care issues: Overview of emerging health services delivery projects. *Health Care Dimensions,* pp. 125-139.

Abdellah, F.G. (1974). A national health strategy for the delivery of long-term health care: Implications for nursing. *Journal of New York State Nurses' Association, 5(4):*7-13.

Abdellah, F.G. (1975, Jan.-Feb.). National library of medicine is official nursing archives. *Nursing Research, 24(1):*64. (Letter).

Abdellah, F.G. (1975, Sept.-Oct.). The nursing archives at the national library of medicine. *Nursing Research, 24(5):*389. (Letter).

Abdellah, F.G. (1975, Nov.). Three views. Patient assessment: Its potential and use (Part 1). *American Health Care Association Journal, 1:*69.

Abdellah, F.G. (1976, March). Nurse practitioners and nursing practice. *American Journal of Public Health, 66(3):*245-246. (Editorial).

Abdellah, F.G. (1976, Aug.). Nursing's role in future health care. *AORN Journal, 24(2):*236-240.

Abdellah, F.G. (1977, July-Aug.). U.S. Public Health Service's contribution to nursing research—past, present, future. *Nursing Research, 26(4):*244-249.

Abdellah, F.G. (1978, July). Long-term care policy issues: Alternatives to institutional care. *American Academy of Political and Social Science Annals, 438:*28-29.

Abdellah, F.G. (1981, Nov.). Nursing care of the aged in the United States of America. *Journal of Gerontological Nursing, 7(11):*657-663.

Abdellah, F.G. (1982, Summer). The nurse practitioner 17 years later: Present and emerging issues. *Inquiry, 19(2):*105-116.

Abdellah, F.G. (1982, Dec.). Keynote address, 75th anniversary of the West Virginia State Nurse's Association. *Weather Vane, 51(6):*10-13, 15.

Abdellah, F.G. (1983, Feb.-March). Future directions: Impact on NSNA 1982 and 2012. *Imprint, 30(1):*66-74.

Abdellah, F.G. (1983, April-May). Future directions of the profession: Impact on NSNA 1982 and 2012 (Part II). *Imprint, 30(2):*91-97.

Abdellah, F.G. (1983, March-April 6-7). 1983-2008: Nursing practice. *Arizona Nurse.*

Abdellah, F.G., & Chow, R.K. (1976, Nov.-Dec.). The long-term care facility improvement campaign: The PACE project. *Association of Rehabilitation Nurses' Journal, 1(7):*3-4.

Abdellah, F.G., & Chow, R.K. (1976, Winter). Long-term care facility improvement—a nationwide research effort. *Journal of Long-Term Care Administration, 4(1):*5-19.

Abdellah, F.G., Foerst, H.V., & Chow, R.K. (1979, June). PACE: An approach to improving the care of the elderly. *American Journal of Nursing, 79(6):*1109-1110.

Abdellah, F.G., & Levine, E. (1954, June). Why nurses leave home. *Hospitals, 28*:80-81.

Abdellah, F.G., & Levine, E. (1957, Feb.). Developing a measure of patient and personnel satisfaction with nursing care. *American Journal of Nursing, 5*:100.

Abdellah, F.G., & Levine, E. (1957, Nov. 1). Polling patients and personnel: What patients say about their nursing care (Part I). *Hospitals, 31*:44.

Abdellah, F.G., & Levine, E. (1957, Nov. 16). What factors affect patients' opinions of their nursing care? (Part 2). *Hospitals, 31*:61.

Abdellah, F.G., & Levine, E. (1957, Dec. 1). What personnel say about nursing care (Part 3). *Hospitals, 31*:53.

Abdellah, F.G., & Levine, E. (1957, Dec. 16). What hospitals have done to improve patient care (Part 4). *Hospitals,* 31:43.

Abdellah, F.G., & Levine, E. (1965, April). Better patient care through nursing research. *International Journal of Nursing Studies, 2*:1.

Abdellah, F.G., & Levine, E. (1965, Winter). The aims of nursing research. *Nursing Research, 14*:27.

Abdellah, F.G., & Levine, E. (1966, Jan.). Future directions of research in nursing. *American Journal of Nursing, 66*:112-116.

Abdellah, F.G., & Levine, E. (1968, Summer). The aims of nursing research. *Comprehensive Nursing Monthly, 3*:12-31. (Japan).

Abdellah, F.G., & Levine, E. (1982, Aug.). Better patient care through nursing research (Part 1). *Kango Tenbo, 7(8)*:714-719. (Japanese Journal of Nursing Science).

Abdellah, F.G., & Strachan, E.J. (1959, May). Progressive patient care. *American Journal of Nursing, 59*:649.

Matarazzo, J.D., Abdellah, F.G. (1971, Sept.-Oct.). Doctoral education for nurses in the U.S. *Nursing Research, 20*:404-414.

Muller, J.E., et al. (1972, March). The Soviet health system: Aspects of relevance for medicine in the U.S. *New England Journal of Medicine, 286*:693-702.

Correspondence

Abdellah, F.G. (1984, March 7). Personal letter.

Secondary Sources
Book Reviews

Abdellah, F.G., & Levine, E. (1957). *Patients and personnel speak: A method of studying patient care in hospitals.* *American Journal of Nursing, 59*:634-635, May 1959.

Abdellah, F.G., & Levine, E. (1965). *Better patient care through nursing research* (1st ed.). *Hospitals, 39*:115, November 1965. *Nursing Outlook, 13*:18, December 1965. *Catholic Nurse, 14*:63, March 1966. *American Journal of Nursing, 66*:828, April 1966. *Nursing Research, 15*:217, Summer 1966. *Nursing Research Reports, 2*:6, June 1967.

Abdellah, F.G., & Levine, E. (1979). *Better patient care through nursing research* (2nd. ed.). *American Journal of Nursing, 80*:67-68, January 1980.

Abdellah, F.G., et al. (1963). *Patient-centered approaches to nursing.* *Hospital Administration, 8*:48, Spring 1963.

Abdellah, F.G., et al. (1973). *New directions in patient-centered nursing.* *American Journal of Nursing, 73*:1439, August 1973. *Nursing Outlook, 22*:555, September 1974.

News Releases

Two Named to Top Nurse Rank in P.H.S. (1970, Nov.). *Nursing Outlook,* 18:10.

Public Health Service Now Has Two Lady Admirals: Jessie Scott and Faye Abdellah. (1970, Nov.). *American Journal of Nursing, 70*:2281.

Appointments. (1971, Jan.). *H.S.M.H.A. Health Report, 36*:27-38.

Department of Health, Education, and Welfare (1971, Jan.-Feb.). Faye C. Abdellah: A New Appointment. *Journal of Continuing Education in Nursing, 2*:9.

Biographic Sources

Directory of Nurses with Doctoral Degrees. (1980, Aug.). American Nurses Association. (ANA Publication No. G-143).

Faye Abdellah Sees Bright Future for Nurses. (1980, September). *American Journal of Nursing, 80*:1671-1672.

The National Nursing Directory. (1982). Rockville, Md.: Aspen Systems.

Who's Who in America: 1982-1983. (42nd ed.). (1982). Chicago, Marquis.

Books

Dolan, J.A., Fitzpatrick, M.L., & Herrmann, E.K. (1983). *Nursing in society: A historical perspective* (15th ed.). Philadelphia: W.B. Saunders.

Griffin, J.G., & Griffin, J.K. (1973). *History and trends of professional nursing.* St. Louis: C.V. Mosby.

Nursing Theories Conference Group, J.B., George, Chairperson. (1980). *Nursing theories: The base for professional practice.* Englewood Cliffs, N.J.: Prentice-Hall.

Orem, D.E. (ed.) (1979). *Concept formalization in nursing, process and product.* Boston: Little, Brown, & Co.

Book Chapters

Falco, S.M. (1980). Faye Abdellah. In Nursing Theories Conference Group, J.B. George, Chairperson, *Nursing theories: The base for professional nursing practice.* Englewood Cliffs, N.J.: Prentice Hall.

Articles

Adebo, E.O. (1974). Identifying problems for nursing research. *International Nursing Review, 21(2):*53.

Alward, R.R. (1983). Patient classification system: The ideal vs. reality. *Journal of Nursing Administration, 13(2):*14-19.

Armiger, B. (1977). Ethics of nursing research: Profile, principles perspective. *Nursing Research, 26(5):*330-336.

Auger, J.A., & Dee, V. (1983). A patient classification system based on the behavioral system model of nursing. *Journal of Nursing Administration, 13(4):*38-43.

Auster, D. (1978). Occupational values of male and female nursing students. *Sociology of Work and Occupations, 5(2):*209-233.

Ballard, S., & McNamara, R. (1983). Qualifying nursing needs in home health care. *Nursing Research, 32(4):*236-241.

Bergman, R., et al. (1981). Role, selection and preparation of unit head nurses (Part I). *International Journal of Nursing Studies, 18(2):*123-152.

Bergman, R., et al. (1981). Role, selection and preparation of unit head nurses (Part II). *International Journal of Nursing Studies, 18(3):*191-211.

Bergman, R., et al. (1981). Role, selection and preparation of unit head nurses (Part III). *International Journal of Nursing Studies, 18(4):*237-250.

Carnegie, M.E. (1975). Financial assistance for nursing research: Past and present. *Nursing Research, 24(3):*163.

Carter, M.D. (1973). Identification of behaviors displayed by children experiencing prolonged hospitalization. *International Journal of Nursing Studies, 10(2):*125-135.

Caterinicccho, R.P., & Davies, R.H. (1983). Developing a client focused allocation statistic of inpatient nursing resource use: An alternative to the patient day. *Social Science and Medicine, 17(5):*259-272.

Chamorro, I.L., et al. (1973). Development of an instrument to measure premature infant behavior and caretaker activities: Time-sampling methodology. *Nursing Research, 22(4):*300-309.

Chamorro, T. (1981). The role of a nurse clinician in joint practice with gynecologic oncologists. *Cancer, 48(2):*622-631.

Chow, R.K. (1974). Significant research and future needs for improving patient care. *Military Medicine, 139(4):*302-306.

Colaizzi, J. (1975). Proper object of nursing science. *International Journal of Nursing Studies, 12(4):*197-200.

Conine, T.A., & Hopper, D.L. (1978). Work sampling: Tool in management. *American Journal of Occupational Therapy, 32(5):*301-304.

Copp, L.A. (1973). Professional change: Which trends do nurses endorse? *International Journal of Nursing Studies, 10(1):*55-63.

Copp, L.A. (1974). Critical concerns and commitments of a new department of nursing. *International Journal of Nursing Studies, 11(4):*203-210.

Cornell, S.A. (1974). Development of an instrument for measuring quality of nursing care. *Nursing Research, 23(1):*103-117.

Craig, S.L. (1980). Theory development and its relevance for nursing. *Journal of Advanced Nursing, 5(4):*349-355.

Crow, R.A. (1981). Research and the standards of nursing care: What is the relationship? *Journal of Advanced Nursing, 6(6):*491-496.

Daeffler, R.J. (1977). Outcomes of primary nursing for the patient. *Military Medicine, 142(3):*204-208.

Delacuestra, C. (1983). The nursing process: From development to implementation. *Journal of Advanced Nursing, 9(5):*365-371.

Denton, J.A., & Wisenbaker, V.B. (1977). Death experience and death anxiety among nurses and nursing students. *Nursing Research, 26(1):*61-64.

Dickoff, J., James, P., & Semradek, J. (1975). Stance for nursing research: Tenacity or inquiry? *Nursing Research, 24(2):*84-88.

Dickoff, J., James, P., & Semradek, J. (1975). Designing nursing research: Eight points to encounter. *Nursing Research, 24(3):*164-176.

Dickson, W.M. (1978). Measuring pharmacist time use: Note on use of fixed interval work sampling. *American Journal of Hospital Pharmacy, 35(10):*1241-1243.

DiMarco, N., et al. (1976). Nursing resources on nursing unit and quality of patient care. *International Journal of Nursing Studies, 13(3):*134-152.

Doerr, B.C., & Jones, J.W. (1979). Effect of family preparation on the state anxiety level of the C.C.U. patient. *Nursing Research, 28(5):*315-316.

Duhart, J., & Chartonb, J. (1973). Hospital reform and health care in medical ordinance. *Revue Francaise De Sociologic, 14:*77-101.

Dungy, C.I., & Mullins, R.G. (1981). School nurse practitioner: Analysis of questionnaire and time-motion data. *Journal of School Health, 51(7):*475-478.

Ellis, R. (1977). Fallibilities, fragments, and frames: Contemplation on 25 years of research in medical-surgical nursing. *Nursing Research, 26(3):*177-182.

Elms, R.R. (1972). Recovery room behavior and postoperative convalescence. *Nursing Research, 21(5):*390-397.

Falcone, A.R. (1983). Comprehensive functional assessment as an administrative tool. *Journal of the American Geriatrics Society, 31(11):*642-650.

Fielder, J.L. (1981). A review of the literature on access and utilization of medical care with special emphasis on rural primary care, social science and medical (Part C). Medical Economics, 15(3c):129-142.

Flook, E. (1973). Health services research and R and D in perspective. *American Journal of Public Health and the Nations Health, 63(8):*681-686.

Fortinsky, R.H., Granger, C.V., & Seltzer, G.B. (1981). The use of functional assessment in understanding home care needs. *Medical Care, 19(5):*489-497.

Foster, S.B. (1974). Adrenal measure for evaluating nursing effectiveness. *Nursing Research, 23(2):*118-124.

Fox, R.N., & Ventura, M.R. (1983). Small scale ad-

ministration of instruments procedures. *Nursing Research, 32(2):*122-125.

Frelick, R.W., & Frelick, J.H. (1976). Coming to grips with main issues. *American Journal of Public Health, 66(8):*795.

French, K. (1981). Methodological considerations in hospital patient opinion surveys. *International Journal of Nursing Studies, 18(1):*7-32.

Golden, A.S. (1975). Task analysis in health manpower development and utilization. *Medical Care, 13(8):*704-710.

Goodwin, J.D., & Edwards, B.S. (1975). Developing a computer program to assist nursing process: Phase 1: From systems analysis to an expandable program. *Nursing Research, 24(4):*299-305.

Gordon, M. (1980). Determining study topics. *Nursing Research, 2:*83-87.

Gordon, M., Sweeney, M.A., & McKeehan, K. (1980). Development of nursing diagnoses. *American Journal of Nursing, 4:*669.

Gortner, S.R., & Nahm, H. (1977). Overview of nursing research in the United States. *Nursing Research, 26(1):*10-33.

Greaves, F. (1980). Objectively toward curriculum improvement in nursing: Education in England and Wales. *Journal of Advanced Nursing, 5(6):*591-599.

Grier, M.R., & Schnitzler, C.P. (1979). Nurses' propensity to risk. *Nursing Research, 28(3):*186-191.

Gunter, L.M., & Miller, J.C. (1977). Toward a nursing gerontology. *Nursing Research, 26(3):*208-221.

Hardy, L.K. (1982). Nursing models and nursing: A restrictive view. *Journal of Advanced Nursing. 7(5):*447-451.

Hayesbautista, D.E. (1976). Classification of practitioners by urban Chicano patients: Aspects of sociology of lay knowledge. *American Journal of Ostometry and Physiological Optics, 53(3):* 156-163.

Heagarty, M.C., et al. (1973). Evaluation of activities of nurses and pediatricians in a university outpatient department. *Journal of Pediatrics, 83(5):* 875-879.

Hodgman, E.L. (1979). Closing the gap between research and practice: Changing the answer to the who, the where and the how of nursing research. *International Journal of Nursing Studies, 16(1):*105-110.

Hooker, B.B. (1977). Diploma school of nursing: Option in post secondary education. *Journal of Nursing Education, 16(3):*36-42.

Hubbard, S.M., & Donehower, M.G. (1980). The nurse in a cancer research setting. *Seminars in Oncology, 1:*9-17.

Jackson, B.S., & Kinney, M.R. (1978). Energy-expenditure, heart rate, rhythm and blood pressure in normal female subjects engaged in common hospitalized patient positions and modes of patient transfer. *International Journal of Nursing Studies, 15(3):*115-128.

Jennings, C.P., & Jennings, T.F. (1977). Containing costs through perspective reimbursement. *American Journal of Nursing, 77(7):*1155-1159.

Ketefian, S. (1975). Application of selected nursing research findings into nursing practice: Pilot study. *Nursing Research, 24(2):*89-92.

Ketefien, S. (1976). Curriculum change in nursing education: Sources of knowledge utilized. *International Nursing Review, 23(4):*107-115.

Krueger, J.C. (1980). Establishing priorities for evaluation and evaluation research: Nursing perspective. *Nursing Research, 2:*115-118.

Kuhn, B.G. (1980). Prediction of nursing requirements from patient characteristics. *International Journal of Nursing Studies, 1:*5-15.

Lanara, V.A. (1976). Philosophy of nursing and current nursing problems. *International Nursing Review, 23(2):*48-54.

Lebow, J.L. (1974). Consumer assessments of quality of medical care. *Medical Care, 12(4):*328-337.

Leininger, M. (1976). Doctoral trends for nurses: Trends, questions, and projected plans. Part I: Trends, questions and issues on doctoral programs. *Nursing Research, 25(3):*201-210.

Lewandowski, L.A., & Kositsky, A.M. (1983). Research priorities for critical care nursing: A study by the American Association of Critical Care Nurses. *Heart and Lung, 12(1):*35-44.

Leyden, D.R. (1983). Measuring patients attitudes in a comprehensive health care setting. *Computers in Biology and Medicine, 13(2):*99-124.

Lindeman, C.A. (1975). Delphi survey of priorities in clinical nursing research. *Nursing Research, 24(6):*434-441.

Majesky, S.J., Brester, M.H., & Nishio, K.T. (1978). Development of a research tool: Patient indications of nursing care. *Nursing Research. 27(6):*365-371.

McGilloway, F.A. (1980). The nursing process: A problem-solving approach to patient care. *International Journal of Nursing Studies, 2:*79-90.

McKinnon, E.L. (1978). Circulation research: Exploring its potential in clinical nursing. *Nursing Research, 21(6):*494-498.

McLane, A.M. (1978). Core competencies of masters-prepared nurses. *Nursing Research, 27(1):*48-53.

Meleis, A.I. (1979). Development of a conceptually based nursing curriculum: International experiment. *Journal of Advanced Nursing, 6:*659-671.

Mickley, B.B. (1974). Physiologic and psychologic responses of elective surgical patients: Early definite or late indefinite scheduling of surgical procedures. *Nursing Research, 23(5):*392-401.

Nunnally, D.M. (1974). Patients' evaluation of their prenatal and delivery care. *Nursing Research, 23(6):*469-474.

Orr, J.A. (1979). Nursing and the process of scientific injury. *Journal of Advanced Nursing, 6:*603-610.

Penchansky, R., & Thomas, J.W. (1981). The concept of access: Definitions and relationship to consumer satisfaction. *Medical Care, 19(2):*127-140.

Rankin, M.A. (1974). Pienschke's theoretical framework for guardedness or openness on cancer unit. *Nursing Research, 23(5):*434.

Risser, N.L. (1975). Development of an instrument to measure patient satisfaction with nurses and nursing care in primary care settings. *Nursing Research, 24(1):*45-52.

Schlotfeldt, R.M. (1975). Research in nursing and research training for nurses: Retrospect and prospect. *Nursing Research, 24(3):*177-183.

Seither, F.G. (1974). Predictive validity study of screening measures used to select practical nursing students: *Nursing Research, 23(1):*60-63.

Sheahan, J. (1980). Some aspects of the teaching and learning of nursing. *Journal of Advanced Nursing, 5(5):*491-511.

Shopa, M.A. (1975). Historical materials in nursing. *Nursing Research, 24(4):*308.

Smoyak, S.A. (1976). Is practice responding to research? *American Journal of Nursing, 76(7):*1146-1150.

Spiegel, A.D., Hyman, H.H., & Gary, L.R. (1980). Issues and opportunities in the regulation of home health care. *Health Policy and Education, 1(3):*237-253.

Taylor, S.D. (1974). Development of a classification system for current nursing research. *Nursing Research, 23(1):*63-68.

Taylor, S.D. (1975). Bibliography on nursing research: 1950-1974. 24(3):207-225.

Temkingreener, H. (1983). Interprofessional perspectives on teamwork in health care: A case study. *Milbank Memorial Fund Quarterly: Health and Society, 61(4):*641-658.

Tornary, R.D. (1977). Nursing research: Road ahead. *Nursing Research, 26(6):*404-407.

Trivedi, V.M., & Hancock, W.M. (1975). Measurement of nursing workload using head nurses' preceptions. *Nursing Research, 24(5):*371-376.

Trivedi, V.M., & Warner, D.M. (1976). Branch and bound algorith for optimum allocation of float nurses. *Management Science, 22(9):*972-981.

Turnbull, E.M. (1978). Effect of basic preventive health practices and mass-media on practice of breast self-examination. *Nursing Research, 27(2):* 98-102.

Ventura, M.R., & Waligoraserofur, B. (1981). Study priorities identified by nurses in mental health setting. International Journal of Nursing Studies, *19(1):*41-46.

Vredevoe, D.L. (1972). Nursing research involving physiological mechanisms: Definitions of variables. *Nursing Research, 21(1):*68-72.

Warner, D.M. (1976). Nurse staffing, scheduling, reallocation in hospital. *Hospital and Health Services Administration, 21(3):*77-90.

White, M.B. (1972). Importance of selected nursing activities. *Nursing Research, 21(1):*4-14.

Wolfer, J.A. (1973). Definition and assessment of surgical patients' welfare and recovery. *Nursing Research, 22(5):*394-401.

Lydia E. Hall

10

Core, Care, and Cure Model

Kim Tippey Peskoe, S. Brook Gumm

CREDENTIALS AND BACKGROUND OF THE THEORIST

Lydia Hall began her prestigious career in nursing as a graduate of the York Hospital School of Nursing in York, Pa. She then earned her B.S. and M.A. degrees from Teacher's College, Columbia University in New York, like many other contemporary nursing theorists.

Hall had faculty positions at the York Hospital School of Nursing and the Fordham Hospital School of Nursing, and was a consultant in Nursing Education to the nursing faculty at State University of New York, Upstate Medical Center. She also was an instructor of Nursing Education at Teacher's College, Columbia University.

Hall's career interests centered around public health nursing, cardiovascular nursing, pediatric cardiology, and nursing of long-term illnesses. She authored 21 publications, with the bulk of articles and addresses regarding her nursing theories published in the early to middle 1960s. In 1967 she received the Award for Distinguished Achievement in Nursing Practice from Columbia University.

Perhaps Hall's greatest achievement in nursing was her design and development of the Loeb Center for Nursing at Montefiore Hospital in New York. Established to apply her theory to nursing practice, the center opened in

January 1963. It demonstrated extreme success and provided empirical evidence to support the major concepts in Hall's theory. Hall served as Administrative Director of the Loeb Center for nursing from its opening until her death in February 1969.

THEORETICAL SOURCES

Hall drew extensively from the schools of psychiatry and psychology in theorizing about the nurse-patient relationship. She was a proponent of Carl Rogers' philosophy of "client-centered therapy." This method of therapy entails establishing a relationship of warmth and safety, conveying a sensitive empathy with the client's feelings and communications as expressed.[8:34] A major premise Hall borrowed from Rogers[8:280] is that patients achieve their maximal potential through a learning process. Rogers[8:47] states that psychotherapy facilitates significant learning by (1) pointing out and labeling unsatisfying behaviors, (2) exploring objectively with the client the reasons for the behaviors, and (3) establishing through reeducation more effective problem-solving habits. In client-centered therapy, changes occur when:

1. The person accepts himself and his feelings more fully
2. He becomes more self-confident and self-directing
3. He changes maladaptive behaviors, even chronic ones
4. He becomes more open to evidence of what is going on both inside and outside of himself[8:280-281]

Extensive documentation indicates the result of this treatment is that physiological and psychological tensions are reduced and that the change lasts.[8:65]

The major therapeutic approach advocated by Hall is also Rogerian. This is the use of reflection, a nondirective method of helping the patient clarify, explore, and validate what he says. Rogers[8:43] states, "The therapist procedure which [clients] had found most helpful was that the therapist clarified and openly stated feelings which the client had been approaching hazily and hesitantly."[8:73]

Hall derived her postulates regarding the nature of feeling-based behavior from Rogers, who repeatedly speaks to the interaction of known feelings and feelings out-of-awareness. Rogers[8:36] hypothesizes that in a client-centered relationship the patient

> will re-organize himself at both the conscious and deeper levels of his personality in such a manner as to cope with life more constructively. . . . He shows . . . more of the characteristics of the healthy, well-functioning person. . . . He is less frustrated by stress, and recovers from stress more quickly.

Hall also adopted Rogers' theory on motivation for change. In this theory Rogers asserts that although the therapist does not motivate the client, neither is the motivation supplied by the client. Alternatively, motivation for change "springs from the self-actualizing tendency of life itself."[8:285] In the proper psychological climate, this tendency is released.

USE OF EMPIRICAL EVIDENCE

Rogers' theories have received wide acclaim in the fields of psychiatry, psychology, and social work. His methods of therapy have been used in caring for clients, and in the area of education, where a nondirective approach is less than common. In *On Becoming a Person,* one of Rogers' students, Samuel Tenenbaum, discussed learning through a nondirective approach and then teaching that way.[8:285]

The application of client-centered therapy in play therapy for children is addressed by Elaine Dorfman in Rogers' book, *Client-Centered Therapy.* In this specialized area, the therapist must work at the child's level of communication. Even with small children, reflection and clarification techniques are instrumental in helping children examine their feelings.[8:299]

Client-centered therapy concepts are also

used in leadership and administration situations. Thomas Gordon has addressed Rogers' concepts as they relate to group dynamics and group-centered leadership.[8:338] Gordon believes a leader can strive to create a nonthreatening psychological climate by conveying warmth and acceptance; clarification statements can be used to link chains of thought.

The multiplicity of applications of Rogerian theory in everyday life is almost endless. Rogers deserves his venerable title of the "founder of nondirective client-centered therapy."[6] His writings would have constituted the most current literature on this topic in the 1960s, when Hall was building her theory of nursing.

While Hall did not actually research her theory, Blue Cross Insurance studies indicated patients at Loeb recovered in half the time, at less than half the cost, and with fewer readmissions than patients who stayed in Montefiore Hospital. Twenty-two home-care programs in the New York area had a readmission rate five times higher than Loeb.[5:91-92] On a follow-up questionnaire, 40 physicians indicated the hospital stay of patients at the Loeb Center ranged from 3 to 43 days shorter than at other hospitals, but the difference was more usually 1 to 3 weeks. Patients and physicians were both pleased with the care.[5:82]

MAJOR CONCEPTS AND DEFINITIONS

BEHAVIOR. Hall broadly defines behavior as everything that is said or done. Behavior is dictated by feelings, both conscious and unconscious.

REFLECTION. Reflection is a Rogerian method of communication in which selected verbalizations of the patient are repeated back

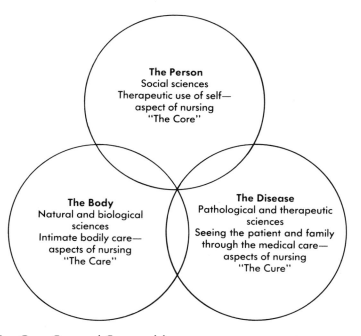

Figure 10-1. Core, Care, and Cure model.
From Hall, L. (1964, Feb.). Nursing: What is it? *The Canadian Nurse, 60(2)*:151. Reproduced with permission from *The Canadian Nurse*.

to him using different phraseology, to invite him to explore his feelings further.[4:88]

SELF-AWARENESS. Self-awareness refers to the state of being that nurses endeavor to help their patients achieve. The more self-awareness a person has of his feelings, the more control he has over his behavior.

SECOND STAGE ILLNESS. Hall[4:84] defines second stage illness as the nonacute recovery phase of illness. This stage is conducive to learning and rehabilitation.[4:84] The need for medical care here is minimal although the need for nurturing and learning is great. Therefore this is the ideal time for wholly professional nursing care.

WHOLLY PROFESSIONAL NURSING. Wholly professional nursing implies nursing care given exclusively by RNs educated in the behavioral sciences who take the responsibility and opportunity to coordinate and deliver the total care of their patients.[4:91] This concept includes the roles of nurturing, teaching, and advocacy in the fostering of healing.

Nursing circles of Care, Core, and Cure are the central concepts of Hall's theory (Figure 10-1). Care alludes to the "hands-on," intimate bodily care of the patient and implies a comforting, nurturing relationship.[4:85] Core involves the therapeutic use of self in communicating with the patient. The nurse reflects questions appropriately and helps the patient clarify motives and goals, facilitating the process of increasing the patient's self-awareness. Cure is the aspect of nursing involved with administration of medications and treatments. The nurse functions in this role as an investigator and potential "painer."[3:152]

MAJOR ASSUMPTIONS

The following assumptions are basic to Hall's theory of nursing. They are explicit and for the most part are adequately defined in her writings.

Nursing

Nursing can and should be professional.[4:81] Hall stipulated patients should be cared for only by professional RNs who can take total responsibility for the care and teaching of their patients. This interesting after-note appears in one of her articles on the Loeb Center:[4:95]

> We hire from 3-year schools, community colleges, baccalaureate, and even master's degree programmes. . . . Although all learn to master satisfactorily, those from the 2 and 3-year programmes reach a plateau. The baccalaureate graduates keep on learning and being and don't seem to stop growing in their ability to gain skills in the nurturing process.

The professional nurse functions most therapeutically when patients have entered the second stage of their hospital stay.[4:84] The second stage is the recuperating or nonacute phase of illness. The first stage of illness is a time of biological crisis, with nursing being ancillary to medicine. After the crisis period the patient is more able to benefit and learn from the teaching that nurses can offer.

Nursing is all complex.[4:84] The patient is certainly complex. Not only is he a human being, bringing with him the influences of his culture and environment, but he may be suffering from an illness that medicine is still struggling to understand and treat. The nurse giving the care is also a unique human being, interacting with the patient in a complex process of teaching and learning.

Nursing expertise centers around the body.[4:85] This refers to Hall's theoretical model because she viewed the patient as composed of Body, Pathology, and Personality. The uniqueness of nursing lies not only in knowing bodily care, but also in knowing how to modify these processes in line with the pathology and treatment, and amend them in line with the personality of the patient.

Person

Patients achieve their maximal potential through a learning process; therefore the chief therapy they need is teaching.[4:82] Rehabilitation is a process of learning to live within limitations. Physical and mental skills must be learned, but a prerequisite to these is learning about oneself as a person, becoming aware of feelings and behaviors, and clarifying motivations. Hall believed this process could best be facilitated by the professional nurse educated in communication skills.

People strive for their own goals, not goals others set for them.[4:82] Hall declared that in the usual medical setting the doctor defines the goals for the patient, but too often these goals do not coincide with the patient's goals for himself. In this situation, effective teaching and learning cannot occur.

A patient is composed of three aspects: Body, Pathology, and Person.[4:84] (These elements are discussed later.) This particular assumption is crucial to Hall's theory of nursing.

People behave on the basis of their feelings, not on the basis of knowledge.[4:89] The evidence that learning has occurred is a resultant change in some behavior. This does not usually happen strictly as a result of knowing information. Actions occur in conjunction with feelings, and feelings are not influenced by rationality.

There are two types of feelings: known feelings and feelings-out-of-awareness.[4:90] When people act on the basis of known feelings, they are *free* and in control of their behavior. When they act on feelings-out-of-awareness, they have no choice as to their behavior and the feelings make them act.

Health

Becoming ill is behavior,[4:90] according to Hall's definition of behavior. Illness is directed by one's feelings-out-of-awareness, which are the root of adjustment difficulties.

Healing may be hastened by helping people move in the direction of self-awareness.[4:90] Once people are brought to grips with their true feelings and motivations, they become free to release their own powers of healing.

Through the process of reflection, "the patient has a chance to move from the unlabeled threat of anxiety . . . through a mislabeled threat of 'phobia' or 'dis-ease' . . . to a properly labeled threat (fear) with which he can deal constructively."[4:91]

Environment

Hospital nursing services are organized to accomplish tasks efficiently.[4:83] Hall viewed these organizations as being an end unto themselves. She did not believe they have patient care and teaching as their goal, but rather that their goal is helping the physicians and administrators get their work done.

Hall was not pleased with the concept of team nursing. She said, "any career that is defined around the work that has to be done, and how it is divided to get it done, is a trade."[4:83] She vehemently opposed the idea of anyone other than educated, professional nurses taking direct care of patients and decried the fact that nursing has trained nonprofessionals to function as practical nurses so that professional nurses can function as practical doctors.

There are two phases of medical care practiced in medical centers: biological crisis and evaluative medicine.[4:84] The biological crisis phase involves intensive medical and diagnostic treatment of the patient. The evaluative medicine phase follows and generally is the time when the patient is observed in order to appraise whether he is meeting the doctor's goals.

THEORETICAL ASSERTIONS

Hall's theory consists of three major tenets. The first is that nursing functions differently in the three interlocking circles which constitute aspects of the patient.[4:81] These three circles are interrelated and are influenced by each other.

They are: the patient's *Body,* the *Disease* affecting the body, and the *Person* of the patient, which is being affected by both of the other circles. Nursing operates in all three circles, but shares them with other professions to different degrees. Because pathologic conditions are treated with medical care (Cure), nursing shares this circle with physicians. The Person aspect (Core) is cared for by therapeutic use of the self. Therefore this arena is shared with psychiatry, psychology, social work, and religious ministry. The body of the patient is cared for exclusively by nursing (Care). This circle includes all intimate bodily care such as feeding, bathing, and toileting the patient.

Hall's second assertion[2:806] is the Core postulate of her theory: As the patient needs less medical care, he needs more professional nursing care and teaching. This inversely proportional relationship alters the ratio of nursing care in the three circles. Patients in the second stage of illness (nonacute phase) are primarily in need of rehabilitation through learning: thus, the Care and Core circles predominate the Cure circle. The Loeb Center was designed for the care of nonacute patients in need of teaching and rehabilitation; the fact that it is staffed and run by nurses with physicians functioning as ancillaries is no surprise.

The third assertion of this theory is that wholly professional nursing care will hasten recovery. Hall decried the concept of team nursing, which gives the care of less complicated cases to caregivers with less training. Nurses are complex people using a complex process of teaching and learning in caring for complex patients with complex diseases. Only professional nurses are inherently qualified to provide the teaching, counseling, and nurturing needed in the second stage of illness.* At the Loeb Center, secretaries and messenger-attendants are employed for the indirect patient care. But they are not permitted to do anything directly related to the patient. The professional nurse is the coordinator for all her patients' therapies, and all disciplines act in a consulting capacity to nursing.[4:82]

LOGICAL FORM

Hall's theory is formulated using inductive logic, moving from specific observations to a generalized concept. For example:

- Nursing care shortens patient recovery time;
- Nursing care facilitates patient recovery;
- Professional nursing improves patient care;
- Therefore "wholly professional nursing will hasten recovery."[5:82]

ACCEPTANCE BY THE NURSING COMMUNITY
Practice

Hall's theory closely resembles the modern nursing model of primary care. Her emphasis on the professional nurse as the primary caregiver parallels primary care nursing to the extent that continuity and coordination of patient care are provided. In addition, Hall's concepts of nurses being accountable and responsible for their own practice are ideas that are pertinent and applicable today. Concern for these concepts demonstrates support for her theory.

Education

Hall's theory delineates definite ideas regarding nursing care being provided for by a professional nursing staff. The acceptance of this philosophy can be seen in the current shift toward professional staffing in many health care facilities, and in the growing trend toward the BSN as the minimum entry level requirement for professional practice. Hall[2:806] also emphasized the concept of nurses practicing nursing while completing their educational programs, instead of practicing as practical doctors. Today's issues

---

*References 3:150;4:83-84.

of narrowing the divide between nursing education and service, and of using nursing diagnoses as a guide for patient care instead of medical diagnoses support Hall's concepts from her theory.

Research

Currently available literature suggests that only at the Loeb Center for nursing is further research on Hall's theories being conducted.

FURTHER DEVELOPMENT

Much research and testing of Hall's theory is needed before it can be applicable and useful to areas of nursing other than long-term illnesses, and rehabilitative nursing. In particular, the theory needs to be adapted to health care facilities that differ from the Loeb Center for Nursing before its true impact and contribution to nursing can be judged. This step would require flexibility and change in several of Hall's main concepts and relationships, particularly those relating to the age and illness orientation of the client. It would be interesting to further develop in a variety of settings the concept of increased nursing care as a means to hasten patient recovery. This tenet has been highly successful at the Loeb Center in reducing both patient days and health care costs. However, other research relating nursing care to patient outcomes has not been based on Hall's model.

CRITIQUE
Simplicity

Hall's theory is simple and easily understood. The major concepts and relationships are limited and clear. The three aspects of professional nursing are identified both individually and as they relate to each other in the total process of patient care. Hall designed basic models to represent the major concepts and relationships of her theory, using individual and interlocking circles to define the three aspects of the patient, and their relationships to the three aspects of nursing. The language used to define and describe the theory is easily understood and is indigenous to nursing.

Generality

Perhaps the most serious flaw in Hall's theory of nursing is its limited generality. Hall's primary target[5:80] in nursing theory is the adult patient who has passed the acute phase of his or her illness and has a relatively good chance at rehabilitation. This concept severely limits application of the theory to a small population of patients of specific age and stage of illness. Although the ideas of Care, Cure, and Core can possibly be applied to patients in the acute phase of their illness, the theory would be most difficult to apply to infants, small children, and comatose patients. In addition, Hall[5:80,82] devotes her theory to adult individuals who are ill. The function of the nurse in preventive health care and health maintenance is not addressed, nor is the nurse's role in community health, even though the model could be adapted.

Hall viewed the role of the nurse as heavily involved in the Care and Core aspects of patient care. Unfortunately, this concept provides for little family interaction with the nurse, as her theory delineates the family aspect of patient care only in the Cure circle.*

The use of therapeutic communication to help the patient look at and explore his feelings regarding his illness and the potential changes the illness might cause is discussed in the Core aspect of nursing care. Therapeutic communication is also thought to motivate the patient by making him aware of his true feelings. However, the only communication technique Hall[4:91] described in her theory as a means to assist the patient toward self-awareness was reflection. This is a very limited approach to therapeutic communication, because not all nurses can effectively use the technique of reflection, and it is not always the most effective and successful communication tool in dealing with patients.[1:47]

---

*References 3:151;4:87

Empirical Precision

Hall's concept of professional nursing hastening patient recovery with increased care as the patient improves has been subjected to a great amount of testing at the Loeb Center for Nursing.[5:80] The fact that the theory is identified with empirical reality cannot be disputed. Evidence obtained through research at the Loeb Center demonstrates that Hall's theory[4:92] does in fact obtain its goal of shortening patient recovery time through concentrated, professional nursing efforts. Currently, the available literature supports the results obtained at the Loeb Center in testing the theory. Although research support has been demonstrated by the success of the Center, a wider range of testing in various settings is necessary to allow for increased empirical precision of the theory.

Derivable Consequences

The theory provides a general framework for nursing, and the concepts are within the domain of nursing although the aspects of Cure and Core are shared with other health professionals and family members. Although the theory does not provide for the resolution of specific issues and problems, it does address itself to the pertinent and contemporary issues of accountability, responsibility, and professionalism. Application of the theory in practice has produced valued outcomes in all three areas. In addition, the theory demonstrates a great impact on the educational preparation of nursing students. Hall[2:806] stated, "With early field experience in a center where nursing rather than medicine is emphasized, the student may emerge a nurse first." Hall believed that in nursing centers the student would benefit from experiencing nursing as it is taught to them in the classroom.

Despite the shortcomings of Hall's theory of nursing, her contribution to nursing practice is tremendous. Her insight into the problems of nursing in the 1960s has provided a base for professional practice in the multidimensional modern domain of nursing in the 1980s.

REFERENCES

1. Hale, K., & George, J. (1980). Lydia E. Hall. In Nursing Theories Conference Group, J.B. George, Chairperson, *Nursing theories: The base for professional practice*. Englewood Cliffs, N.J.: Prentice-Hall.
2. Hall, L.E. (1963, Nov). Center for nursing. *Nursing Outlook, 11*:805-806.
3. Hall, L.E. (1964, Feb.). Nursing: What is it? *Canadian Nurse, 60*:150-154.
4. Hall, L.E. (1969). The Loeb Center for nursing and rehabilitation. *International Journal of Nursing Studies, 6*:81-95.
5. Henderson, C. (1964, June). Can nursing care hasten recovery? *American Journal of Nursing, 64:80-83.*
6. Knech, D., et al. (1976). *Psychology: A basic course*. New York: Alfred Knopf.
7. Rogers, C. (1951). *Client-centered therapy*. Boston: Houghton Mifflin.
8. Rogers, C. (1961). *On becoming a person*. Boston: Houghton Mifflin.

BIBLIOGRAPHY
Primary Sources
Book Chapters

Hall, L. (1965). Nursing—what is it? In H. Baumgarten, Jr., *Concepts of nursing home administration*. New York: Macmillan.
Hall, L. (1966). Another view of nursing care and quality. In M.K. Straub, *Continuity of patient care: The role of nursing*. Washington, D.C.: Catholic University of America Press.

Articles

Hall, L. (1955, June). Quality of nursing care. *Public Health News*. (New Jersey State Department of Health.) *36*(6):212-215.
Hall, L. (1963, Nov.). Center for nursing. *Nursing Outlook, 11*:805-806.
Hall, L. (1964, Feb.). Nursing: What is it? *Canadian Nurse, 60*:150-154.
Hall, L. (1969). The Loeb Center for nursing and rehabilitation. *International Journal of Nursing Studies, 6*:81-95.
Hall, L., Hauck, M., & Rosenson, L. (1949, March). The cardiac child in school and community. *New York Heart Association Publication*.

Pamphlets

Hall, L. (1951). *What the classroom teacher should know and do about children with heart disease.* American Heart Association.

Reports

Hall, L. (1960). *Report of a work conference on nursing in long-term chronic disease and aging.* National League for Nursing as a League Exchange #50. New York: National League for Nursing.

Hall, L. (1963, June). *Report of Loeb Center for nursing and rehabilitation project report.* Congressional Record Hearings before the Special Subcommittee on Intermediate Care of the Committee on Veterans' Affairs. Washington, D.C., pp. 1515-1562.

Secondary Sources
Book Chapters

Chinn, P.L., & Jacobs, M.K. (1983). Theory in nursing: A current overview. In P.L. Chinn, & M.K. Jacobs, *Theory and nursing.* St. Louis: C.V. Mosby.

Griffith, J. (1982). Other frameworks and models. In J. Griffith, & P. Christenson, *Nursing Process: Application of theories, frameworks, and models.* St. Louis: C.V. Mosby.

Hale, K., & George, J. (1980). Lydia E. Hall. In Nursing Theories Group Conference, J.B. George, Chairperson, *Nursing theories: The base for professional practice.* Englewood Cliffs, N.J.: Prentice Hall.

Articles

Alfano, G. (1964, June). Administration means working with nurses. *American Journal of Nursing, 64*:83-85.

Bernardin, E. (1964, June). Loeb Center: As the staff nurse sees it. *American Journal of Nursing, 64*:85-86.

Bowar-Ferres, S. (1975, May). Loeb Center and its philosophy of nursing. *American Journal of Nursing, 65*:810.

Henderson, C. (1964, June). Can nursing care hasten recovery? *American Journal of Nursing, 64*:80-83.

Isler, C. (1964, June). New concepts in nursing therapy: More care as the patient improves. *RN, 27*:58-70.

Correspondence

Alfano, G.J. (1984, Jan. 26). Personal correspondence.

Alfano, G.J. (1984, Feb. 15). Personal correspondence.

Wender, B. (1984, Jan. 25). (Secretary of the Loeb Center) Telephone interview.

Other Sources

Chinn, P.L., & Jacobs, M.K., (1983). *Theory and nursing.* St. Louis: C.V. Mosby.

Rogers, C. (1951). *Client-centered therapy.* Boston: Houghton Mifflin.

Rogers, C. (1961). *On becoming a person.* Boston: Houghton Mifflin.

Dorothea E. Orem

11

Self-Care Deficit Theory of Nursing

Jeanne Donohue Eben, Margaret J. Nation, Ann Marriner,
Sherry B. Nordmeyer

CREDENTIALS AND BACKGROUND OF THE THEORIST

Dorothea Orem was born in Baltimore, the second of her parents' two children, both of whom were daughters. She attended Providence Hospital School of Nursing in Washington, D.C., where she was influenced by the Daughters of Charity of St. Vincent de Paul and a scholarly

The authors wish to express appreciation to Dorothea E. Orem for critiquing the chapter.

aunt. After graduating in the early 1930s, she continued her education by obtaining her Bachelor of Science degree in nursing education in 1939 and her Masters of Science degree in nursing education in 1945 from the Catholic University of America. During that time she did private duty, staff nursing, teaching, and was assistant to the Director of the Providence Division of the School of Nursing, The Catholic University of America. After earning her Master's degree, Orem became the Director of the Providence Hospital School of Nursing and Director of Nursing Service of the Hospital in

117

Detroit, a position she held from 1945 to 1948.

From 1949 to 1957, Orem was a nurse consultant in the Division of Health and Institutional Service of the Indiana State Board of Health. During this time Orem began to redevelop her definitions of nursing and nursing practice.

Orem left Indiana in 1957 to serve as a curriculum consultant to the Office of Education in the U.S. Department of Health, Education, and Welfare in Washington, D.C. She held the position from 1958 until 1960. While at HEW she worked on a project to upgrade practical nurse training that stimulated a need to address the question, "What is the subject matter of nursing?" This experience resulted in her 1959 publication, *Guides for Developing Curricula for the Education of Practical Nurses.*

In 1959 Orem became an Assistant Professor of Nursing Education at The Catholic University of America. She subsequently served as Acting Dean of the School of Nursing and as an Associate Professor of Nursing Education. She continued to develop her concept of nursing and self-care while at Catholic University, and in 1971, published her book, *Nursing: Concepts of Practice.*[13,14] The second and third editions, published in 1980 and 1985, further refined the self-care deficit concept of nursing practice.

In 1965 interested faculty members formed the Nursing Model Committee of the Nursing Faculty of The Catholic University of America to explore and develop a model for guiding nursing research. "They recognized the need to isolate the general conceptual elements of nursing that would give direction to the recognition of problems that are specifically nursing problems and to the organization of knowledge accruing from research in problem areas."[37]

Three years later five of these committee members and six colleagues of varying backgrounds formed the Nursing Development Conference Group because of their "dissatisfactions with and concerns for the development of nursing as a discipline. The absence of an organizing framework for nursing knowledge and the Group's conviction that the use of a general concept of nursing would aid in formalizing such a framework provided the base for action."[33:ix] Although the composition of the groups changed over time, the work initiated by the Nursing Model Committee and continued by the Nursing Development Conference Group resulted in *Concept Formalization in Nursing: Process and Product.* The first edition, published in 1973, identified and described the conceptual structure of nursing. In 1979 the second edition further developed the conceptual structure.*

In 1970 Orem resigned from the faculty at Catholic University and established her own consulting firm of Orem & Shields in Chevy Chase, Md. Currently she works as a consultant in nursing and nursing education.

Orem has been the recipient of several honorary degrees. She received an honorary doctorate from Georgetown University, Washington, D.C., in 1976 and from Incarnate Word College, San Antonio, Texas, in 1980. In 1980 she was awarded The Catholic University of America's Alumni Achievement Award for Nursing Theory.[37,38,40]

In 1956 Orem wrote, "The art of nursing is practiced by 'doing for' the person with the disability, by 'helping him to do for himself' and/or by 'helping him to learn to do for himself.' "[32;35:208] This is as true now as it was then as it described the essence of nursing.

THEORETICAL SOURCES

Although Orem cites Eugenia K. Spaulding as a great friend and teacher, she indicates that no particular nursing leader was a direct influence on her work. She believes association with many nurses over the years provided many learning experiences and she views her work with graduate students and collaborative works

---

*References 33:ix-x; 36; 38; 40.

with colleagues as valuable endeavors.[38] While crediting no one as a major influence, she does cite many other nurses' works in terms of their contributions to nursing including, but not limited to, Abdellah, Henderson, Johnson, King, Levine, Nightingale, Orlando, Peplau, Riehl, Rogers, Roy, Travelbee, and Wiedenbach.* She also cites numerous authors in other disciplines including, but not limited to, Gordon Allport, Chester Barnard, René Dubos, Erich Fromm, Gartly Jaco, Robert Katz, Kurt Lewin, Ernest Nagel, Talcott Parsons, Hans Selye, and Ludwig von Bertalanffy.‡

USE OF EMPIRICAL EVIDENCE

In 1958, Orem had a spontaneous insight about why individuals required and could be helped through nursing that enabled her to formulate and express her concept of nursing. Her knowledge of the features of nursing practice situations was acquired over many years.[38]

MAJOR CONCEPTS AND DEFINITIONS

Orem labels her self-care deficit theory of nursing as a general theory. This general theory is composed of three related theories: (1) the theory of self-care (describes and explains self-care); (2) the theory of self-care deficit (describes and explains why people can be helped through nursing); and (3) the theory of nursing systems (describes and explains relationships that must be brought about and maintained for nursing to be produced).§ The major concepts of these theories are identified here and discussed more fully in Orem's book *Nursing: Concepts of Practice* (Figure 11-1).

SELF-CARE. Self-care is an adult's continuous contribution to his or her own continued exis-

Figure 11-1. Conceptual framework for nursing. *R*, relationship; <, deficit relationship, current or projected.
Used with permission from Orem, D.E. (1980). *Nursing: Concepts of practice*. New York: McGraw-Hill.

tence, health, and well-being.[33:13] "Self-care is the practice of activities that individuals initiate and perform on their own behalf in maintaining life, health and well-being."[33:35]

Self-care requisites. Self-care requisites are "the purposes to be attained through the kinds of actions termed self-care."[36:37;39:85] They may be broken down into three categories.

Universal self-care requisites. Universal self-care requisites are common to all human beings and include the maintenance of air, water, food, elimination, activity and rest, and solitude and social interaction, prevention of hazards, and promotion of human functioning.*

---

*References 9:38, 39, 61, 100-103.
‡References 39:222-225
§References 34:209; 35:214.

*References 36:42; 39:90-91.

These eight requisites represent the kinds of human actions that bring about the internal and external conditions that maintain human structure and functioning, which in turn support human development and maturation. When it is effectively provided, self-care or dependent care organized around universal self-care requisites fosters positive health and well being.[39:91]

Developmental self-care requisites. Developmental self-care requisites were separated from universal self-care requisites in the second edition of *Nursing: Concepts of Practice*. They promote processes for life and maturation and prevent conditions deleterious to maturation or mitigate those effects.[34:47]

Health deviation self-care requisites. Orem* defined health deviation self-care requisites in the following way.

> Disease or injury affects not only specific structures and physiological or psychological mechanisms but also integrated human functioning. When integrated functioning is seriously affected . . . the individual's power of agency are seriously impaired either permanently or temporarily. . . . When a change in health state brings about total or almost total dependence on others for the needs to sustain life or well-being, the person moves from the position of self-care agent to that of patient or receiver of care. . . . Evidence of health deviations leads to demands for determining what should be done to restore normalcy. . . . Seeking and participating in medical care for health deviations are self-care actions. . . . Pain, discomfort, and frustration resulting from medical care also create requisites for self-care to bring relief. . . . If persons with health deviations are to become competent in managing a system of health-deviation self-care, they must also be able to apply relevant medical knowledge to their own care.

THERAPEUTIC SELF-CARE DEMAND. Therapeutic self-care demand is "the totality of self-care actions to be performed for some duration in order to meet self-care requisites by using valid methods and related sets of operations or actions."[36:39]

SELF-CARE AGENCY. Self-care agency is "the power of an individual to engage in estimative and production operations essential for self-care."[33:118] There are three subsidiary terms.

Agent. An agent is the "person taking action."*

Self-care agent. A self-care agent is "the provider of self-care."*

Dependent-care agent. A dependent-care agent is "the provider of infant care, child care, or dependent adult care."*

SELF-CARE DEFICIT. Self-care deficit is "a relationship between self-care agency and therapeutic self-care demand in which self-care agency is not adequate to meet the known therapeutic self-care demand."[39:31] It determines when and why nursing is needed.[34:26]

NURSING AGENCY. Nursing agency is the characteristic that qualifies persons to fill the status of nurse in social groups. "The provision of nursing to individual men, women, and children or to multiperson units such as families requires that nurses have specialized abilities that enable them to provide care that compensates for or aids in overcoming the health-derived or health-related self-care or dependent-care deficits of others."[34:87] The specialized abilities are the nursing agency.[34:87]

NURSING SYSTEMS. "Nursing systems are formed when nurses use their abilities to prescribe, design, and provide nursing for legitimate patients (as individuals or groups) by performing discrete actions and systems of action. These actions or systems regulate the value of or the exercise of individuals' capabilities to engage in self-care and meet the self-care requisites of the individual therapeutically."[34:29]

*References 36:48-50; 39:98-99.

*References 34:35; 39:84.

Types of nursing systems. Three types of nursing systems are identified (Figure 11-2). Whether the nursing system is wholly compensatory, partly compensatory, or supportive-educative depends on "who can or should perform those self-care actions."*

Wholly compensatory nursing systems. Wholly compensatory nursing systems are needed when the "nurse should be compensating for a patient's total inability for (or prescriptions against) engaging in self-care activities that require ambulation and manipulation movements."†

Partly compensatory systems. Partly compensatory systems exist when "both nurse and patient perform care measures or other actions involving manipulative tasks or ambulation."‡

Supportive-educative systems. Supportive-educative systems are "for situations where the patient is able to perform or can and should learn to perform required measures of externally or internally oriented therapeutic self-care but cannot do so without assistance."‡

Methods of assistance. Methods of assistance include: "(1) acting or doing for; (2) guiding; (3) teaching; (4) supporting; and (5) providing a developmental environment."[34:61]

MAJOR ASSUMPTIONS

Assumptions basic to the general theory were formalized in the early 1970s and were presented at Marquette University School of Nursing in 1973.[38] Orem[34:33-34] lists the five assumptions underlying the general theory of nursing as:

1. Human beings require continuous deliberate inputs to themselves and their environments in order to remain alive and function in accord with natural human endowments.
2. Human agency, the power to act deliberately, is exercised in the form of care of self and others in identifying needs for and in making needed inputs.
3. Mature human beings experience privations in the form of limitations for action in care of self and others involving the making of life-sustaining and function-regulating inputs.
4. Human agency is exercised in discovering, developing, and transmitting to other ways and means to identify needs for and make inputs to self and others.
5. Groups of human beings with structured relationships cluster tasks and allocate responsibilities for providing care to group members who experience privations for making required deliberate input to self and others.

Orem lists presuppositions for the theory of Self-Care, the theory of Self-Care Deficit, and the theory of Nursing Systems in *Nursing: Concepts of Practice.*[39:33-38]

THEORETICAL ASSERTIONS

The model shows that when an individual's self-care capabilities are less than the therapeutic self-care demand, the nurse compensates for the self-care or dependent-care deficits. The relational structure is discussed in Orem's book, *Nursing: Concepts of Practice,* as central ideas and propositions of the three related theories of self-care, self-care deficits, and nursing systems.*

Self-Care

Self-care and care of dependent family members are learned behaviors that purposely regulate human structural integrity, functioning, and human development. The theory of self-care denotes the relationship between the deliberate self-care actions of mature and maturing members of social groups and their own development and function-

---

*References 34:96-97; 39:152.
†References 34:97-98; 39:154.
‡References 34:101; 39:156.

*References 34:26-30; 39:33-38.

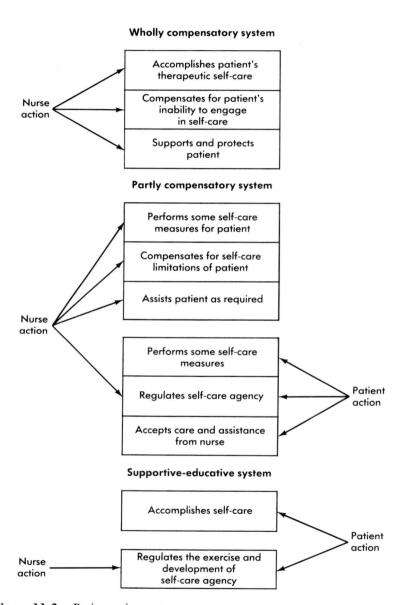

Figure 11-2. Basic nursing systems.
Used with permission from Orem, D.E. (1980). *Nursing: Concepts of practice*. New York: McGraw-Hill.

ing as well as the relationship of the continuing care of dependent members to their functioning and development.*

Self-Care Deficit

Individuals experience a self-care deficit when they are unable to care for themselves.

People can benefit from nursing because they are subject to health-related or health-derived limitations that render them incapable of continuous self-care or dependent care or that result in ineffective or incomplete care.†

Nursing Systems

Nursing systems are formed when nurses use their abilities to prescribe, design, and provide nursing for legitimate patients (as individuals or groups) by performing discrete actions and systems of action. These actions or systems regulate the value of or the exercise of individuals' capabilities to engage in self-care and meet the self-care requisites of the individual therapeutically.‡

LOGICAL FORM

Orem's spontaneous insight led to her initial formalization and subsequent expression of a general concept of nursing. That generalization then made possible deductive thinking about nursing.[38]

Susan and Thomas Taylor from the University of Missouri at Columbia have worked with Orem's general theory of nursing using a mathematical logic approach to explicate its syntactical structure or internal logic as a step toward identifying rules and modes of inquiry.[38,40]

ACCEPTANCE BY THE NURSING COMMUNITY

Orem's self-care theory has achieved a greater level of acceptance by the nursing community than the works of the majority of other theorists.

*References 34:28; 39:36.
†References 34:27; 39:34-36.
‡References 34:29; 39:37-38.

Practice

Many articles document the use of the self-care theory as a basis for clinical practice. In 1971 Lucille Kinlein established an independent nurse practice in College Park, Md. Although Kinlein's concepts differ from Orem's, her practice was stimulated by Orem's self-care theory. In 1977 Kinlein[25,26] published *Independent Nursing Practice with Clients* in which she documented her experience in setting up an independent practice and her use of self-care.

At Johns Hopkins Hospital in Baltimore the self-care theory was used in several outpatient clinics. Nurse specialists managed three of those units—two cardiac clinics and a diabetic clinic. These clinics were managed separately from the standard medically managed clinics. Although there was a mechanism for referral to a medical doctor, the nurse specialists controlled the clinics and used Orem's self-care theory in their daily practice.[1]

A group of graduate students at the University of Texas School of Nursing, as part of their course work, applied Orem's theory in a nursing home to specific patients. Their conclusions were "that through the employment of the self-care conceptual framework the nurses developed a greater respect for the patient, the patient realized his right of choice as a consumer of health care and participated in care geared to re-establishing his self-sufficiency."[2:11]

An article by Virginia Mullin states that implementation of Orem's self-care theory faces many constraints within the acute care setting. Mullin[31:183] wrote that "these constraints can be dealt with effectively in nursing by each individual nurse internalizing the beliefs about self-care and translating those beliefs into practice."

Orem's self-care concept has been used in work with adolescent alcohol abusers,[30] employees with rheumatoid arthritis,[9] women recovering from radical mastectomies,[28] families and children with cystic fibrosis,[27] patients with congestive heart failure,[7] pretransfer teaching for cardiac patients,[45] diabetic patients,[1,3,15] persons receiving enterostomal therapy,[5] renal transplant recipients,[21] and patients receiving peritoneal dialysis.[41] It has been related to family-centered maternity care,[19] hospitalized children,[13] and hospice care.[46] Orem's self-care deficit theory has been used in the context of the nursing process to teach patients to increase their self-care agency,[23] to evaluate nursing practice,[43] and to differentiate nursing from medical practice.[29]

Education

Orem's self-care deficit theory has been used as a basis for the focus of the curriculum in nursing education at many schools of nursing, such as Thornton Community College, South Holland, Illinois[14]; Georgetown University, Washington, D.C.; University of Southern Mississippi at Hattiesburg[20]; and Southern Missouri State at Springfield.[44]

At Georgetown University School of Nursing Orem's self-care deficit theory was introduced as early as the freshman year. This establishes the theory early in the educational process, which allows the student to have a broader perspective on nursing.[42]

The curriculum for the Southwest Missouri State School of Nursing RNBSN program uses the self-care theory extensively. Students are taught to incorporate the theory in nursing care plans, patient teaching, and everyday nursing practice.[44] Goodwin[18] proposed a model of the nursing process for faculty to use to have students apply models incorporating theories to clinical practice.

Orem's self-care concept provided the conceptual framework for Dickerson and Lee-Villasenor's[15] research[11] and for Gallant and McLane's outcome criteria.[16] Denyes[10] developed a Likert scale questionnaire for clinical nursing assessment and studies with adolescents and Crockett[8] described the self-reported development of coping beliefs and practices of adult psychiatric and nonpsychiatric subjects.

Research

Several research projects have incorporated Orem's self-care theory. Kearney and Fleischer developed an instrument to measure a person's exercise of self-care agency and administered it to nursing students in an associate degree program and to students in two psychology courses. Findings concluded that people who exercise a high degree of self-care agency describe themselves as a self-controlled, dependable, assertive, intelligent, confident, responsible, helpful, and adaptable. Kearney and Fleischer recommended that the scale be administered to other populations to further validate the results of the study.[24]

Barbara J. Horn, Mary Ann Swain, and their associates have developed criteria measures of nursing care around the universal self-care requisites and health-deviation self-care requisites along with instruments and procedures to measure the quality of nursing care provided.[22]

In a study done at the University of Michigan, the authors, who were research assistants on the Horn and Swain study, developed eight categories of patient outcomes related to health-deviation self-care actions. The study had not been concluded when the article was published because a method of data collection still needed to be determined. The ultimate goal of the study was to establish an instrument that could be used to measure the health status of hospitalized patients along dimensions related to their requirements for universal and health-deviations self-care.[6]

FURTHER DEVELOPMENT

Orem's work has been used most with ill adults. However, Orem defined dependent care agent as the provider of infant or child care and identified early on developmental as one of the three types of self-care requisites. She added a section on "age-specific factors in nursing children" in the 1980 edition of her book *Nursing: Concepts of Practice** and a section on multiperson units in the 1985 edition.† She had addressed the

---

*References 34:155-159; 39:259-262.
†Reference 34:251-256.

multiperson unit in a table in the 1980 edition.[34] Orem[36] discussed her conceptual model and community health nursing at the eighth annual community health nursing conference at the University of North Carolina at Chapel Hill, and has addressed the relationship of her model to rehabilitation in Cincinnati.[40]

CRITIQUE
Simplicity

Orem identified six major concepts in the self-care deficit theory of nursing. They are self-care, therapeutic self-care demand, self-care agency, self-care deficit, nursing agency, and nursing system. She uses these six concepts to express the three constituent theories of the general theory of nursing.[38,39] The conceptual framework appears simple. Subconcepts are identified to express the substantive structure of the six broad conceptual elements of the theory.

Generality

The self-care deficit theory of nursing as expressed is universal. It is a theory of nursing as nursing regardless of time or place. Its use as a guide to practice was initially and at present most commonly applied in the care of ill adults. From the beginning, it has been applied in the care of both well and sick children. The universality of the theory should be differentiated from its application in terms of time, place, and individuals.[38]

Empirical Precision

This theory identifies concepts, provides definitions, describes relationships, and states assumptions. It can be, and has been, used for research.

Derivable Consequences

Orem's self-care deficit theory of nursing provides a general framework to direct nursing action. Orem[34:92-103] views nursing within the framework of the theory as related to patients' therapeutic self-care demands, their self-care agency, and the relationships between them. She sees three types of nursing systems: doing self-care for the individual (wholly compensatory), assisting the individual with self-care (partially compensatory), and educating and supporting the individual to help him or her better perform self-care.

Orem believes her self-care theory applies to other groups in addition to nurses.

> The self-care theory component of the general theory of nursing is common to the health professions and to all members of social groups. Physicians as well as paramedical groups help people with aspects of self-care and with development of capabilities to engage in self-care. Persons helped may or may not be in need of nursing or may or may not be under nursing care.[38]

The assumptions used in this theory are logically sound and accepted by the nursing community. The concepts are relevant for nursing. The relationships explained and implied are useful in explaining patiency and the nurse-patient relationship.

Orem's theory does direct nursing practice, the stated goal. Her nursing systems provide a framework for nursing practice, based on the amount and kind of nursing agency needed. In her books Orem also addresses educational needs for nurses to be able to practice as well as the use of various levels of nursing practice. Additional research is desirable.

REFERENCES

1. Allison, S. (1973). A framework for nursing action in a nurse-conducted diabetic managed clinic. *Journal of Nursing Administration, 3(4):*53-60.
2. Anna, D., et al. (1978, Nov.). Implementing Orem's conceptual framework, *Journal of Nursing Administration,* 8:8-11.
3. Bachschieder, J. (1974). Self-care requirements, self-care capabilities and nursing systems in the diabetic nurse managed clinic. *American Journal of Public Health,* 64(12):1138-1146.
4. Bennett, J.G. (Ed.) (1980). Symposium on the self-care concept of nursing. *Nursing Clinics of North America,* 15:129-217.
5. Bromley, B. (1980, Feb.). Applying Orem's self-care theory in enterostomal therapy. *American Journal of Nursing,* 80:245-249.

6. Clinton, J.E., et al. (1977, Sept.). Developing criterion measures of nursing care: Case study of a process. *Journal of Nursing Administration, 7(7):*41-45.

7. Crews, J. (1972). Nurse-managed cardiac clinics. *Cardiovascular Nursing, 8:*15-18.

8. Crockett, M.S. (1982). Self reported coping histories of adult psychiatric and nonpsychiatric subjects and controls. *Nursing Research,* 31:122. (Abstract).

9. Dear, M.R., & Keen, M.F. (1982). Promotion of self-care in the employee with rheumatoid arthritis. *Occupational Health Nursing, 30(1):*32-34.

10. Denyes, M.J. (1982). Measurement of self-care agency in adolescents. *Nursing Research, 31:*63. (Abstract).

11. Dickson, G.L., & Lee-Villasenor, H. (1982). Nursing theory and practice: A self-care approach. *Advances in Nursing Science, 5(1):*29-40.

12. Eichelberger, K.M., et al. (1980). Self-care nursing plan: Helping children to help themselves. *Pediatric Nursing 6(3):*9-13.

13. Facteau, L.M. (1980). Self-care concepts and the care of the hospitalized child. *Nursing Clinics of North America,* 15:145-155.

14. Fenner, K. (1979). Developing a conceptual framework. *Nursing Outlook,* 27:122-126.

15. Fitzgerald, S. (1980). Utilizing Orem's self-care nursing model in designing an educational program for the diabetic. *Topics in Clinical Nursing, 2(2):*57-65.

16. Gallant, B.W., & McLane, A.M. (1979). Outcome criteria: A process for validation at the unit level. *Journal of Nursing Administration, 9(1):*14-21.

17. Garavan, P., et al. (1980). Self-care applied to the aged. *New Jersey Nurse, 10(1):*3-5.

18. Goodwin, J.O. (1980, Nov.-Dec.). A cross-cultural approach to integrating nursing theory and practice. *Nurse Educator, 5(6):*15-20.

19. Harris, J.K. (1980). Self-care is possible after Cesarean delivery. *Nursing Clinics of North America.* 15:191-204.

20. Herrington, J.V., & Houston, S. (1984, Jan.). Using Orem's theory: A plan for all seasons. *Nursing and Health Care, 5(1):*45-47.

21. Hoffart, N. (1982, June). Self-care decision making by renal transplant recipients. *AANNT Journal, 9(3):*43-47.

22. Horn, B.J., & Swain, M.A. (1977). *Development of Criterion Measures of Nursing Care* (Vols. 1 and 2). Springfield, Va.: University of Michigan and National Center for Health Services Research, U.S. Department of Commerce. (NTIS Nos. 267-004 and 267-005).

23. Joseph, L.S. (1980). Self-care and the nursing process. *Nursing Clinics of North America,* 15:131-143.

24. Kearney, B., & Fleischer, B.L. (1979). Development of an instrument to measure exercise of self-care agency. *Research in Nursing and Health, 2(1):*25-34.

25. Kinlein, M. (1977). *Independent nursing practice with clients.* Philadelphia: J.B. Lippincott.

26. Kinlein, M.L. (1977, April). The self-care concept, *American Journal of Nursing,* 77:598-601.

27. Kruger, S., Shawver, M., & Jones, L. (1980). Reactions of families to the child with cystic fibrosis. *Image,* 12:67-72.

28. Martin, L. (1980). Self-care nursing model for patients experiencing radical change in body image. *Journal of Obstetric, Gynecologic, and Neonatal Nursing, 7(6):*9-13.

29. McIntyre, K. (1980). The Perry model as a framework for self-care. *Nurse Practitioner, 5(6):*34-38.

30. Michael, M.M., & Sewall, K.S. (1980). Use of adolescent peer group to increase the self-care agency of adolescent alcohol abusers. *Nursing Clinics of North America,* 15:157-176.

31. Mullin, V.I. (1980, March). Implementing the self-care concept in the acute care setting. *Nursing Clinics of North America, 15(1):*183.

32. Orem, D.E. (1956). *Hospital nursing service: An analysis and report of a study of administrative positions in one hospital nursing service.* Indianapolis: Indiana State Board of Health.

33. Orem, D.E. (1979). *Concept formalization in nursing: Process and product.* Boston: Little, Brown.

34. Orem, D.E. (1980). *Nursing: Concepts of practice.* New York: McGraw-Hill.

35. Orem, D.E. (1983). The self-care deficit theory of nursing: A general theory. In I. Clements & F. Roberts (Eds.), *Family health: A theoretical approach to nursing care.* New York: Wiley.

36. Orem, D.E. (1984, May). Orem's conceptual model and community health nursing. In M.K. Asay, C.C. Ossler (Eds.), *Proceedings of the Eighth Annual Community Health Nursing Conference: Conceptual Models of Nursing Applications in Community Health Nursing.* Chapel Hill: University of North Carolina Press.

37. Orem, D. (1984). Vitae.
38. Orem, D. (1984). Personal correspondence.
39. Orem, D. (1985). *Nursing: Concepts of practice.* New York: McGraw-Hill.
40. Orem, D. (1985). Telephone interviews.
41. Perras, S.T., & Zappacosta, A.R. (1982, June). The application of Orem's theory in promoting self-care in a peritoneal dialysis facility. *AANNT Journal, 9(3):*37-40.
42. Piemme, J.A., & Trainor, M.A. (1977). A first-year nursing course in a baccalaureate program. *Nursing Outlook, 25(3):*185-186.
43. Runtz, S.E., & Urtal, J.G. (1983, March). Evaluating your practice via a nursing model. *Nurse Practitioner, 8(3):*30-40.
44. Schumacher, L. (1984, April). Interview.
45. Toth, J.C. (1980). Effects of structured preparation for transfer on patient anxiety on leaving coronary care unit. *Nursing Research, 29:*28-34.
46. Walborn, K.A. (1980). A nursing model for the hospice: Primary and self-care nursing. *Nursing Clinics of North America, 15:*205-217.

BIBLIOGRAPHY
Primary Sources
Books

Orem, D.E. (Ed.) (1959). *Guides for developing curricula for the education of practical nurses.* Vocational Division #274, Trade and Industrial Education #68. Washington, D.C., U.S. Department of Health, Education, and Welfare.

Orem, D.E. (1971). *Nursing: Concepts of practice.* Scarborough, Ontario: McGraw-Hill.

Orem, D.E. (Ed.) (1973). *Concept formalization in nursing: Process and product.* Boston: Little, Brown.

Orem, D.E. (Ed.) (1979). *Concept formalization in nursing: Process and product* (2nd ed.). Boston: Little, Brown.

Orem, D.E. (1980). *Nursing: Concepts of practice.* (2nd ed.). New York: McGraw-Hill.

Orem, D.E. (1985). *Nursing: Concepts of practice* (3rd ed.). New York: McGraw-Hill.

Orem, D.E., & Parker, K.S. (Eds.). (1963). *Nurse education workshop proceedings.* Washington, D.C.: Catholic University of America.

Orem, D.E., & Parker, K.S. (Eds.). (1964). *Nursing content in preservice nursing curriculum.* Washington, D.C.: The Catholic University of America Press.

Book Chapters

Orem, D.E. (1966). Discussion of paper—Another view of nursing care and quality. In K.M. Straub, & K.S. Parker *Continuity of patient care: The role of nursing.* Washington, D.C.: The Catholic University of America Press.

Orem, D.E. (1969). Inservice education and nursing practice forces affecting nursing practice. In D.K. Petrowski, & K.M. Staub (Eds.), *School of Nursing Education.* Washington, D.C.: The Catholic University of America Press.

Orem, D.E. (1981). Nursing: A triad of action systems. In G.E. Lasker (Ed.), *Applied systems and cybernatics* (Vol. IV). Systems research in health care, biocybernatics and ecology. New York: Pergaman Press.

Orem, D.E. (1982). Nursing: A dilemma for higher education. In Sister A. Power (ed.), *Words commemorated: Essays celebrating the centennial of Incarnate Word College.* San Antonio, Tex.: Incarnate Word College.

Orem, D.E. (1983). The self-care deficit theory of nursing: A general theory. In I. Clements, and F. Roberts (Eds.), *Family health: A theoretical approach to nursing care.* New York: Wiley Medical Publications.

Orem, D.E. (1984). Orem's conceptual model and community health nursing. In M.K. Asay and C.C. Ossler, *Proceedings of the Eighth Annual Community Health Nursing Conference: Conceptual models of nursing applications in Community Health Nursing.* Chapel Hill: University of North Carolina, Dept. of Public Health Nursing, School of Public Health.

Articles

Orem, D.E., & O'Malley, M. (1952, Aug.). Diagnosis of hospital nursing problems. *Hospitals, 26:*63.

Orem, D.E. (1962, Jan.). The hope of nursing. *Journal of Nursing Education, 1:*5+.

Orem, D.E. (1979, March). Levels of nursing education and practice. *Alumnae Magazine, The Johns Hopkins School of Nursing, 68:*2-6.

Reports

Orem, D.E. (1955). *Indiana hospitals: a report.* Author of three sections of ten-year report of status and problems of Indiana hospitals. The Indiana State Board of Health.

Orem, D.E. (1956). *Hospital nursing service: An analysis and report of a study of administrative positions in one hospital nursing service.* The Indiana State Board of Health.

Orem, D.E., Dear, M., & Greenbaum, J. (1976). *Organization of nursing faculty responsibilities.* (Project Report, Public Health Service Grant No. 03D-005-3666). Washington, D.C.: Georgetown University School of Nursing.

Audiotape

Orem, D.E. (1978, Dec.). Paper presented at the Second Annual Nurse Educator Conference, New York. Audio tapes available from Teach 'em, Inc., 160 E. Illinois Street, Chicago, Ill. 60611.

Correspondence

Orem, D. (1983) Vitae.
Orem, D. (1984) Personal correspondence.
Orem, D. (1984) Telephone interviews.
Orem, D. (1985) Telephone interviews.

Secondary Sources
Book Reviews

Orem, D.E. (1971). *Nursing: Concepts of practice.*
Canadian Nurse, 67:47, December 1971.
Supervisor Nurse, 3:45-6, January 1972.
American Journal of Nursing, 72:1330, July 1972.

Orem, D.E. (1980). *Nursing: Concepts of practice* (2nd ed.).
Registered Nurse Association of British Columbia, 12:25, November 1980.
AORN Journal, 24:776, October 1981.
Nursing Times, 78:1671, October 6-12, 1982.
Journal of Advanced Nursing, 8(1):89, January 1983.

Dissertations

Laurin, J. (1979). *Development of a nursing process-outcome model based on Orem's concepts of nursing practice for quality nursing care evaluation.* Doctoral dissertation. Catholic University of America.

Sullivan, T.J. (1979). *A self-care model of nursing practice for nursing the aged.* Doctoral dissertation. Columbia University Teachers College.

Underwood, P.R. (1978). *Nursing care as a determinant in the development of self-care behavior by hospitalized adult schizophrenics.* Doctoral dissertation. University of California, San Francisco.

Books

Chinn, P.L., & Jacobs, M.K. (1983). *Theory and nursing: A systematic approach.* St. Louis: C.V. Mosby.

Fitzpatrick, J.J., et al. (1982). *Nursing models and their psychiatric mental health applications.* Bowie, M.D.: Robert J. Brady.

Horn, B.J., & Swain, M.A. (1977). *Development of criterion measures of nursing care* (Vols. 1 and 2). University of Michigan and National Center for Health Services Research. U.S. Department of Commerce. (NTIS Publication No. 267-004 and 267-005).

Kin, H.S. (1983). *The nature of theoretical thinking in nursing.* Norwalk, Conn.: Appleton-Century-Crofts.

National League of Nursing (1978). *Theory development: What, why, how?* New York: N.L.N. Publication 15-1708, pp. 73-74.

Book Chapters

Calley, J.M., et al. (1980). The Orem self-care nursing model. In J.P. Riehl, and C. Roy, *Conceptual models for nursing practice.* New York: Appleton-Century-Crofts, pp. 302-314.

Coleman, L.J. (1980). Orem's self-care nursing model. In J.P. Riehl, and C. Roy, *Conceptual models for nursing practice.* New York: Appleton-Century-Crofts, pp. 315-328.

Fawcett, J. (1984). Orem's self-care model. In J. Fawcett, *Analysis and evaluation of conceptual models in nursing.* Philadelphia: F.A. Davis, pp. 175-210.

Foster, P.C., & Janssens, N.P. (1980). Dorothea E. Orem. In Nursing Theories Conference Group, J.B. George, Chairperson, *Nursing theories: The base for professional practice.* Englewood Cliffs, N.J.: Prentice-Hall, pp. 91-106.

Goldstein, N., et al. (1983) Self-care: A framework for the future. In P.L. Chinn (Ed.). *Advances in nursing theory development.* Rockville, Md.: Aspen Systems, pp. 107-121.

Horn, B.J, & Swain, M.A. (1976). An approach to development of criterion measures for quality patient care. In *Issues in evaluation research.* Kansas City: American Nurses' Association.

Horn, B.J (1978). Development of criterion measures of nursing care. (Abstract). In *Communicating nursing research* (Vol. 11: New approaches to communicating nursing research). Boulder, Col. Western Interstate Commission for Higher Education.

Johnson, R.L. (1982). Individual psychotherapy: Relationships of theoretical approaches to nursing conceptual models. In J. Fitzpatrick, et al., *Nursing models and their psychiatric mental health applications*. Bowie, Md., Robert J. Brady, pp. 56-60.

Johnston, R.L. (1983). Orem self-care model of nursing. In J. Fitzpatrick, & A. Whall, *Conceptual models of nursing, analysis and application*. Bowie, Md: Robert J. Brady, pp. 137-156.

Kinlein, M.L. (1977). *Independent nursing practice with clients*. Philadelphia, J.B. Lippincott, pp. 15-24.

Meleis, A.I. (1985). Dorothea Orem. In A.I. Meleis, *Theoretical nursing: development and progress*. Philadelphia: J.B. Lippincott, pp. 284-296.

Roy, C. (1980). A case study viewed according to different models. In J.P. Riehl, and C. Roy, *Conceptual models for nursing practice*. New York: Appleton-Century Crofts, pp. 385-386.

Spangler, Z.S., & Spangler, W.O. (1983). Self-care: A testable model. In P.L. Chinn (Ed.), *Advances in nursing theory development*. Rockville, Md.: Aspen Systems, 89-105.

Stanton, M. (1980). Nursing theories and the nursing process. In Nursing Theories Conference Group, J.B. George, Chairperson, *Nursing theories: The base for professional practice*. Englewood Cliffs, N.J.: Prentice-Hall, pp. 213-217.

Sullivan, T.J. (1980). Self-care model for nursing. In *Directions for nursing in the 80's*. Kansas City: American Nurses' Association.

Underwood, P.R. (1980). Facilitating self-care. In P. Potheir (Ed.), *Psychiatric nursing: A basic text*. Boston: Little, Brown.

Thibodeau, J.A. (1983). An eclectic model: The Orem model. In J.A. Thibodeau, *Nursing models: Analysis and evaluation*. Monterey, Cal.: Wadsworth Health Sciences Division, pp. 125-140.

Articles

Allison, S. (1973). A framework for nursing action in a nurse-conducted diabetic management clinic. *Journal of Nursing Administration, 3(4)*:53-60.

Anna, D.J., et al. (1978, Nov.). Implementing Orem's conceptual framework. *Journal of Nursing Administration, 8*:8-11.

Bachscheider, J. (1974). Self-care requirement, self-care capabilities, and nursing systems in the diabetic nurse management clinic, *American Journal of Public Health, 64(12)*:1138-1146.

Bennett, J.G. (1980, March) Symposium on the self-care concept of nursing. *Nursing Clinics of North America, 15*:129-217.

Bilitski, J.S. (1981). Nursing science and the laws of health as a step in the process of theory development. *Advances in Nursing Science, 4(1)*:15-29.

Bromley, B. (1980, Feb.). Applying Orem's self-care theory in enterostomal therapy. *American Journal of Nursing, 80(2)*:245-249.

Chang, B. (1980). Evaluation of health care professionals in facilitating self-care: Review of the literature as a conceptual model, *Advances in Nursing Science, 3(1)*:43-58.

Clinton, J.F., et al. (1977, Sept.). Developing criterion measures of nursing care: Case study of a process. *Journal of Nursing Administration, 7(7)*:41-45.

Crews, J. (1972). Nurse-managed cardiac clinics. *Cardiovascular Nursing, 8*:15-18.

Crockett, M.S. (1982). Self-reported coping histories of adult psychiatric and non-psychiatric subjects and controls. *Nursing Research, 31*:122. (Abstract).

Dear, M.R., & Keen, M.F. (1982). Promotion of self-care in the employee with rheumatoid arthritis. *Occupational Health Nursing, 30(1)*:32-34.

Denyes, M.J. (1982). Measurement of self-care aging in adolescents. *Nursing Research, 31*:63. (Abstract).

Dickson, G.L., et al. (1982, Oct.). Nursing theory and practice: A self-care approach. *Advances in Nursing Science, 5(1)*:29-40.

Eichelberger, K.M., et al. (1980). Self-care nursing plan: Helping Children to help themselves. *Pediatric Nursing, 6(3)*:9-13.

Elstad, I. (1981, Nov. 20). A critique of the theory on self-care. *Sykepleien, 68(20)*:16-19.

Facteau, L.M. (1980, March). Self-care concepts and the care of the hospitalized child. *Nursing Clinics of North America, 15(1)*:145-155.

Fitzgerald, S. (1980, July). Utilizing Orem's self-care nursing model in designing an educational program for the diabetic. *Topics of Clinical Nursing, 2(2)*:57-65.

Fleener, K. (1979). Developing a conceptual framework. *Nursing Outlook, 27*:122-126.

Gallant, B.W., & McLane, A.M. (1979). Outcome criteria: A process for validation at the unit level. *Journal of Nursing Administration, 9(1)*:14-21.

Garvan, P., et al. (1980). Self-care applied to the aged. *New Jersey Nurse, 10(1)*:3-5.

Goodwin, J.O. (1980, Nov-Dec.). A cross-cultural approach to integrating nursing theory and practice. *Nurse Educator 5(6)*:15-20.

Harper, D.C. (1984, April). Application of Orem's theoretical construct to self-care medication behaviors in the elderly. *Advances in Nursing Science, 6(3)*:29-46.

Harris, J.K. (1980, March). Self-care is possible after cesarean delivery. *Nursing Clinics of North America, 15*:191-204.

Herrington, J.V., & Houston, S (1984, Jan). Using Orem's theory: A plan for all seasons. *Nursing and Health Care, 5(1)*:45-47.

Hoffart, N. (1982, June). Self-care decision-making by renal transplant recipients. *AANNT Journal, 9(3)*:39-47.

Joseph, L.S. (1980, March). Self-care and the nursing process. *Nursing Clinics of North America, 15(1)*:131-143.

Kearney, B., & Fleischer, B. (1979). Development of an instrument to measure exercise of self-care agency. *Research in Nursing Health, 2*:25-34.

Kinlein, M.L. (1977). The self-care concept. *American Journal of Nursing, 4*:598-601.

Kruger, S., Shawver, M., & Jones, L. (1980). Reactions of families to the child with cystic fibrosis. *Image, 12*:67-72.

McFarland, E.A. (1980, Jan). Nursing theory: The comparison of four theoretical proposals. *Journal of Advanced Nursing, 5(10)*:3-19.

McIntyre, K. (1980). The Perry model as a framework for self-care. *Nurse Practitioner, 5(6)*:34-38.

Marten, L. (1978). Self-care nursing model for patients experiencing radical change in body image. *Journal of Obstetric, Gynecologic and Neonatal Nursing, 7(6)*:9-13.

MeInyk, K.A. (1983, May-June). The process of theory analysis: An examination of the nursing theory of Dorothea E. Orem. *Nursing Research, 32(3)*:170-174.

Michael, M.M., & Sewall, K.S. (1980, March). Use of the adolescent peer group to increase the self-care agency of adolescent alcohol abusers. *Nursing Clinics of North America, 15(1)*:157-176.

Mullin, V.I. (1980, March). Implementing the self-care concept in the acute care setting, *Nursing Clinics of North America, 15(1)*:177-190.

Nordentoft, L.S. (1981, Oct. 21). The concept of self-care defined and applied in a nursing model. *Sygeplejerskon, 81(41)*:4-6.

Perras, S.T., et al. (1982, June). The application of Orem's theory in promoting self-care in a peritoneal dialysis facility. *AANNT Journal, 9(3)*:37-39.

Piemme, J.A., & Trainor, M.A. (1977). A first-year nursing course in a baccalaureate program. *Nursing Outlook, 25(3)*:184-187.

Porter, D., & Shamian, J. (1983, Sept.). Self-care in theory and practice. *Canadian Nurse, 79(8)*:21-23.

Runtz, S.E., & Urtel, J.G. (1983, March). Evaluating your practice via a nursing model. *Nurse Practitioner, 8(3)*:30-32, 37-40.

Smith, M.C. (1979, Oct.). Proposed metaparadigm for nursing research and theory development: An analysis of Orem's self-care theory. *Image, 11(3)*:5-9.

Smith, S.R. (1981, Oct.). Sound off: "Oremization," the curse of nursing. *R.N., 10*:83.

Symposium on self-care concept of nursing (1980, March). *Nursing Clinics of North America, 15(1)*:129-217.

Toth, J.C. (1980). Effects of structured preparation for transfer on patient anxiety on leaving coronary care unit. *Nursing Research, 29*:28-34.

Valsat, S., et al. (1983, Jan. 20). Report from an Orem seminar. *Sykepleien, 70(2)*:18-19.

Walborn, K.A. (1980, March). A nursing model for the hospice: Primary and self-care nursing. *Nursing Clinics of North America, 15(1)*:205-217.

Correspondence

Schumacher, Lawrence (1984, April 3). Interview.

Evelyn Adam

12

Conceptual Model for Nursing

Terri Creekmur, Janet DeFelice, Anne Hodel, Cheryl Y. Petty

CREDENTIALS AND BACKGROUND OF THE THEORIST

Evelyn Adam was born April 9, 1929, in Lanark, Ontario, Canada. She graduated from Hotel Dieu Hospital in Kingston, Ontario, in 1950 with a Diploma in Nursing. She received a B.Sc. degree in 1966 from the University of Montreal and an M.N. degree from the University of California at Los Angeles in 1971. At

U.C.L.A. she met Dorothy Johnson, who she feels has "definitely been the most important influence" on her professional life.[6]

In 1979 she published her first book, *Être Infirmière* and in 1980 wrote the English version of *To Be A Nurse*. Since then, her book has been translated into Dutch (1981) and Spanish (1982). Adam has also written numerous articles on conceptual models for nursing and has coauthored several others. Professional journals publishing her articles include *Infirmière Canadienne, Canadian Nurse, Journal of Advanced Nursing, Nursing Papers: Perspectives in Nursing,* and *Journal of Nursing Education.*

The authors wish to express appreciation to Evelyn Adam for editing the chapter.

131

Adam has been a visiting professor at several universities. She has functioned as a resource person and speaker for various professional corporations, clinical and educational settings, and national and international conventions. Since 1983, she has been a member of the review board for *Nursing Papers* and has directed the research of many graduate students since 1974. She is currently Professor of Nursing at both undergraduate and graduate levels and secretary of the nursing faculty at the University of Montreal.

Whereas nursing care of the elderly is a recent professional interest, promoting conceptual models for nursing has predominated since 1970. She strongly feels that "nursing practice, education, and research must be based on an explicit frame of reference specific to nursing."[6]

Adam's work makes an important distinction between a conceptual model and a theory. "A [conceptual] model is usually based on, or derives from, a theory. . . . A model, emerging from a theory, may become the basis for a new theory."[1:40] "A conceptual model, for whatever discipline, is not reality; it is a mental image of reality or a way of conceptualizing reality. A conceptual model *for* nursing is therefore a conception *of* nursing."[5:42]

Adam[4,6] accepts Roy and Roberts' definition[10:5] of a theory as "a system of interrelated propositions used to describe, predict, explain, understand, and control a part of the empirical world."

Therefore a theory is useful to more than one discipline. A conceptual model for a discipline is useful only to that particular discipline. Adam[7] believes "The day may come when nursing theory will be as useful to related disciplines as existing theories, developed in other fields, are today useful to nursing."

Adam[2:5] writes that "a conceptual model is an abstraction, a way of looking at something, an invention of the mind."

A conceptual model for a discipline is a very broad perspective, a global way of looking at a discipline. Most of the conceptual models for nursing that we know have come from two sources: one, a theory, chosen by the author, and the other, her professional experience.[6]

A conceptual model is the precursor of a theory. The model specifies the discipline's focus of inquiry, identifies those phenomena of particular interest to nursing and provides a broad perspective for nursing research, practice, and education. The study of phenomena that concern nursing, that is, nursing research, may lead to theories that will describe, explain, or predict those phenomena. Such theories will not be theories *of nursing* but theories *of the phenomena* that are nursing's focus of inquiry.[4:12]

Many nurses are unable to communicate clearly and explicitly their conception of the service they offer to society. Adam contends this is not because they do not have a conception of nursing but because their conceptual base is not clear. If the nurse's mental image of nursing is vague or blurred, it will therefore be difficult to put into words. The nurse will then be unable to articulate her particular role in health care and may well find that her professional activities are based on a perspective borrowed from another discipline.

Adam[1:41] states that "a model indicates the goal of our [nursing] profession—an ideal and limited goal, because it gives us direction for nursing practice, nursing education, and nursing research." Nurses who have a clear, concise conceptual base specific to nursing will be able to identify areas for theory development, prepare future practitioners of nursing, and demonstrate in their own practice nursing's contribution to health care. In this way health care will improve and the nursing profession will grow.

Although it is not necessary for every nurse to adopt the same conceptual model, it is essential that every nurse have a concise and explicit framework on which to base her work. The conceptual model is "the conceptual departure point" for her teaching, research or nursing care. Speaking figuratively, Adam places the conceptual model in the nurse's occipital lobe, known also as her visual lobe. The nurse uses a great deal of scientific knowledge as well as her experience, intuition, and creativity. In drawing on this knowledge, she is guided by her conceptual model, that is her mental image of nursing.[7]

The abstraction that is the conceptual model is linked to the reality that is nursing practice through the nursing process.[2] The data we collect depend on our conceptual base. The way we interpret the data, the plan we develop, the nursing action we choose, and the evaluation of our intervention also depend on our model. The number of steps in the nursing process is not significant because the difference is the conceptual base.[6]

In addition to the conceptual model and the nursing process, the nurse must also establish with the client what will be perceived to be a helping relationship. Adam considers this perhaps the most important component of being a nurse. It is the climate of empathy, warmth, mutual respect, caring, and acceptance that determines the effectiveness of nursing care.[2:50;7]

Key

▨ Conceptual model

☰ Nursing process

▢ Helping relationship

Figure 12-1. Pictorial representation of nursing practice.
From: Adam, E. (1980). *To be a nurse*. Philadelphia, W.B. Saunders Company. Reprinted by permission.

Adam feels that three components constitute nursing practice: the client, the nurse (with her conceptual model as a base for the nursing process), and the relationship between the client and nurse. She has created a pictorial representation of nursing practice in her books (Figure 12-1).[2:43;2:55;7]

Adam insists the helping relationship and the systematic process (which nurses have, perhaps wrongly, labeled the "nursing" process) are important to all health professionals. Nursing fits into the whole of health care as an integral component of the interdisciplinary health team. Each discipline makes a unique contribution to the promotion and preservation of health and to the prevention of health problems. Although some services overlap within this interdisciplinary health team, each discipline is present because of its distinct and specific contribution to health.

This relationship can be illustrated with a schematic flower (Figure 12-2). Each petal rep-

resents a distinct health discipline: nursing, medicine, physical therapy, speech therapy, or nutrition, for example. The center of the flower indicates the shared functions. A part of each petal is separate and distinct from the others, and the largest part of each petal represents the unique contribution of each discipline. Our conceptual model clarifies and makes explicit nursing's "petal."

Nurses currently have several conceptual models from which to choose. The decision to adopt one of the conceptual models for (not *of*) nursing is often made by considering the eventual evaluation of that particular model. Adam insists that conceptual models must be evaluated by criteria different from those used to evaluate theories. She quotes the three criteria established by Dorothy Johnson[8]:

1. Social significance: clients would be asked if the service (nursing) was significant to their health.
2. Social congruence: clients would be asked if the service (nursing) was congruent with their expectations.
3. Social utility: nurses would be asked if the conceptual model provided useful direction for education, practice, and research.

Such criteria are extrinsic to the model itself. However, in order to use these criteria the conceptual model in question must already have been adopted in practice, education, and research settings. A vicious cycle may develop because some nurses may hesitate to adopt a model until it has been evaluated and it cannot be evaluated until it has been adopted.* Adam recognizes a model can be evaluated intrinsically for content, logic, and other criteria that will help nurses choose one model rather than another. However, the social decisions (extrinsic criteria) constitute the definitive evaluation of the conceptual base of a service profession.[3]

Adam's conviction that every nurse should

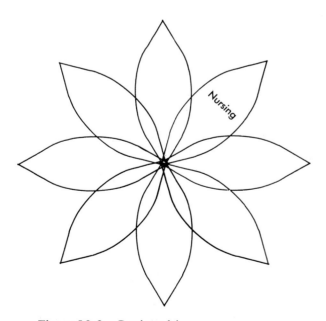

Figure 12-2. Petal model.

Used with permission from Adam, E. (1983). *Être infirmière* (2nd ed.). Montreal: Editions HRW Ltie.

*References 3:11; 4:16-18; 5:44;7.

have a conceptual base specific to nursing rather than one borrowed from another discipline has led her to publish many articles and books, to speak at professional meetings, and to teach courses on this subject. She feels that the existing models are often viewed as being too abstract or too complex and therefore beyond the understanding of many nurses. Adam published *Être Infirmière* and *To Be A Nurse* to help nurses understand the writings of Virginia Henderson. She accomplished this by placing Henderson's concept of nursing within the structure of a conceptual model and by developing and refining the subconcepts identified by Henderson.

This chapter evaluates the conceptual model Adam developed in her book. The model is not a theory, but it does suggest areas for theory development.

SUMMARY OF THE CONCEPTUAL MODEL FOR NURSING

In *To Be A Nurse,* Adam explains the essential elements of a conceptual model as presented by Dorothy Johnson. She then develops Virginia Henderson's concepts within the structure of a conceptual model.*

Assumptions

The assumptions that form the theoretical foundation of Virginia Henderson's vision of nursing are drawn in part from the works of Edward Thorndike, an American psychologist, and in part from Henderson's experience in rehabilitation. There are three assumptions:

1. Every individual strives for and desires independence.
2. Every individual is a complex whole, made up of fundamental needs.

3. When a need is not satisfied, it follows that the individual is not complete, whole, or independent.

Values

The beliefs underlying Virginia Henderson's conception of nursing are also three in number.

1. The nurse has a unique function, although she shares certain functions with other professionals.
2. When the nurse takes over the physician's role, she delegates her primary function to inadequately prepared personnel.
3. Society wants and expects this service (nursing) from the nurse and no other worker is as able, or willing, to give it.

Major Units

The major units of Henderson's model[2:13-15] are:

1. The goal of nursing is to maintain or restore the client's independence in the satisfaction of his fundamental needs.
2. The client or beneficiary of the nurse's service is a whole being made up of 14 fundamental needs:
    a. Breathe normally.
    b. Eat and drink adequately.
    c. Eliminate body wastes.
    d. Move and maintain desirable postures.
    e. Sleep and rest.
    f. Select suitable clothes—dress and undress.
    g. Maintain body temperature within normal range [by adjusting clothing and modifying the environment].
    h. Keep the body clean and well groomed and protect the integument.
    i. Avoid dangers in the environment and avoid injuring others.
    j. Communicate with others in expressing emotions, needs, fears, or opinions.
    k. Worship according to one's faith.

---

*The following summary material is reprinted with permission from Adam, E. (1980). *To Be A Nurse*. Philadelphia: W.B. Saunders. pp. 13-15.

    l. Work in such a way that there is a sense of accomplishment.

    m. Play or participate in various forms of recreation.

    n. Learn, discover, or satisfy the curiosity that leads to normal development and health, and use the available health facilities.

3. The role of the nurse is a complementary-supplementary one.

4. The source of difficulty, or the probable origin of those problems known as nursing problems, is either a lack of knowledge, will, or strength.

5. The intervention: The focus, or centre of attention of the nurse's action is the client's deficit or area of dependence [lack of knowledge, will, or strength].

6. The desired consequences are maintained or increased independence in the satisfaction of the 14 basic needs or, in some cases, a peaceful death.

THEORETICAL SOURCES

Adam[6] says she chose to work with Henderson's concept of nursing for two reasons. First, she felt that Henderson's work was "partly known but badly known," that is, incompletely known or understood, even though many nurses were acquainted with it. She hoped that her own publications would contribute to the recognition of Henderson's work as a useful conceptual base for nursing practice, research, and education. In addition, she felt that Henderson's work was more immediately accessible than other works, because the language was already familiar to nurses. Adam[6] "is not saying that Henderson's frame of reference is any better, or more useful, or more significant or more congruent than others. Such an evaluation has not yet been done . . . but it seems more immediately accessible."

Adam's concern for the need of an explicit conceptual model for nursing was developed when she was a student of Dorothy Johnson. It was also through Johnson that Adam became familiar with the structure of a conceptual model: assumptions, values, and major units. Adam[6;8:7-15] believes Johnson was the first nurse to avail herself of that structure, which was already being used in fields such as sociology, psychology, and mathematics.

USE OF EMPIRICAL EVIDENCE

In choosing Virginia Henderson's writings as the basis of her conceptual model, Adam accepted the scientific principles on which Henderson based her work. The chapter on Virginia Henderson discusses the contribution of Claude Bernard's principle of physiological balance and Abraham Maslow's hierarchy of needs. Because Adam did not change the basic content but merely developed it further, this empirical foundation also is unchanged.

In the previous section of this chapter the source of the structure (assumptions, values, and six major units) was identified as sociology, mathematics, and other sciences. This structure has been extensively used in several sciences so it has good reliability.

MAJOR CONCEPTS AND DEFINITIONS*

    Assessment tool: instrument the professional uses in collecting information about the beneficiary; the nursing history tool; the data collection tool.

    Assumption: the theoretical or scientific basis of a conceptual model; the premises which support the major units of the model.

    Beneficiary: the second major unit of a conceptual model; the person or group of persons, toward whom the professional directs her activities; the client; the patient.

    Change: a substitution of one thing in place of another; an alteration.

    Collection of data: the first step of the nursing process; the collecting of information about the client; the client's nursing history.

    Concept: an idea; a mental image; a generaliza-

---

*Reprinted with permission from Adam, E. (1980). *To Be A Nurse.* Philadelphia: W.B. Saunders. pp. 116-118.

tion formed and developed in the mind.

Conception: a way of conceptualizing a reality; an invention of the mind; a mental image. Depending on its level of abstraction, a conception may be a philosophy, a theory or a conceptual model.

Conceptual Model: an abstraction or a way of conceptualizing a reality: a theoretical frame of reference sufficiently explicit as to provide direction for a particular discipline; a conception made up of assumptions, values, and major units.

Conceptual model for nursing: a mental representation, concept, or conception of nursing which is sufficiently complete and explicit as to provide direction for all fields of activity of the nursing profession.

Consequences: the sixth major unit of a conceptual model; the results of the professional's efforts to attain the ideal and limited goal.

Goal of the profession: the first major unit of a conceptual model; the end which the members of the profession strive to achieve.

Helping relationship: the interaction between the beneficiary (the helpee) and the professional (the helper) which aids the helpee to live more fully: the interpersonal exchange in which the helper illustrates such facilitating qualities as empathy, respect, and others.

Intervention: the fifth major unit of a conceptual model; the focus and modes of the professional's intervention. [In the context of the nursing process, the intervention is the fourth step (implementation of the plan of action or the nursing action itself).]

Intervention focus: part of the fifth major unit of a model; the focus or centre of the professional's attention at the moment he intervenes with a client.

Intervention modes: part of the fifth major unit; the means or ways of intervening at the professional's disposal.

Major units: the six essential components of a complete and explicit conception.

Need: a requirement, a necessity.

Need, fundamental: a requirement common to all human beings, well or ill.

Need, individual: a specific, particular or personal requirement which derives from a fundamental need.

Nursing care plan: a written plan of action; the written communication that comes from the second and third steps of the nursing process; a plan to be followed; a projection of what is to be done.

Nursing process: a methodical, systematic way of proceeding towards an action: a dynamic and logical method; a five step process.

Practice: one of the three fields of activity of a service profession (the other two being education and research); the field of activity of the administrator and the practitioner of the service.

Problem: a difficulty to be reduced or removed.

Problem-solving method: the scientific process of solving problems; the systematic manner of proceeding used to solve problems.

Role: the third major unit of a conceptual model; the part played by the professional; the societal function of the professional.

Source of difficulty: the fourth major unit of a conceptual model; the probable origin of the client difficulty with which the professional is prepared to cope.

Values: the value system underlying a conceptual model.

MAJOR ASSUMPTIONS

In developing Henderson's work into a conceptual model, Adam[2:14] described the goal of nursing as maintaining or restoring the client's independence in the satisfaction of his 14 fundamental needs. The nurse plays a complementary-supplementary role, complementing and supplementing the client's strength, knowledge, and will.

The nurse has a unique province, although she shares certain functions with other health professionals. Society wants and expects the nurse to provide her unique service.

In Adam's model the person is portrayed as a complex whole, made up of 14 fundamental needs. Each need has biological, physiological, and psychosociocultural dimensions. When a need is not satisfied, the person is not complete, whole, or independent. The nurse's client may also be a family or a group.[7:97-100] The concept of environment is specifically addressed in only one of the fundamental needs. However, environment is implicit in all the fundamental needs because the sociocultural dimension is integral to each need.

Health is not defined separately in *To Be A Nurse*. But Adam uses this term in discussing the goal of nursing. She says, "The goal of nursing is to maintain or to restore the client's independence in the satisfaction of his fundamental needs. This goal, congruent with the goal common to the entire health team, makes clear the nurse's specific contribution to the preservation and improvement of health."[2:14] Since an entirely satisfactory definition of health is still a subject of debate, it behooves each health discipline to make explicit its particular contribution to health.[3:95]

THEORETICAL ASSERTIONS

In the description of the conceptual model's major units, the relationships among the basic concepts can be seen in the elements Adam has labeled beliefs and values. She feels these constitute the *why* of the model and must be shared by all who use the model. Values are not subject to the criteria of *truths*, but must reflect the values of the larger society nursing wishes to serve.

1. "The nurse has a unique function, although she shares certain functions with other professionals."[2:13] The nurse must have a conceptual model in order to have a distinct professional identity and to assert herself as a colleague of the other health team members.
2. "When the nurse takes over the physician's role, she delegates her primary function to inadequately prepared personnel."[2:13] The nurse who strives to assume the physician's role will relinquish the nurse's role to some other care provider who may not have the skills and the knowledge base required for nursing.
3. "Society wants and expects this service (nursing) from the nurse and no other worker is as able, or willing to give it."[2:14] Nursing owes its existence to the fact that it fulfills a societal need, as does any service profession.

ACCEPTANCE BY THE NURSING COMMUNITY
Practice

Basing her practice on this conceptual model, the nurse is seen in a complementary-supplementary role and her goal is client independence in the satisfaction of his needs. The model serves as a guide for using the nursing process and the problem-solving method. Guided by the 14 fundamental needs, the practitioner, in whatever setting, will assess the independence of the client in need satisfaction. She will then identify his specific needs, determine the source of difficulty, and plan the intervention to complement client strength, will, or knowledge. After the care is given, it is evaluated in reference to the client objectives—have the specific needs been satisfied and has client independence been increased? A nursing problem—a client's health problem requiring a nurse's intervention—is a dependency problem in need satisfaction.[2:40] A nursing diagnosis is a specific need that is unsatisfied because of insufficient strength, will, or knowledge. Criteria for identifying specific needs have been developed.[2:73] According to Adam, the nurse "carries out the social mission of contributing to the public's improved health by working toward greater client independence."[2:66]

Education

Adam discusses the educational objectives and goals, and the program content in *To Be A Nurse*. She states, "Following Henderson's concept of nursing, the nursing curriculum is planned to prepare a health worker capable of maintaining and restoring the client's independence in the satisfaction of his fundamental needs."[2:57] With this concept, a student learns the complementary-supplementary role. Adam divides the program into official and unofficial content, both of equal importance. Unofficial content "covers everything that is learned in an educational program without being taught."[2:58] Official content "is formally recognized and actually taught."[2:58] Official content is further divided into nursing and nonnursing.

According to Henderson's frame of reference, nursing content includes:

1. the goal of nursing, which is to preserve or re-establish the client's independence in the satisfaction of his basic needs.
2. the detailed description of the 14 fundamental needs, each with its biological, physiological, psychological, social and cultural dimensions.
3. the individual variations in fundamental needs.
4. the various problems of dependence originating from a lack of strength, will, or knowledge.
5. the explanation of the complementary-supplementary role.
6. the description of the various needs of intervention.
7. the study of the desired consequences: continued or increased independence and, in certain circumstances, a peaceful death.
8. the study of the systematic process and the problem-solving method as applied to nursing[2:58-59]

Essential subject matters, regardless of the conceptual model for nursing, are "the helping relationship, . . . the concept of health, . . . and the history."[2:59]

The theoretical courses, in the nonnursing content, include anatomy, physiology, pathology, psychology, sociology, and anthropology. In relation to Henderson's model, the first three relate to the biophysiological dimension and the last three to the psychosociocultural aspect of the fundamental needs.

Subject matter derived from the conceptual model's assumptions is "the concepts of independence and dependence; the concepts of universal and individual human needs, hierarchy of human needs, and need satisfaction; and the concept of wholeness."[2:60]

The practical aspect of nursing content consists of technical procedures and clinical experiences. Techniques are important in the complementary-supplementary role because the nurse is assisting the client in those activities that cannot be completed because of insufficient strength, will, or knowledge. Techniques help pursue the goal of client independence in the satisfaction of his needs. Adam[2:62] feels "The goal of clinical experiences is to provide the student with opportunities to help a client recover his independence in the satisfaction of his basic needs."

Although the level of education may increase, the model remains the conceptual base. The baccalaureate student's formal education will help her identify complex and subtle specific needs, find new ways of complementing and supplementing, and form and continue a helping relationship. Master's level students learn to be specialists in independence nursing or in the teaching and administration of independence nursing. Doctoral students may use the concept of independence in need satisfaction as a basis of research for theory development.

Research

Adam posed 12 questions from the conceptual model for research development. These include:

1. How can client independence be measured?
2. How can his degree of dependence be quantified?
3. What dependency problems are solved by what nursing interventions?
4. At what point must the intervention be discontinued if independence is to be promoted?
5. How can certain interventions be made more easily acceptable?
6. How can the nurse determine how much intervention is enough?
7. What dependency problems are most often encountered among selected groups—e.g., cancer patients, the aged, the mentally confused?
8. How does pain, anxiety, etc. affect independence?
9. How can linguistic barriers be overcome?

10. How can the nurse help certain ethnic or socio-economic groups to be independent?
11. How can the nurse increase client participation in health care?
12. Is the conceptual model socially useful, significant, and congruent?[2:66-67]

Adam[4] states that various clinical and educational settings in Canada are at varying stages of basing nursing care and teaching on her model and research for a small number of master's theses has been based on it. Correspondence received from Canada, the United States, and abroad indicates her books have received very favorable reviews.

LOGICAL FORM

Adam has used the structure of a conceptual model that was useful in various other sciences before being introduced into nursing. The essential elements of a model for a helping or service profession follow.

ASSUMPTIONS. The assumptions are "the suppositions that are taken for granted by those who wish to use the model; they are the 'how' of the model, its foundation."[2:6]

BELIEFS AND VALUES. The beliefs and values "constitute the 'why' of the model and are not subject to the criteria of truth." They must "reflect the value system of the larger society that the profession wishes to serve" and "be shared by the members of the profession who wish to use the model."[2:7]

MAJOR UNITS. The major units "are the 'what' of the conceptual model." They "make clear what nursing is in any setting and at any time."[2:7]

Ideal and limited goal. The ideal and limited goal of the profession is "*ideal* because it represents the ideal that all members of the profession would like to achieve and *limited* because it delineates the parameters of the profession."[2:7]

Beneficiary. The beneficiary of the professional service is "that person or group of persons toward whom the professional directs his attention." "The nurse must have a clear mental image of her client—whether he is well or ill."[2:8]

Role of the professional. The role of the professional is "the role in society played by the members of the discipline."[2:8]

Source of difficulty of the beneficiary. The source of difficulty of the beneficiary "refers to the probable origin of the client's difficulty; one with which the professional, because of his education and experience, is prepared to cope."[3:8] "The probable origin of those client problems which the nurse is prepared to solve must be made explicit."[2:9]

Intervention.

Intervention focus. The focus or center of the intervention is "the focus of the professional's attention at the moment he intervenes with the client. The patient or beneficiary is perceived as an extremely complex individual; however, within that complexity only one aspect can receive all the professional's attention at any given moment. . . . No one person can do everything at the same time."[2:9]

Intervention modes. The modes of intervention "are the means the professional has at his disposal to intervene. . . . A conceptual model for nursing will indicate what means are at the nurse's disposal when she intervenes as a health professional."[2:9]

Consequences. The consequences "are the desired results of the professional activities and must be congruent with the ideal goal."[2:10]

Adam has developed Henderson's concept of nursing into a conceptual model for nursing by placing Henderson's writings in the structure of a model. She has supplied the logical form that was less apparent in Henderson's work. Through the logical form of the resulting conceptual model, clear direction is provided to nursing practitioners, educators, and researchers.

Through the use of the structure that comprises a conceptual model and Henderson's writings, it may be said that Adam used the deductive form of logical reasoning.

FURTHER DEVELOPMENT

Although no empirical evidence has been collected for theories deriving from this model, Adam feels it could be the basis for theory development. As with other conceptual models for nursing, this one specifies nursing's focus of inquiry. From the conceptual departure point of independence in need satisfaction, descriptive and experimental studies could be carried out resulting in the identification of descriptive terms peculiar to the concept under scrutiny. That identification of descriptive terms is the first step in theory development. Possible developments might be a theory of need satisfaction, a theory of independence in need satisfaction, or a theory complementing the knowledge or the motivation of specific client populations. Such theories would not be theories of nursing, but theories of the phenomena that concern nursing.[4]

CRITIQUE
Simplicity

The essential elements listed by Adam give the appearance of a simple conceptual model. However, on closer inspection the number of subconcepts produces a complex picture. The interrelatedness of the components necessary for the care of the whole client also adds to the complexity of the model. The concepts presented are clearly defined and easy to follow.

Generality

The assumptions, values, and major units involve nursing and clients in all aspects of society. They are not limited to age, medical diagnosis, or health care setting. Each of the 14

basic needs has biophysiological and psychosociocultural aspects.

Empirical Precision

Although testing of the model is unavailable at this time, it appears to have the potential for a high degree of empirical precision. This is related to its reality base and designated subconcepts.

Derivable Consequences

Because of the empirically based concepts and broad scope, the model is potentially applicable to nursing practice, education, and research.

Conclusion

Adam's work in developing the conceptual model is unique in that she has taken a previously existing concept of nursing and presented it within the previously existing structure of a model. The result is something more than the sum of the two. It is a complete, concise, explicit conceptual model. Adam then clarified the interrelatedness of the model, the process, and the client-nurse relationship. Making a clear distinction between model and theory, Adam explained the impact of the model on nursing research, practice, and education.

Adam[6] states that "the adoption of a conceptual model will not solve all of nursing's problems." A conceptual model makes explicit nursing's particular contribution to health care and provides nurses a professional identity and a conceptual point of departure.

It would seem that every nurse who adopts a concise and explicit conceptual model is a potential nursing theorist. A nurse who is able to articulate the scope of nursing practice would be more likely to identify areas for nursing theory development and nursing research. Imagine that the majority of nurses have an explicit conceptual model and are able and willing to provide written documentation that would become the basis for empirical evidence. This opens the door to a marked increase in nursing theory and knowledge.

REFERENCES

1. Adam, E. (1975, Sept.). A conceptual model for nursing. *Canadian Nurse, 71*:40-41.
2. Adam, E. (1980). *To be a nurse.* Philadelphia: W.B. Saunders.
3. Adam, E. (1983). *Être infirmière* (2 e éd.). Montréal: Editions HRW Ltée.
4. Adam, E. (1983). Modèles conceptuels. *Nursing Papers: Perspectives en Nursing, 15(2)*:10-21.
5. Adam, E. (1983). Frontiers of nursing in the 21st century: Development of models and theories on the concept of nursing. *Journal of Advanced Nursing, 8*:41-45.
6. Adam, E. (1984, Dec. 4). Personal interview.
7. Adam, E. (1985, April). Toward more clarity in terminology—frameworks, theories and models. *Journal of Nursing Education* 24(4):151-155.
8. Johnson, N. (1974, Sept.-Oct.). Development of theory: A requisite for nursing as a primary health profession. *Nursing Research, 23(5)*:372-377.
9. Riehl, J.P., & Roy, C. (1974). *Conceptual models for nursing practice.* New York: Appleton-Century-Crofts, pp. 7-15.
10. Roy, C., & Roberts, S.L. (1981). *Theory construction in nursing: An adaptation model.* Englewood Cliffs, N.J.: Prentice-Hall.

BIBLIOGRAPHY
Primary Sources
Books

Adam, E. (1979). *Être infirmière.* Montréal: Editions HRW Ltée.
Adam, E. (1980). *To be a nurse.* Philadelphia: W.B. Saunders.
Adam, E. (1981). *To be a nurse.* (Dutch translation). Holland: De Tÿdstroom.
Adam, E. (1982). *To be a nurse.* (Spanish translation). Madrid: Editora Inportecnica.
Adam, E. (1983). Être infirmière (2nd, ed.). Montréal: Editions HRW Lteé.

Book Chapters

Adam, E. (1983). Development of models and theories on the concept of nursing, In *Health care for all: Challenge for nursing* (17th quadrennial Congress, ICN 1981). Geneva: ICN.
Adam, E. (1983). The shape of the nursing world to come: The nursing process. In *Health care for all: Challenge for nursing,* (17th quadrennial Congress, ICN 1981). Geneva: ICN.
Adam, E. (1984). Modèles conceptuels. In M. McGee (Ed.), *Theoretical pluralism in nursing science.* Ottawa: University of Ottawa Press.

Articles

Adam, E. (1975, Sept.). Un modèle conceptuel: à quoi bon? *L'infirmière Canadienne, 19*(9):22-23.
Adam, E. (1975, Sept.). A conceptual model for nursing. *Canadian Nurse, 71*(9):40-41.
Adam, E. (1981, Sept.), Les normes de la pratique infirmière de l'A.I.I.C.: Une interprétation. *L'Infirmière Canadienne, 23*(9):28-29.
Adam, E. (1981, Sept.). CNA's standards for nursing practice: An interpretation. *Canadian Nurse, 77*(8):32-33.
Adam, E. (1983). Frontiers of nursing in the 21st century: Development of models and theories on the concept of nursing. *Journal of Advanced Nursing, 8*:41-45.
Adam, E. (1983). Modèles conceptuels. *Nursing Papers: Perspectives en nursing, 15(2)*:10-21.
Adam, E. (1984). Questions et réponses relatives au schème conceptuel de Virginia Henderson. *L'Infirmière Canadienne, 26*(3):27-31.
Adam, E. (1985, April). Toward more clarity in terminology: Frameworks, theories, and models. *Journal of Nursing Education. 24*(4):151-155.

Reports

Adam, E. (1980). *Programmes s'inspirant d'un modèle nursing.* Dans Retour aux sources. Ottawa: A.I.I.C., pp. 27-33.
Adam, E. (1980). *Implementing the curriculum based on a nursing model.* In Back to basics. Ottawa: A.I.I.C., pp. 22-28.
Adam, E., et al. (1980). *Normes de la pratique infirmière.* Ottawa: A.I.I.C.
Adam, E., et al. (1980). *Standards for nursing practice.* Ottawa: A.I.I.C.
Adam, E. (1981). *L'application d'un modele conceptuel au programme de'études collegial.* Dans Rapport du Colloque des Techniques infirmières Partie I. Gouvernement du Québec, pp. 49-55.
Adam, E. (1981). *Leadership in nursing: The case for a conceptual model.* In Report of Annual Meeting, CAUSN, Western Region, University of Saskatchewan. Saskatoon, Saskatchewan, pp. 1-15.
Adam, E. (1981). *The case for a conceptual model.* In

Proceedings from Nursing Explorations 1980, School of Nursing, McGill University, 9 pp.

Correspondence

Adam, E. (1984, Oct. 2). Personal correspondence.
Adam, E. (1984, Nov. 1). Telephone interview.
Adam, E. (1984, Nov. 4). Telephone interview.
Adam, E. (1984, Nov. 6). Personal correspondence.
Adam, E. (1984, Nov. 12). Telephone interview.
Adam, E. (1984, Nov. 26). Telephone interview.
Adam, E. (1984, Dec. 4). Personal interview (Videotape)

Secondary Sources
Books

Chinn, P., & Jacobs, M. (1983). *Theory and nursing: A systematic approach.* St. Louis: C.V. Mosby.
Henderson, V. (1966). *The nature of nursing.* New York: Macmillan.

Articles

Henderson, V. (1964). The nature of nursing. *American Journal of Nursing, 64*:62-68.
Henderson, V. (1982). The nursing process: Is the title right? *Journal of Advanced Nursing, 7*:103-109.
Winkler, J. (1983). Conceptual models (a response to "Modèles conceptuels," by E. Adam). *Nursing Papers: Perspectives en nursing, 15(4)*:69-70.

Book Reviews

Adam, E. (1980). *Être infirmière.*
Infirmière Canadienne, 21:46, April 1979.
Infirmière Canadienne, 21:10, June 1979. Revue de l'infirmière (Paris), 6:75, June 1979.
Revue de l'infirmière (Paris), 8:8-9, October 1979.
Infirmière enseignante (Paris), 10:11, February 1980.
Le Devoir (daily newspaper, Montreal), March 19, 1979.
Adam, E. (1980). *To be a nurse.*
Canadian Nurse, 77:50, March 1981.
Nursing Times, 77:1041, June 1981.
The Australian Nurses Journal, 11:28, October 1981.
Continuing Education in Nursing, 12:39, November-December 1981.

Other

Riehl, J.P., & Roy, C. (1974). *Conceptual models for nursing practice.* New York: Appleton-Century-Crofts.
Riehl, J.P., & Roy, C. (1980). *Conceptual models for nursing practice* (2nd ed.) New York: Appleton-Century-Crofts.
Roy, C., & Roberts, S.L. (1981). *Theory construction in nursing: An adaptation model.* Englewood Cliffs, N.J.: Prentice-Hall.

Madeleine Leininger

13

Transcultural Care Theory

Sr. Judith Alexander, Carolyn J. Beagle, Pam Butler,
Deborah A. Dougherty, Karen D. Andrews Robards

CREDENTIALS AND BACKGROUND OF THE THEORIST

Madeleine M. Leininger, the first professional nurse anthropologist, is the founder of transcultural nursing and a pioneer of transcultural nursing care theory. Born in Sutton, Nebraska, she began her nursing career by graduating from a diploma program at St. Anthony's School of Nursing in Denver. In 1950 she ob-

The authors wish to express appreciation to Jeanette Adam and Kathy McGregor for assistance with data collection, and to Dr. Madeleine Leininger for critiquing the chapter.

tained a B.S. degree in biological science from Benedictine College, Atchison, Kansas. After graduation she served as an instructor, a staff and head nurse on a medical-surgical unit, and as the nursing director of the psychiatric unit at St. Joseph's Hospital in Omaha. During this time she worked on graduate studies in administration, teaching and curriculum, and test and measurement at Creighton University in Omaha.[9]

In 1954 Leininger obtained an M.S.N. in psychiatric nursing from Catholic University of America in Washington, D.C. She then moved to the University of Cincinnati, where she began the first clinical specialist graduate program in child psychiatric nursing in the country. In 1955 she began 3 years of graduate work at the University of Cincinnati in curriculum and social sciences. Meanwhile, she initiated and directed the first graduate program in psychiatric nursing at the university's College of Nursing.

While working with children in the middle 1950s Leininger identified a lack of understanding by the staff of cultural factors influencing the behavior of children. She observed and experienced both cultural differences and a few common expressions among the children. The obvious differences among the children's cultural lifeways deeply concerned her. When psychoanalytic theories were not effective in explaining these diversities and planning nursing interventions, she became increasingly concerned and frustrated that the children's behaviors and her interventions seemed inappropriate. Leininger posed many questions to herself and her staff. But when she found no means to understand the children she began looking toward other fields.

During the 1950s Margaret Mead began a visiting professorship at the Department of Psychiatry at the University of Cincinnati, and Leininger discussed with Mead the potential interrelationships between nursing and anthropology. In 1959 Leininger began doctoral work and in 1965 obtained a Ph.D. in anthropology from the University of Washington in Seattle with a focus on cultural and psychological anthropology and general ethnology. As a doctoral student Leininger studied the Gadsup people of the eastern highlands of New Guinea. Beginning in 1960 she lived alone with the Gadsup for 1½ years and conducted an ethnographic, ethnocare, and ethnohealth study.[4:21-44] She was able to observe not only unique features of the culture, but also a number of marked differences between western and nonwestern cultures. From her in-depth study and firsthand experiences with the Gadsup, she began to develop her theory of culture care. As a result of this research Leininger[4:23] was able to influence nursing students to "understand the

why of the cultural and biological differences" and to interest nurses in the study of anthropology.

During the 1950s and 1960s, Leininger identified several common areas of linkage and interest between nursing and anthropology. From this knowledge came *Nursing and Anthropology: Two Worlds to Blend,* the first book in transcultural nursing. The ideas presented in the book laid the foundation for developing the field of transcultural nursing and health care. Her second book, *Transcultural Nursing: Concepts, Theories and Practices,* provided definitive ways of how the disciplines of anthropology and nursing are complementary, yet different. Leininger[4:21-44] has spent the past 30 years developing transcultural care theory and practices.

The first course in transcultural nursing was offered in 1966 at the University of Colorado, where Leininger was a Professor of Nursing and Anthropology. This marked the first joint appointment of a professor of nursing and another discipline in the United States. In 1969 Leininger was appointed Dean and Professor of Nursing and Lecturer in Anthropology at the University of Washington in Seattle. There she established one of the first academic departments in the nursing school called "Comparative Nursing Care Systems" to support the master and doctoral programs in transcultural nursing. Five years later she was appointed Dean and Professor of Nursing at the College of Nursing and Adjunct Professor of Anthropology at the University of Utah in Salt Lake City and again initiated master and doctoral programs in transcultural nursing.[9] These were graduate programs with substantive courses focused specifically on transcultural nursing.

In 1981 Leininger was recruited to Wayne State University where she serves as Professor of Nursing and Adjunct Professor of Anthropology, and as Director of the Center for Health Research in the city of Detroit, Michigan. At Wayne State she once again initiated master and doctoral courses in transcultural nursing. In addition to serving as Director of the transcultural nursing offerings at Wayne State, Leininger also teaches transcultural nursing courses for baccalaureate, master's, and doctoral students and conducts several research studies in this area.

With the growing interest in transcultural nursing and health care, Leininger[9] annually gives several keynote addresses, and conducts workshops and conferences nationally and internationally and has done so since 1965. Her academic vitae records nearly 500 such conferences, keynote addresses, and workshops in the United States, Canada, Europe, Pacific Islands, and Asia. Many education and practice settings request her consultation with cultures.

As the first professional nurse to complete a doctoral degree in anthropology and to initiate several master and doctoral nursing education programs, Leininger has many areas of expertise and interests. She has studied at least six major cultures in depth and has done several ethnographic and enthnonursing studies. Besides transcultural nursing care, other related areas of interest are comparative education and administration, nursing theory, politics of nursing and health care, cross-cultural caring, nursing research, futurology of nursing and health care, and nursing leadership. She has initiated and chaired nine National Transcultural Nursing Conferences and seven National Research Caring Conferences.[5] Leininger has gained international recognition in nursing and other related fields by her work. She has energetically worked to persuade nurse educators to incorporate transcultural nursing concepts and research into nursing curricula and nursing practices. While very active in nursing, she has been involved in anthropology in teaching and research since the early 1960s. She is one of the few nurses to keep active in two disciplines and to contribute to both fields.

Leininger has published numerous films, research projects, books, book chapters, and articles on culture, care, and health phenomena and other topics relevant to nursing and anthropology. She has authored or edited 18 books and more than 250 published articles, and is viewed by some nurses as one of the most creative and productive authors in nursing, providing fresh and substantive ideas.

Examples of her books include *Nursing and Anthropology: Two Worlds to Blend* (1970), *Transcultural Nursing: Concepts, Theories and Practices* (1978), *Caring: An Essential Human Need* (1981), *Care: The Essence of Nursing and Health* (1984), *Qualitative Research Methods in Nursing* (1985), and *Transcultural Care Diversity and Universality: A Theory of Nursing* (1985).

Leininger has received many awards and recognition of her accomplishments. She is listed in *Who's Who of American Women, Who's Who in Health Care, Who's Who in Community Leaders, The World's Who's Who of Women in Education,* and *The International Who's Who in Community Service.* Her name appears on *The National Register of Prominent Americans and International Notables, International Women,* and *The National Register of Prominent Community Leaders.* She received an Honorary Doctorate of Human Letters from Benedictine College, Atchison, Kansas, in 1975, and in 1976 was presented an Award of Recognition for unique and significant contributions to the American Association of Colleges of Nursing. Leininger is a Fellow in the American Academy of Nursing and a Fellow of the American Anthropological Society. Other affiliations include Sigma Theta Tau, the National Honor Society of Nursing; Delta Kappa Gamma, the National Honorary Society in Education; and the Society for Applied Anthropology. She has served as distinguished visiting scholar or lecturer in 24 universities in this country and abroad.

THEORETICAL SOURCES FOR THEORY DEVELOPMENT

Leininger has developed a derived theory from the discipline of anthropology and has conceptualized the theory in a new and unique way to be relevant to nursing (Figure 13-1). She has defined transcultural nursing as:

a major area of nursing which focuses upon a comparative study and analysis of different cultures and subcultures in the world with respect to their caring behavior; nursing care; and health-illness values, beliefs, and patterns of behavior with the goal of developing a scientific and humanistic body of knowledge in order to provide culture-specific and culture-universal nursing care practices.[4:8]

The goal of transcultural nursing extends beyond an open appreciation of differing cultures, "to make professional nursing knowledge and practices culturally based, culturally conceptualized, culturally planned, and culturally operationalized."[4:12] Leininger[4:13] has stated that in time there will be "a new taxonomy of nursing

practice which will reflect different kinds of nursing care which are culturally defined, classified, and tested as a guide to provide nursing care." In addition, she states that "transcultural nursing is becoming one of the most important, relevant, and highly promising subfields of study, research, and practice for the future of nursing."[4:14] She predicts that for nursing to be relevant to the world, transcultural nursing knowledge will be as imperative as broad and specific knowledge and skills are for all nursing education and practice.

Leininger[4:32] defines theory as "a set of logically interrelated concepts, hypotheses or propositions which can be tested for the purpose of explaining or predicting an event, phenome-

Figure 13-1. Leininger's conceptual theory and generating model to study transcultural and ethnocaring constructs. Model was developed in 1968 and reflects revisions and additions since that time. (The ethnocaring definitions are not presented here.) Data come from 30 cultures using a modified ethnoscience and ethnonursing research approach.

Used with permission from Leininger, M.M. (1981). *Caring: An essential human need.* Thorofare, N.J.: Charles B. Slack.

non, or situation." Transcultural nursing theory is defined as:

> a set of interrelated cross-cultural nursing concepts and hypotheses which take into account individual and group caring behaviors, values, and beliefs based upon their cultural needs, in order to provide effective and satisfying nursing care to people; and if such nursing practices fail to recognize culturological aspects of human needs, there will be signs of less efficacious nursing care practices and some unfavorable consequences to those served.[4:33]

Leininger[4:34] developed the theory "based upon the belief that cultures can determine most of the care they desire or need from professional care-givers." Her theory is directed toward consumers of care to get *their* viewpoints, world views, knowledge, and practices as bases for sound professional actions and decisions. It may be considered a comprehensive and holistic nursing theory because it takes into account social structure, world view, values, environment, language expressions, and folk-professional systems to discover nursing knowledge.

USE OF EMPIRICAL EVIDENCE

Leininger[2:13] believes "The most unifying, dominant and central intellectual and practice focus of nursing is care." She goes on to say "The construct of care is complex and varied in that it includes concepts related to caring behaviors, caring processes, caring needs, caring consequences, caring conflicts, and caring gaps, both in universal and nonuniversal practice."[2:13] Leininger favors ethnomethods as the sound and logical approach to study care because they are directed toward people's views and lifeways. Ethnoscience is one of the ethnomethods used in anthropology to discover nursing knowledge. She defines *ethnonursing* as "the systematic study and classification of nursing care beliefs, values, and practices as cognitively perceived by a designated culture through their local language, experiences, beliefs, and value

system."[4:15] Although nursing has used the words care and caring to describe itself and its practice for more than a century, definitions and clear understanding of these terms have been lacking. "Indeed, the concepts about caring are some of the least understood and least studied of all human knowledge and research areas."[4:33] By means of transcultural nursing theory, a systematic study of such interrelated concepts can be done in order to know, explain, and predict cultural behavior and nursing care behaviors of diverse groups from a cross-cultural view. An important goal is to be able to document, know, "predict, and explain whether this general transcultural nursing theory is valid, and if so, under what conditions and external and internal forces."[4:34]

Leininger holds that "caring behavior and practices uniquely distinguish nursing from the contributions of other disciplines."[5:4] The reasons she gives for studying care may be distilled into four. "First, the construct of care appears critical to human growth, development, and survival for human beings for millions of years."[5:7] The second reason is to explicate and understand the roles of the caregiver and care recipient in different cultures. Third, "to preserve and maintain care as this human attribute is essential for the survival of humans and cultures through time."[5:8] Fourth, the nursing profession has never systematically studied care in relation to nursing care, and Leininger contends care is an elusive phenomenon with embedded knowledge that can provide a sound basis for nurses to use care in specific and unique ways to maintain health, prevent illnesses, and for healing or to alleviate human discomforts. Care is viewed by Leininger as one of the most powerful concepts and unique phenomenon to nursing, but care concepts of each culture must be documented, understood, and used in a therapeutic way so that *care is the therapy*.

To date Leininger has studied six cultures in depth and approximately 30 cultures from a miniethnomethodological approach. From those 58 care constructs have been identified with linguistic terms, meanings, and uses by the people of diverse cultures. A taxonomy of care constructs, several theoretical statements, and hypotheses are being generated.[5:12]

Leininger believes the goal of health care personnel should be to work toward an understanding of care and health of different cultures so that each culture's care, values, beliefs, and lifeways will provide a basis for planning and effectively implementing culture-specific care. She maintains that nursing cannot separate social structure factors from health, wellness, illness, or care when working with cultures, because they tend to be closely interrelated and interdependent. Social structure factors such as religion, politics, culture, economics, and kinship are significant forces affecting health, care, and cure.

Leininger[4:56] contends that cultural blindness, shock, imposition, and ethnocentrism can be significantly reduced and transcultural health care more effectively rendered if an individual's or group's culture is understood. She feels care is the human services quality that makes health consumers either satisfied or unsatisfied with health services and it is the *care, not* the *cure,* that health consumers consciously or unconsciously value.[7:8]

MAJOR CONCEPTS AND DEFINITIONS

In discussing Leininger's theory several terms are relevant, but only a few major ones are defined here. The reader can study her full theory from her book *Transcultural Care Diversity and Universality: A Theory in Nursing.*

CARE. Care in a generic sense refers to those assistive, supportive, or facilitative acts toward or for another individual or group with evident or anticipated needs to ameliorate or improve a human condition or lifeway.[7:4]

CARING. Caring refers to the direct (or indirect) nurturant and skillful activities, processes, and decisions related to assisting people in such a manner that reflects behavioral attributes which are empathetic, supportive, compassionate, protective, succorant, educational, and others dependent upon the needs, problems, values, and goals of the individual or group being assisted."[7:4]

CULTURE. "Culture is the learned and transmitted cultural values, beliefs, rules of behavior, and lifestyle practices of particular people."[8] Leininger considers culture the blueprint for thought and action as a dominant force in determining health-illness caring patterns and behaviors. Cultural values and behaviors vary enormously between and among all humans and groups of humans.

Cultural values. "Cultural values are the powerful directive forces which give order and meaning to people's thinking, decisions, and actions."[8]

Cultural variations. "Cultural variations are the slight or marked variability among or between cultures or subcultures that make them different or unique with respect to traditional or non-traditional lifestyles."[8]

NURSING. Leininger[7:4-5] defines nursing as:

> a learned humanistic art and science that focuses upon personalized (individual and group) care behaviors, functions, and processes directed toward promoting and maintaining health behaviors or recovery from illness which have physical, psychocultural, and social significance or meaning for those being assisted generally by a professional nurse or one with similar role competencies.

MAJOR ASSUMPTIONS

A few major assumptions to support Leininger's transcultural care theory[7:5-6] can be stated:

1. Human caring is a universal phenomenon, but the expressions, processes, and patterns of caring vary among cultures.
2. Caring acts and processes are essential for human birth, development, growth, and survival, and for a peaceful death.

3. Caring is the essence and unifying intellectual and practical dimension of professional nursing.
4. Care has biophysical, cultural, psychologic, social, and environmental dimensions that must be explicated and verified to provide truly holistic care to people.
5. Nursing acts are transcultural and require nurses to identify and use intercultural nurse-client and system data.
6. Care behaviors, goals, and functions vary with social structure and specific values of people from different cultures.
7. Self and other care practices vary in different cultures and in different care systems.
8. The identification of universal and non-universal folk and professional caring behaviors, beliefs, and practices is essential to advancing the body of nursing and generic care knowledge.
9. Care is largely culturally derived and requires culturally based knowledge and skills for efficaciousness.
10. There can be no curing without caring, but there may be caring without curing.

In *Transcultural Nursing: Concepts, Theories, and Practices,* published in 1978, Leininger[4:35-36] lists 10 basic assumptions. These are very similar to the 10 assumptions in her 1984 publication *Care: The Essence of Nursing and Health.*[7:5-6] The terms *culture* and *transcultural* are more prevalent in her earlier works because she was in the process of discovering ethnocare data. But nine of the ten assumptions in *Care: The Essence of Nursing and Health* include the term *care*—revealing greater discovery and emphasis on care.

THEORETICAL ASSERTIONS

Leininger has developed several formulations from her transcultural nursing theory as examples to stimulate further research by nurses. These formulations are based on her ongoing inquiry, research studies, and other anthropological and nursing investigations from mainly ethnomethod studies. From her field studies, she has identified and made some relationship statements. Others are available in her theory book, *Transcultural Care Diversity and Universality: A Theory of Nursing.*

In *Transcultural Nursing: Concepts, Theories, and Practices* several hypotheses and propositions are stated recognizing that her theory continues to be developed and refined. For example:

1. Identifiable differences in caring values and behaviors between and among cultures leads to differences in the nursing care expectations of care-seekers.
2. Differences in caring values and norms of behavior exist between technologically dependent and nontechnologically dependent societies.
3. Professional people working in strange cultures with different values about nursing care or caring behaviors can create obvious cultural conflicts and problems unless they are willing to recognize and adapt to indigenous caring values and expectations.
4. The greater the dependence of nursing personnel upon technological caring tools and activities, the greater the interpersonal distance and the fewer the client's satisfactions.
5. Nursing care interventions which provide culture-specific caring practices will show greater signs of satisfactions from clients than will noncultural oriented caring services.[4:37]

In *Care: The Essence of Nursing and Health*[7:6-7] Leininger lists nine theoretical statements and hypotheses.

1. Intercultural differences in care beliefs, values, and practices reflect identifiable differences in nursing care practices.
2. Cultures that highly value individualism with independence modes will show signs of self-care practices and values; whereas cultures that do not value individualism with independence modes will show limited signs of self-care practices and more signs of other-care practices.

3. There is a close relationship between caregiver and care receiver behaviors.

4. People from different cultures can identify caring and noncaring behaviors and attitudes.

5. The greater the differences between folk care values and professional care values, the greater the signs of cultural conflict and stresses between professional caregivers and nonprofessional care receivers.

6. Technologic caring acts, techniques, and practices differ cross-culturally and have different outcomes for health and nursing care practices.

7. The greater the signs of dependency upon technology to give care, the greater the signs of depersonalized human care to clients.

8. Symbolic and ritual forms of nursing care behaviors have different meanings in different cultures, which necessitates knowledge of the meaning and functions of care symbols and rituals.

9. There is a close relationship between political, religious, economic, and cultural values and the quality of health care services rendered.

A sample of other relationship statements from Leininger's *Transcultural Nursing: Concepts, Theories, and Practices*[4:45-46] includes:

1. Cultures that perceive illness to be largely a personal and internal body experience (i.e., caused by physical, genetic, and intrabody stresses) tend to use more technical and physical self-care control methods (pills and physical techniques) than cultures that view illness as an extrapersonal experience.

2. Cultures which strongly emphasize caring behaviors and processes tend to have more females in caring roles and less males.

3. Cultures that emphasize curing behaviors and treatment processes tend to have more male curers and less female carers.

4. Clients needing caring services tend to seek first the local (nonprofessional) caring persons, such as family members or friends, and later may seek professional caregivers if their condition is aggravated or if death is feared.

5. Ritualized ethnocaring activities which have therapeutic benefits to clients and their families tend to be viewed as less therapeutic by Western professional nurses.

6. Where there is a marked evidence of nurturant caring behaviors in a culture, there will be less curing and more health maintenance activities.

LOGICAL FORM

Most of Leininger's approach to the study of transcultural care has been derived from anthropological research methods and from her development of the ethnonursing method. From the beginning, she has emphasized studying people from their *emic* or local knowledge and experiences and using qualitative research methodologies. A recent book provides substantive knowledge about qualitative methods in nursing.[10]

In her own research, Leininger has been skilled in using ethnonursing, ethnographic participant-observation methods that provide a holistic approach to study human behavior in context. With this method, the researcher moves with the people in their daily living activities. The nurse researcher inductively obtains data of documented descriptive accounts of actually observed and verified behavior that reveals "the essence, nature, process, and attributes of caring behavior and therapeutic nursing care" within a culture.[4:47] This approach is important for all nursing studies, but especially for identifying substantive nursing knowledge.[4:46-47]

Leininger[10] also uses the ethnoscience method as a formal and rigorous method to study nursing and human phenomenon. "Ethnoscience refers to the systematic study of the way of life of a designated cultural group in order to obtain an accurate account of the people's behavior and how they perceive and know their universe.[4:76] This method involves classifying data as it reflects the people's views. Through checking and rechecking data, a high degree of validity and reliability can be obtained about the characteristics of a culture, and theoretical formulations are made from the data. The ethnoscience method provides data that will help nurses know meanings and explain, and predict human behavior within a culture.[4:76] In order to refine the empirical data obtained through ethnoscientific research, the researcher must analyze data from *emic* and *etic* approaches. "An *emic* analysis reveals the native's or a local culture's way of classifying and knowing their world."[4:78] An *etic* analysis searches for features that may be found in more than one culture. Universal features may be discovered through *emic* analysis of data.[4:78]

There are other methods of research, such as hypothesis-testing and descriptive-survey methods, that can be applied to transcultural care theory development. The method of choice depends on the phenomena to be studied and the creativity and willingness of the nurse researcher to try different research methods to discover nursing knowledge.[4:49]

Figure 13-1 depicts the phases involved in obtaining ethnographic data and to generate nursing theory. Phase I identifies the major sources used to derive ethnocaring and ethnonursing data. First, general lifeways are observed and studied. Next, the social structure features, such as the educational, cultural, political, economic, kinship, religious, and health systems that influence behavior in a culture are examined. The third step involves explication of cultural values and beliefs, including those related to health and illness. Finally, the health-illness caring system is assessed by the nurse researcher observing, listening, and participating in the system. It is important to look at both folk and professional health care systems.[4:42-43]

Phase II involves classifying specific and general caring constructs. The term *caring constructs* is used for the listed behaviors because each has subcategories that must be examined in relation to a specific culture. Not every identified construct is found in every culture. The order in which the constructs are ranked differs from one culture to another. For example, in a study Leininger[7:146] conducted on southern/rural black and white American lifeways, the black villagers ranked *concern for "brothers and sisters"* as the most important care construct, while the

white villagers ranked *concern for social or community folks* as the highest care construct. Validation of care was essential in the identification of different care constructs.[4:43-44]

Phase III involves the analysis and testing of the care constructs previously identified. First, research hypotheses are developed and tested. Next, the results of the ethnocaring research data are analyzed and nursing interventions are determined based on the research data.[4:44]

Leininger continues to refine and develop her theory of transcultural diversity and universality of care and health, having recently developed the Sunrise Conceptual Model for Culturologic Interviews, Assessments and Therapy Goals. This model and the full theory of transcultural diversity and universality of care and health are not addressed here and only selected ideas are offered to introduce the reader to Leininger's pioneering and creative work of evolving theory through time. The Sunrise Conceptual Model is introduced in *Care: The Essence of Nursing and Health* and explained more fully in *Transcultural Care Diversity and University: Theory of Nursing.*

ACCEPTANCE BY THE NURSING COMMUNITY
Practice

Leininger gives several reasons for the slowness of nurses to recognize and value culture factors in nursing practices and education, and hence, the acceptance of transcultural nursing and her theory. First, there were virtually no nurses prepared in anthropology to understand transcultural concepts, models, and theories. Most nurses had no idea about the nature of anthropology and how anthropological knowledge could contribute to health care behaviors. Second, although patients had long-standing and inherent cultural needs, many were reluctant to push health personnel to meet their cultural needs, and therefore did not demand that their cultural and social needs be recognized or met.[4:42-43] Third, transcultural nursing articles submitted for publication were rejected because editors did not know, value, or understand the relevance of anthropology to nursing.

Nurses are now gradually realizing the importance of transcultural nursing, and the need to understand cultures. Leininger[4:123] believes, "We are entering a new phase of health emphasis as we examine the impact of cultural factors upon health and illness behavior." There is an increased display of cultural identity, which is accompanied by increased demands for culture specific care and general health services. The world is strongly multicultural and health personnel are expected to respond to clients' diverse cultural needs.

Education

The inclusion of culture in nursing curricula began in 1966 at the University of Colorado, where Leininger was a professor of nursing and anthropology. Awareness of the relationship between culture and nursing began to appear in the middle 1970s, but there were few nurse educators adequately prepared to teach courses on culture and nursing and too few qualified faculty. The world's first doctoral program in transcultural nursing was approved and implemented in 1977 at the University of Utah. Today, with heightened public awareness of health care costs, different cultures, and human rights, there is a greater demand for comprehensive, holistic, and multicultural client care. Leininger[4:18-21] suggests these demands allude to culture-specific care and that there is an urgent need for nurses to be educated in this aspect of nursing care.

There are a few nursing curricula that emphasize transcultural nursing and care. One such program was recently developed at Cuesta College in California. An Associate Degree program, it was developed with care as the central theme and cultural care diversity. Course titles include Caring Concepts I and II, Caring of Families, and Professional Self-Care.[7] Currently there are five master's and four doctoral programs in the United States offering transcul-

tural nursing courses and field experiences. This is an encouraging trend, but more programs and courses are needed to make transcultural nursing both a specialty and general area of study. More research related to care concepts is being generated by faculty and graduate students. Despite the encouraging outcomes, using care as the central theme for nursing curriculum needs further research with respect to validation of its usefulness and effectiveness.[12:245-248]

Research

"Several nurses are testing transcultural theories and conducting basic and advanced research studies in transcultural nursing in the United States and other countries."[4:24] There is a heightened interest on the part of consumers who are providing funding to continue research in transcultural nursing care. "Nurse anthropologists and other interested nurses have also been active contributors to international, national, regional, and local workshops and to the development of conferences and instructional programs on the topic of transcultural nursing."[4:24] Through ethnographic studies transcultural nurses have "stimulated and maintained a stream of humanistic conscious-raising to people who know little about unfamiliar cultures in the world."[4:46]

FURTHER DEVELOPMENT

"It is reasonable to predict that all professional nurses in this country and abroad will come to recognize the need to know and use cultural concepts in their practice, teaching, research, and consultation."[4:26] Currently, the demand for prepared transcultural nurses exceeds the number of specialists in the field. Transcultural nurse theorists, researchers, and scholars are needed to develop and synthesize the new nursing knowledge, and to change the norms of nursing practice. "By the year 2000, it is hoped that most nurses will have a basic knowledge of a number of cultural groups in the world and an in-depth knowledge of two or three cultures."[4:28] Leininger believes transcultural nursing research will lead to new theories and conceptualizations for nursing practice and education. "Health disciplines will gradually become involved in transcultural studies and practices in the near future as health science courses and programs of study become established."[4:28] Because of the increased need for international understanding and nursing care, there will be an increasing demand for transcultural nurses, prepared as educators, researchers, and consultants. "It is reasonable to predict that transcultural nurse specialists . . . will be tomorrow's leaders in national and international teaching, research, and service programs."[4:28]

The present and future research in the field of transcultural nursing will enhance theoretical development and will continue to identify culture-specific and universal care constructs. Eventually universal care constructs may be identified to establish a true scientific and humanistic body of nursing knowledge with a care focus.

CRITIQUE
Simplicity

Because the concepts of transcultural nursing theory are complex and multiple, the theory is not simple. Many questions are proposed in pursuit of a scientific body of nursing knowledge based on systematic investigation. The theoretical development and the research goals are to seek both universal and specific culturally defined care phenomena from diverse cultures and from the culture of nursing. The theory is truly transcultural or global in scope and highly complex. Leininger's theory is an evolving one with different, but related models to guide the researcher in conceptualizing the theory and research approaches. Because of its holistic and comprehensive nature, several concepts and constructs related to social structure, environment, and language influencing care and health are included in the theory and conceptual model. The theory shows multiple interrelationships of concepts and diversity of key concepts of the theory. It is a theory that requires anthropological and transcultural nursing knowledge be used fully and accurately by nursing researchers.

Generality

The transcultural nursing theory does purport to demonstrate the criterion of generality, as it is a qualitative-oriented theory and is broad, comprehensive, and worldwide in scope. In fact, transcultural nursing theory addresses nursing care from a multicultural and world view perspective. It is useful and applicable to both groups and individuals with the goal of rendering culture-specific nursing care. The broad or generic concepts are organized and operationalized for study in specific cultures. The research has lead to a taxonomy of care, with many subsets. However, many more aspects of culture, care, and health, as these factors impact upon nursing, are yet to be discovered. From this culture-specific data, a few universal care constructs are being identified. More research is needed, and a greater number of the world's cultural groups need to be studied to validate the caring constructs. The theoretical model is a guide for the study of any culture and for comparative study of several cultures. Empirical findings from ethnographic, ethnonursing, and ethnoscience methods are evident.

Empirical Precision

The transcultural nursing theory is researchable, and much qualitative research has been evident. This qualitative approach differs from the traditional quantitative research method and renders the precision of the research more difficult to achieve. However, the ethnoscience research method is extremely rigorous and linguistically exacting in nature and outcomes. Fifty-eight care constructs have been identified thus far, and more are being discovered. The important attribute is that empirical precision is evident with the use of ethnomethods or from an *emic* or people's viewpoint leading to high validity and reliability of data. It is hoped that ongoing and future research will lead to additional care and health findings and the implications for ethnonursing practices and education to fit specific cultures as well as universal features.

Derivable Consequences

Transcultural nursing theory has outcomes that are very important for nursing. Rendering culture-specific care is a necessary and essential new goal in nursing. It places the transcultural nursing theory well within the domain of the nursing knowledge acquisition and use. The theory is useful and applicable to nursing practice, education, and research. The concept of care as the primary focus of nursing, and the base of nursing knowledge and practice, is long overdue and essential to advance nursing knowledge and practices. Leininger notes that although nursing has always made claims to concept of care, rigorous research has been limited on care. Because of its broad and multicultural focus this theory could be the means for establishing nursing as a discipline and a profession.

REFERENCES

1. Leininger, M. (1969). Conference on the nature of science and nurisng. *Nursing Research, 18(5)*.
2. Leininger, M. (1970). *Nursing and anthropology: Two Worlds to blend*. New York: John Wiley & Sons.
3. Leininger, M. (1977). Cultural diversities of health and nursing care. *Nursing Clinics of North America, 12(1)*:5-18.
4. Leininger, M. (1978). *Transcultural nursing: Concepts, theories, and practices*. New York: John Wiley & Sons.
5. Leininger, M. (1981). *Caring: An essential human need* (Proceedings of the three national caring conferences). Thorofare, N.J.: Charles B. Slack, Inc.
6. Leininger, M. (1983). Academic and professional vitae. (Current through December 1983.)
7. Leininger, M. (1984). *Care: The essence of nursing and health*. Thorofare, N.J.: Charles B. Slack, Inc.
8. Leininger, M. (1984, Oct. 19). *Transcultural care: Nursing for tomorrow*. Workshop presentation by Indiana University Alumni Association, Indiana University School of Nursing, Indianapolis.
9. Leininger, M. (1984, Oct. 19). Personal interview.
10. Leininger, M. (1985). *Qualitative research methods in nursing*. New York: Brune & Stratton.
11. Leininger, M. (1985). *Transcultural care diversity and universality: A theory of nursing*. Thorofare, N.J.: Charles B. Slack, Inc.
12. MacDonald, M.R. (1984). The central construct for an associate degree nursing curriculum. In M. Leininger (Ed.), *Care: The essence of nursing and health*. Thorofare, N.J.: Charles B. Slack, Inc.

BIBLIOGRAPHY
Primary Sources
Books

Hofling, C.F., & Leininger, M. (1960). *Basic psychiatric concepts in nursing*. Philadelphia: J.P. Lippincott.

Leininger, M. (1970). *Nursing and anthropology: Two worlds to blend*. New York: John Wiley & Sons.

Leininger, M. (1973). *Contemporary issues in mental health nursing*. Boston: Little, Brown.

Leininger, M. (Ed.). (1974). *Health care dimensions (Vol. 1): Health care issues*. Philadelphia: F.A. Davis.

Leininger, M. (Ed.). (1975). *Health care dimensions (Vol. 2): Barriers and facilitators to quality health care*. Philadelphia: F.A. Davis.

Leininger, M. (Ed.). (1976). *Health care dimensions (Vol. 3): Transcultural health care issues and conditions*. Philadelphia: F.A. Davis.

Leininger, M. (Ed.). (1976). *Transcultural nursing care of infants and children*. Salt Lake City: University of Utah College of Nursing.

Leininger, M. (1978). *Transcultural nursing care of the elderly*. Salt Lake City: University of Utah College of Nursing.

Leininger, M. (1978). *Transcultural nursing: Concepts, theories and practices*. New York: John Wiley & Sons.

Leininger, M. (Ed.). (1979). *Transcultural nursing care of the adolescent and middle age adult*. Salt Lake City: University of Utah College of Nursing.

Leininger, M. (Ed.). (1979). *Transcultural nursing: Proceedings from four transcultural nursing conferences*. New York: Masson.

Leininger, M. (Ed.). (1980). *Cultural change, ethics*

and the nursing care implications. Salt Lake City: University of Utah College of Nursing.

Leininger, M. (Ed.). (1980). *Transcultural nursing: Teaching, practice, and research*. Salt Lake City: University of Utah College of Nursing.

Leininger, M. (Ed.). (1981). *Caring: An essential human need*. Thorofare, N.J.: Charles B. Slack, Inc.

Leininger, M. (Ed.). (1984). *Care: The essence of nursing and health*. Thorofare, N.J.: Charles B. Slack, Inc.

Leininger, M. (Ed.). (1985). *Transcultural care diversity and universality: A theory of care and nursing*. New York: Grune & Stratton.

Leininger, M. (Ed.). (1985). *Qualitative research methods in nursing*. New York: Grune & Stratton.

Smith, C.M., Wolf, V.C., & Leininger, M. (Eds.). (1973). *Nursing at the University of Washington, 1973-1975*. Seattle: University of Washington, Office of Publications and Department of Printing, 1973.

Book Chapters

Leininger, M. (1968). The research critique: Nature, function and art. In M. Batey (Ed.), *Communicating nursing research: The research critique*. Boulder, Col.: Western Interstate Commission on Higher Education, pp. 20-23.

Leininger, M. (1969). The young child's response to hospitalization: Separation anxiety or lack of mothering care? In M. Batey (Ed.), *Communicating nursing research*. Boulder, Col.: Western Interstate Commission on Higher Education, pp. 26-39.

Leininger, M. (1971). Anthropological approach to adaptation: Case studies from nursing. In J. Murphy (Ed.), *Theoretical issues in professional nursing*. New York: Appleton-Century-Crofts, pp. 77-102.

Leininger, M. (1973). The culture concept and its relevance to nursing. In M. Auld, & L. Birum (Eds.), *The challenge of nursing: A book of readings*. St. Louis: C.V. Mosby, pp. 39-46.

Leininger, M. (1973). Primex. In M. Auld, & L. Birum (Ed.), *The challenge of nursing: A book of reading*. St. Louis: C.V. Mosby, pp. 237-242.

Leininger, M. (1973). Nursing in the context of social and cultural systems. In P. Mitchell (Ed.), *Concepts basic to nursing*. New York: McGraw-Hill, pp. 37-60.

Leininger, M. (1974, Fall). Humanism, health and cultural values. In *Health care dimensions* (Vol. 1): *Health care issues*. Philadelphia: F.A. Davis, pp. 37-60.

Leininger, M. (1975, Spring). Health care delivery systems for tomorrow: Possibilities and guidelines. In *Health care dimensions* (Vol. 2): *Barriers and facilitators to quality health care*. Philadelphia: F.A. Davis, pp. 83-95.

Leininger, M. (1976, Spring). Conflict and conflict resolutions: Theories and processes relevant to the health professions. In *Health care dimensions* (Vol. 3): *Transcultural health care issues and conditions*. Philadelphia: F.A. Davis, pp. 165-183.

Leininger, M. (1976, Spring). Toward conceputalization of transcultural health care systems: Concepts and a model. In *Health care dimensions* (Vol. 3): *Transcultural health care issues and conditions*. Philadelphia: F.A. Davis, pp. 3-22.

Leininger, M. (1976). Transcultural nursing: A promising subfield of study for nurse educators and practitioners. In A. Reinhardt (Ed.), *Current practice in family centered community nursing*. St. Louis: C.V. Mosby, pp. 36-50.

Leininger, M. (1978). Futurology of nursing: Goals and challenges for tomorrow. In N. Chaska (Ed.), *Views through the mist: The nursing profession*. New York: McGraw-Hill, pp. 379-396.

Leininger, M. (1978). Professional, political, and ethnocentric role behaviors and their influence in multidisciplinary health education. In A. Hardy, & M. Conway (Ed.), *Role theory: Perspectives for health professionals*. New York: Appleton-Century-Crofts.

Leininger, M. (1981). Transcultural nursing issues for the 1980's. In J. McCloskey, & H. Grace (Ed.), *Current issues in nursing*. Boston: Blackwell Scientific Publications.

Leininger, M. (1981). Women's role in society in the 80's. In *Maternal child nursing in the 80's*. Nursing perspective: A forum in honor of Katherine Kendall. College Park, Md.: University of Maryland School of Nursing.

Leininger, M. (1983). Intercultural interviews, assessments and therapy implications. In P. Pederson, (Ed.), *Interviews and assessments*. Beverly Hills, Cal.: Sage.

Articles

Leininger, M. (1961, Oct.). Changes in psychiatric nursing. *Canadian Nurse, 57*:938-948.

Leininger, M. (1964, June). A Gadsup Village experiences its first election. *Journal of Polynesian Society, 73*:29-34.

Leininger, M. (1967, April). The culture concept and its relevance to nursing. *Journal of Nursing Education, 6*:27-39.

Leininger, M. (1967, Spring). Nursing care of a patient from another culture: Japanese-American patient. *Nursing Clinics of North America, 2*:747-762.

Leininger, M. (1968, Sept.-Oct.). The research critique: Nature, function, and art. *Nursing Research, 17(5)*:444-449.

Leininger, M. (1968, Nov.). Cultural differences among staff members and the impact on patient care. *Minnesota League for Nursing Bulletin, 16*:5-9.

Leininger, M. (1968, Nov.). The significance of cultural concepts in nursing. *Minnesota League for Nursing Bulletin, 16*:3-4.

Leininger, M. (1969, Jan.). Community psychiatric nursing: Trends, issues and problems. *Perspectives in Psychiatric Care, 7*:10-20.

Leininger, M. (1969, Jan.). Ethnoscience: A new and promising research approach for the health sciences. *Image, 3*:2-8.

Leininger, M. (1969, Sept.-Oct.). Conference on the nature of science in nursing. Introduction: Nature of science in nursing. *Nursing Research, 18*:388-389.

Leininger, M. (1970). Witchcraft practices and nursing therapy. *ANA Clinical Conferences*. New York: Appleton-Century-Crofts, p. 76.

Leininger, M. (1970). Some cross-cultural universal and non-universal functions beliefs and practices of food. In J. Dupont (Ed.), *Dimensions of Nutrition*. Proceedings of the Colorado Dietetic Association Conference [held in Fort Collins, Colorado, 1969]. Colorado Associated Universities Press, 1970, pp. 153-179.

Leininger, M. (1971, March). Anthropological issues related to community mental health programs in the United States. *Community Mental Health Journal, 7*:50-62.

Leininger, M. (1971, Nov.). Dean proposes educational teamwork. *Health Science Review, 1*:4.

Leininger, M. (1971, Dec.). This I believe . . . about interdisciplinary health education for the future. *Nursing Outlook, 19*:787-791.

Leininger, M. (1972). Using cultural styles of people: Conflicts and changes in the subculture of nursing. *Psychiatric Nursing Bulletin*, pp. 43-61.

Leininger, M. (1972, July). This I believe . . . about interdisciplinary health education for the future. *AORN Journal*, pp. 89-104.

Leininger, M. (1973, Winter). Health care delivery systems for tomorrow: Possibilities and guidelines. *Washington State Journal of Nursing, 45*:10-16.

Leininger, M. (1973, Spring). Witchcraft practices and psychocultural therapy with urban United States families. *Human Organization, 32*:73-83.

Leininger, M. (1973, March). An open health care system model. *Nursing Outlook, 21*:171-175.

Leininger, M. (1973, July). Primex: Its origins and significance. *American Journal of Nursing, 73*:1274-1277.

Leininger, M. (1973, Aug.). Witchcraft practices and psychocultural therapy with U.S. urban families. *Mental Health Digest, 5*:33-40.

Leininger, M. (1973, Fall). A new model: Working model for future nurse participation and utilization. *Washington State Journal of Nursing, 45*:7-15.

Leininger, M. (1973). Becoming aware of types of health practitioners and cultural imposition. *Speeches presented during the 48th Convention.* American Nurses' Association.

Leininger, M. (1974, March-April). The leadership crisis in nursing: A critical problem and challenge. *Journal of Nursing Administration, 4*:28-34.

Leininger, M. (1974, Spring). Scholars, scholarship and nursing scholarship. *Image, 6*:1-14.

Leininger, M. (1974, Dec.). Conflict and conflict resolution: Theories and processes relevant to the health professions. *American Nurse, 6*:17-21.

Leininger, M. (1974). Leadership in nursing: Challenges, concerns, and effect. *The Challenge: Rational administration in nursing and health care services,* University of Arizona, pp. 35-53.

Leininger, M. (1975, Feb.). Conflict and conflict resolution. *American Journal of Nursing, 75*:292-296.

Leininger, M. (1975, May). Transcultural nursing presents exciting challenge. *American Nurse, 5*:4.

Leininger, M. (1976, May-June). Doctoral programs for nurses: Trends, questions and projected plans. *Nursing Research, 25*:201-210.

Leininger, M. (1976, Fall). Two strange health tribes: Gnisrun and Enicidem in the United States. *Human Organization, 35*:253-261.

Leininger, M. (1976, Feb.). Caring: The essence and central focus of nursing. *American Nurses' Foundation, 12*:2-14.

Leininger, M. (1977). Cultural diversities of health and nursing care. *Nursing Clinics of North America, 12*(1):5-18.

Leininger, M. (1977). Roles and directions in nursing and cancer nursing. *Proceedings of the Second National Conference on Cancer Nursing.* American Cancer Society.

Leininger, M. (1977). *Territoriality, power and creative leadership in administrative nursing contexts.* (Publication No. 52-1675:6-18). National League for Nursing.

Leininger, M. (1977, Nov.). Issues in nursing: A learning challenge. *Vital Signs,2*:3. (Publication of the Student Nurses' Association, University of Utah.)

Leininger, M. (1978, March). Nursing in the future: Some brief glimpses (Part I). *Vital Signs, 2*:7.

Leininger, M. (1978, April). Nursing in the future: Some brief glimpses (Part II). *Vital Signs, 2*:8.

Leininger, M. (1978, May). Nursing in the future: Some brief glimpses (Part III). *Vital Signs,2*:9.

Leininger, M. (1978, June). Changing foci in nursing education: Primary and transcultural care. *Journal of Advanced Nursing,* pp. 155-166.

Leininger, M. (1978, Spring). Political nursing: Essential for health and educational systems of tomorrow. *Nursing Administration Quarterly, 2* (3):1-16.

Leininger, M. (1978, Oct.). Transcultural nursing: A new subfield to generate nursing and health care knowledge. *Scholarly Lecture Series.* University of Manitoba.

Leininger, M. (1978, Dec.). Creating and maintaining a nursing research support center. *Adelphi Report,* Adelphi University, pp. 35-60.

Leininger, M. (1978, Dec.). Transcultural nursing for tomorrow's nurse, *Imprint.*

Leininger, M. (1979, April). Health promotion and maintenance: An old transcultural challenge and a new emphasis for the health professions. Health Promotion: In *Health and Illness, Monograph #4.* Series 1978. Sigma Theta Tau.

Leininger, M. (1979). Consumer health care needs, nursing leadership and future directions. *Proceedings of the Leadership Conference.* Seattle: University of Washington, School of Nursing.

Leininger, M. (1979). Principles and guidelines to assist nurses in cross-cultural nursing and health practices. *Hope Conference Report.* Millwood, Va.: International Nursing Project Hope Health Sciences Education Center.

Leininger, M. (1979, Oct.). *Sociocultural forces impacting upon health care and the nursing profession.* NIH Annual Meeting of Nursing Departments. Washington, D.C.: National Institutes of Health.

Leininger, M. (1980, Winter). University of Utah nursing clinics. *Western Journal of Nursing Research, 2*:411.

Leininger, M. (1980, Aug.). Transcultural nursing: A new subfield. *Health Clinics International, 2*:3-4.

Leininger, M. & Shubin, S. (1980, June). Nursing patients from different cultures. *Nursing, 80*:10.

Leininger, M. (1980, Oct.). Caring: A central focus for nursing and health care services. *Nursing and Health Care, 1*:135-143, 176.

Leininger, M. (1981, July-Aug.). Woman's role in society in the 1980s. *Issues in Health Care of Women, 3(4)*:203-215.

Leininger, M. (1981, Sept.). Transcultural nursing: Its progress and its future. *Nursing and Health Care, 2(7)*:365-371.

Leininger, M. (1982, Jan.). Creativity and challenges for nurse researchers in this economic recession. *Center for Health Research News, 1*:1. (Publication of the College of Nursing, Wayne State University.)

Leininger, M. (1982, Nov.). Getting to 'Truths' or mastering numbers and research designs. *Center for Health Research News, 1*:2. (Publication of the College of Nursing, Wayne State University.)

Leininger, M. (1983, March). Creativity and challenges for nurse researchers in this economic recession. *Journal of Nursing Administration, 13*:21-22.

Leininger, M. (1983, May). Qualitative research methods: A new direction to document and discover nursing knowledge. *Center for Health Research News, 3*:2. (Publication of the College of Nursing, Wayne State University.)

Leininger, M. (1983, Aug.). Cultural care: An essential goal for nursing and health care. *Journal of Nephrology Nursing, 10*:11-17.

Leininger, M. (1983, Oct.-Dec.). Community psychiatric nursing in community mental health: Trends, issues, and problems. *Perspective Psychiatric Care, 21(4)*:139-146.

Leininger, M. (1984, March-April). Transcultural nursing: An overview. *Nursing Outlook, 32(2)*:72-73.

Leininger, M. (1985, April). Transcultural care diversity and universality: A theory of nursing. *Nursing and Health Care, 6(4)*:209-212.

Book Prefaces and Forewords

Leininger, M. (1972). Introduction. In K. Leahy, M. Cobb, & M. Jones, *Community Health Nursing*. New York: McGraw-Hill.

Leininger, M. (1972). Introduction. In L. Schwartz, & J. Schwartz, *Psychodynamic concepts of patient care*. Englewood Cliffs, N.J.: Prentice-Hall, Inc.

Leininger, M. (1973, July). Foreword. In M. Disbrow (Ed.), *Meeting consumers' demands for maternity care*. Seattle: University of Washington Press.

Leininger, M. (1974, Fall). Preface. In M. Leininger (Ed.), *Health care issues: Health care dimensions*, Second issue, Philadelphia: F.A. Davis.

Leininger, M. (1975, Spring). Preface. In M. Leininger (Ed.), *Transcultural health care issues and conditions: Health care dimensions*, Second issue, Philadelphia: F.A. Davis.

Leininger, M. (1976, Spring). Preface. In M. Leininger (Ed.), *Transcultural health care issues and conditions: Health care dimensions*, Third issue, Philadelphia: F.A. Davis.

Leininger, M. (1978). Foreword. In J. Watson, *Nursing: The philosophy and science of caring*. Boston: Little, Brown.

Leininger, M. (1979). Foreword. In L.S. Bermosk, & S.E. Porter, *Womens' health and human wholeness*. New York: Appleton-Century-Crofts.

Leininger, M. (1979). Preface. In M. Leininger, (Ed.)., *Proceedings of the national transcultural nursing conferences*. New York: Masson.

Leininger, M. (1980). Foreword. *Transcultural nursing: Teaching, research, and practice*. Salt Lake City.

Leininger, M. (1981). Introduction. *Six proceedings of the transcultural nursing conferences in 1976, 1977, 1978, 1979, 1980, 1981*. New York: Masson International Press.

Leininger, M. (1981). Preface. *Caring: An essential human need*. Thorofare, N.J.: Charles B. Slack, Inc.

Leininger, M. (1981). Preface. *Maternal child nursing in the 80's*. Nursing perspective: A forum in honor of Katherine Kendall. College Park, Md.: University of Maryland, School of Nursing.

Leininger, M. (1983). Preface. *Transcultural health and nursing references*. Thorofare, N.J.: Charles B. Slack, Inc.

Leininger, M. (1983). Preface. *Care: The essence of nursing and health*. Thorofare, N.J.: Charles B. Slack, Inc.

Leininger, M. (1983). Preface. In K. Vestal, & C. McKenzie (Eds.), *High risk perinatal nursing*. Philadelphia: W.B. Saunders.

Secondary Sources

Chinn, P.L., & Jacobs, M.K. (1983). Theory and nursing: A systematic approach. St. Louis: C.V. Mosby.

Jean Watson

14

Philosophy and Science of Caring

Beverly D. Porter, Rebecca S. Sloan

CREDENTIALS AND BACKGROUND OF THE THEORIST

Jean Watson was born July 21, 1940, the youngest of eight children. She grew up in a small town in West Virginia in a large family with a strong belief system. She is married and has two children.

Watson received a Bachelor of Science in Nursing from the University of Colorado at

The authors wish to express appreciation to Dr. Jean Watson for critiquing the chapter.

Boulder in 1964 and began her nursing career as a psychiatric–mental health nurse therapist for a private group. She also continued her education and in 1966 received a Master's in psychiatric–mental health nursing from the University of Colorado at Denver. In 1973 Watson received a Ph.D. in educational psychology and counseling, with a special cognate emphasis in social and clinical psychology, from the University of Colorado at Boulder.

After graduation, Watson accepted a faculty position at the University of Colorado. She also served as a clinical consultant to the Boulder County Hospice and was active in crisis intervention and bereavement studies. She received several research grant awards to study cognitive systems of nurses and the influence of conceptual system on education, especially in psychosocial nursing. In addition she was involved in developing the doctoral nursing program at the University of Colorado.

Watson has been the recipient of numerous awards and honors during her career. She received a Kennedy Foundation Award for a special short-term study in bioethics in Georgetown University's Kennedy Institute in 1977 and the Sigma Theta Tau National Honorary Nursing Society Award for Creativity in Nursing in 1980. In 1981 she was admitted as a fellow in the American Academy of Nursing. Watson was awarded a Visiting Kellogg Fellowship for study at the Western Australian Institute of Technology in 1981-1982 and a faculty fellowship in the Lincoln Institute of Health Sciences in the Royal College of Nursing in Melbourne during 1981-1982. She also received a National Science Council Award to serve as visiting lecturer-consultant at the National Taiwan University in 1982.

A member of the University of Colorado School of Nursing faculty since 1973, Watson has been associate dean of the baccalaureate program and was director of the doctoral program and coordinator of the psychosocial mental health nursing doctoral program from 1979 to 1981. During that time she also chaired the University of Colorado Faculty Council, the academic governing body for the four-campus system. She became Dean of the School of Nursing in 1983.

Watson has published on a variety of topics. She has authored book chapters and many articles in the nursing literature. While working with a group of colleagues on curriculum development, Watson was approached to publish a textbook for an integrated baccalaureate nursing curriculum. The result was what she refers to as a treatise on nursing. Published in 1979, *Nursing: the Philosophy and Science of Caring* is now treated as a theory of nursing. It was fol-

lowed in 1985 by a second major work, *Nursing: Human Science and Human Care, A Theory of Nursing*.

There has long been a discrepancy in nursing between theory and practice. To reduce this dichotomy, Watson proposes a philosophy and science of caring. Caring is central to nursing practice.[3:xii] It is more than a task-oriented behavior and includes such illusive aspects of health as the interpersonal relationship between the nurse and client. Watson[6:xiii] believes ultimate nursing care is the result of combined study of the sciences and the humanities culminating in a therapeutic nurse-client relationship. The process is based on 10 carative factors of nursing.

THEORETICAL SOURCES

In addition to traditional nursing knowledge and the works of Nightingale, Henderson, Krueter, Hall, and Leininger, Watson drew heavily on the sciences and the humanities in developing her framework. Her work has a phenomenological existential perspective.

The views of Carl Rogers appear often in Watson's work. Rogers describes several incidents leading to the formulation of his thoughts on human behavior. One such episode involves his learning "that it is the *client* who knows what hurts and that the facilitator should allow the direction of the therapeutic process to come from the client."[4:11-12] Rogers[4:18-19] believed that through understanding the client would come to accept himself, an initial step toward a positive outcome. The therapist helps by clarifying and stating feelings about which the client has been unclear. To do this the therapist must be able to understand the meanings, feelings, and attitudes of the client. A warm interest has been found to facilitate understanding. Rogers presents an unpublished thesis by R.D. Quinn who studied recorded therapists' statements both in and out of context. Degree of understanding was judged to be high in both contexts and Quinn[4:44] concluded that understanding is primarily a desire to understand.

Another concept of Rogerian theory is that the therapist-client relationship is more important to the outcome than adherence to traditional methods. Rogers[4:32] states:

> In my early professional years I was asking the question, How can I treat, or cure, or change this person? Now I phrase the question in this way: How can I provide a relationship which this person may use for his own personal growth?

To support his concept Rogers notes a study by Betz and Whitehorn[1] describing the differences in degree of improvement for schizophrenic patients treated by two methods. Those patients treated by physicians who endeavored to understand the personal meaning of their patients' behavior fared better than patients of doctors who saw their clients as symptomatic of a specific diagnosis.* Additionally, J. Seeman's study[5:272-299] describes the effectiveness of psychotherapy when characterized by mutual affection and respect between the therapist and client.

Watson believes a strong liberal arts background is essential to the process of holistic care for clients. She sees the study of the humanities as an experience resulting in mind expansion, increased thinking skills, and personal growth. But Watson‡ describes the current status of nursing by using as an analogy the mythological Danaides, who attempted to fill a broken jar with water, only to see the water flow through the cracks. Until nursing merges theory and practice through combined study of the sciences and the humanities, similar cracks will be evident in the scientific basis of nursing knowledge.

Yalom's 11 carative factors stimulated Watson's thinking[6:xvi] about the psychodynamic and human components that could apply to nursing

and caring and, consequently, to the 10 carative factors in nursing.

USE OF EMPIRICAL EVIDENCE

Watson and her colleagues have attempted to study the concept of caring by collecting data to use in classifying caring behaviors, to describe the similarities and differences between what nurses consider care and what clients consider care, and to generate testable hypotheses around the concept of nursing care. They studied responses from registered nurses, student nurses, and clients to the same open-ended questionnaire covering a variety of aspects of "(a) taking care of and (b) caring about" patients. Their findings revealed a discrepancy in the values considered most important to clients versus the student nurses versus the registered nurses. Their conclusions stressed the need for further study in order to clarify what behaviors and values are important from each viewpoint. Their study also raised a question regarding differences in values for persons in different situations, as well as the question of meeting minimum care needs before the quality of care can be evaluated.[9:32-44]

MAJOR CONCEPTS AND DEFINITIONS

Watson[6:9-10] bases her theory for nursing practice on the following 10 carative factors. Each has a dynamic phenomenological component that is relative to the individuals involved in the relationship as encompassed by nursing.

FORMATION OF A HUMANISTIC-ALTRUISTIC SYSTEM OF VALUES. Humanistic and altruistic values are learned early in life, but can be greatly influenced by nursing educators. This factor describes satisfaction through giving and extension of the sense of self.[6:10-12]

---

*References 1:89-117; 7:321-331.
‡References 7:413-416; 8:244-249

INSTILLATION OF FAITH-HOPE. This factor describes the nurse's role in promoting wellness by helping the client adopt health-seeking behaviors, by using the power of suggestion positively to support the client, and by developing effective nurse-client interrelationships.[6:12-16]

CULTIVATION OF SENSITIVITY TO ONE'S SELF AND TO OTHERS. Recognition of feelings leads to self-actualization through self-acceptance for the nurse and client. If a nurse is able to express her feelings, she is better able to allow others to express theirs.[6:16-19]

DEVELOPMENT OF A HELPING-TRUST RELATIONSHIP. A helping-trust relationship promotes and accepts the expression of positive and negative feelings. It involves congruence, empathy, nonpossessive warmth, and effective communication.[6:23-41]

Congruence. Congruence involves being real, honest, genuine, and authentic.[6:26-28]

Empathy. Empathy is the ability to experience, and thereby understand, the other person's perceptions and feelings and to communicate those understandings.[6:28-30]

Nonpossessive warmth. Nonpossessive warmth is demonstrated by a moderate speaking volume, a relaxed, open posture, and facial expressions that are congruent with other communications.[6:30-33]

Effective communication. Effective communication has cognitive, affective, and behavioral response components.[6:33-41]

PROMOTION AND ACCEPTANCE OF THE EXPRESSION OF POSITIVE AND NEGATIVE FEELINGS. The sharing of feelings is a risk-taking experience for both the nurse and the client. The nurse must be prepared for negative feelings. The nurse must understand that intellectual and emotional understanding of a situation are different.[6:17-48]

SYSTEMATIC USE OF THE SCIENTIFIC PROBLEM-SOLVING METHOD FOR DECISION MAKING. Use of the nursing process brings a scientific problem-solving approach to nursing care, dispelling the traditional image of nurses as the "doctor's handmaiden." The nursing process is similar to the research process.[6:51-66]

PROMOTION OF INTERPERSONAL TEACHING-LEARNING. This factor is an important concept for nursing in that it separates *caring* from *curing*. It allows the patient to be informed and thus shifts responsibility for wellness to the client. The nurse facilitates this with teaching-learning techniques to enable the client to provide self-care, determine his own needs, and provide for his own growth.[6:69-79]

PROVISION FOR A SUPPORTIVE, PROTECTIVE OR CORRECTIVE MENTAL, PHYSICAL, SOCIOCULTURAL, AND SPIRITUAL ENVIRONMENT. Nursing must recognize that the client's environment includes external and internal variables. Change can be experienced in any aspect and requires coping. The nurse assesses and facilitates the client's coping abilities. Comfort, privacy, safety, and clean, aesthetic surroundings are important.[6:81-101]

ASSISTANCE WITH THE GRATIFICATION OF HUMAN NEEDS. The nurse recognizes the biophysical, psychophysical, psychosocial, and intrapersonal needs of herself and her client. Clients must attain the lower order needs before attaining those higher in the needs hierarchy. Food, elimination, and ventilation are lower order biophysical needs. Activity-inactivity and sexuality are lower order psychophysical needs. Achievement and affiliation are higher order psychosocial needs. Self-actualization is a higher order intrapersonal-interpersonal need.[6:105-203]

ALLOWANCE FOR EXISTENTIAL-PHE-NOMENOLOGICAL FORCES. Phenomenology describes data of the immediate situation that help people understand the phenomena in question.[6:208] Existential psychology is a science of human existence that employs the method of phenomenological analysis.[6:209] Watson considers this factor to be difficult to understand. It is included to provide a thought-provoking experience leading to a better understanding of ourselves and others.[6:205-215]

Watson believes nurses have the responsibility to go beyond the 10 carative factors and develop the areas of health promotion through preventive actions. This is accomplished by teaching clients behavioral changes to promote health, providing situational support, teaching problem-solving methods, and recognizing coping skills and adaptation to loss.[6:217-305]

MAJOR ASSUMPTIONS

Watson[6:8-9] states the major assumptions of her theory are:

1. Caring can be effectively demonstrated and practiced only interpersonally.
2. Caring consists of carative factors that result in the satisfaction of certain human needs.
3. Effective caring promotes health and individual or family growth.
4. Caring responses accept a person not only as he or she is now, but for what he or she may become.
5. A caring environment offers the development of potential while allowing the person to choose the best action for himself or herself at a given point in time.
6. Caring is more healthogenic than is curing. The practice of caring integrates biophysical knowledge with knowledge of human behavior to generate or promote health and to provide ministrations to

those who are ill. A science of caring is therefore complementary to the science of curing.
7. The practice of caring is central to nursing.

THEORETICAL ASSERTIONS

According to Watson, nursing tries to understand how health, illness, and human behavior are interrelated. With her philosophy and science of caring, she tries to define an outcome of scientific activity in regard to the humanistic aspects of life. In other words, she attempts to make nursing an interrelationship of quality of life and death, as well as the prolongation of life.[6:xvii]

Watson believes nursing is concerned with promoting and restoring health and preventing illness. But *health* is more than the absence of illness and is an illusive concept because it is subjective.[6:219] *Caring* is a nursing term, representing all the factors the nurse uses to deliver health care to her client. The nurse provides care to her clients through Watson's 10 carative factors.[6:6] Each carative factor describes the caring process of how a client attains, or maintains, health or dies a peaceful death. On the other hand, Watson describes *curing* as a medical term referring to elimination of disease.[6:7]

In *Nursing: The Philosophy and Science of Caring* Watson[6:8] writes that the basic premises of a science for nursing are:

1. Caring (and nursing) has existed in every society. Every society has had some people who have cared for others. A caring attitude is *not* transmitted from generation to generation by genes. It is transmitted by the culture of the profession as a unique way of coping with its environment. Nursing has always held a caring stance in regard to other human beings. That stance has been threatened by a long history of procedure-oriented demands and the development of different levels of nursing. However, the opportunities for

nurses to obtain advanced education and engage in higher-level analyses of problems and concerns in their education and practice have allowed nursing to combine its humanistic orientation with the relevant science.

2. There is often a discrepancy between theory and practice or between the scientific and artistic aspects of caring, partly because of the disjunction between scientific values and humanistic values.

LOGICAL FORM

The framework is presented in a logical form. It contains broad ideas, but a focused framework. It is derived from many disciplines and addresses many situations on the health-illness continuum. Watson's definition of caring as opposed to curing delineates nursing from medicine. This concept is helpful in classifying the body of nursing knowledge as a separate science.

Watson's theory has concrete support from theorists in other disciplines, such as Rogers, Erickson, and Maslow. She is adamant in her support for the Bachelor of Science in Nursing as the minimum requirement for entry into nursing. This stems from her strong belief that a broad liberal arts background increases the nurse's communication and problem-solving skills.[6:xv]

ACCEPTANCE BY THE NURSING COMMUNITY
Practice

When considering practice using Watson's framework, it must be assumed that a limited number of graduates have been formally educated in these concepts. However, many components of Watson's framework are practiced in other institutions that seek to use a holistic approach to nursing care. Examples are those 4-year schools requiring considerable liberal arts education. It is possible that nurses already practice many of her concepts, but Watson has formally organized these components of nursing care and attached labels to the behaviors.

Education

Watson has been active in curriculum planning at the University of Colorado. Her framework is being taught in the 4-year nursing curriculum at Bellarmine College in Louisville, Kentucky. Assumption College in Worcester, Massachusetts, and other undergraduate programs also use the framework. In addition, the concepts are now widely used in nursing programs in Australia and in some programs in Sweden, Finland, and Great Britain. Watson[10] believes her theory will have more acceptance through a liberal arts college with a religious background than through the large university setting, unless the university curriculum is committed to a liberal education along with the professional nursing education.

Critics of the author's work have concentrated on the use of undefined terms, incomplete treatment of subject matter when describing the 10 carative factors, and a lack of attention to the pathophysiological aspects of nursing. Watson[6:xv] addresses these charges in the preface of her book, where she defines her intent to describe the *core* of nursing—those aspects of the nurse-client relationship resulting in a therapeutic outcome—rather than the *trim* of nursing—the procedures, tasks, and techniques employed by various practice settings. Using this focus, the framework is not limited to any nursing specialty. The concepts could be incorporated into nursing education programs as a philosophical guideline. A study of Watson's framework leads the reader through a thought-provoking experience by emphasizing communication skills, use of self, and growth.

Research

Watson has attempted to research her framework and to arrive at empirical data amenable to research techniques. However, this very abstract framework is difficult to study concretely.

As with much research, some questions have been answered and new questions raised. Additional research will be needed to define these concepts. Watson would like to see her framework used as a catalyst for hypothesis formation resulting in additional study. The body of nursing knowledge has much to gain from this undertaking.

FURTHER DEVELOPMENTS

Nursing research has traditionally followed the *received view* format in which single-factor methodology is compared against rigorous standards of truth, operational definitions, and observational criteria.[7:413-416] Watson concludes that this methodology does not apply to the multifactorial study of nursing care. She proposes that as nursing advances in its own doctoral programs, the process of scientific development will be used on itself. Nursing research will adopt the received view, reject it, and synthesize new ideas, which will result in a new nursing model for the 1980s and 1990s.

Continued research of Watson's theory may promote widespread acceptance of her views. To provide further development of the theory, it is vital that those who have studied Watson's work share it with their peers. This largely untested theory should lend itself to hypothesis formation.[2:139] Hypothesis formation should then result in additional research attempts to define, refine, and advance her concepts for the betterment of nursing care.

CRITIQUE
Clarity

On the surface, Watson's theory is easily read and uses nontechnical language providing clarity. Semantic clarity could be improved by employing precise definitions of terms. For example, nursing is defined in a variety of ways in various portions of the book. One broad definition of nursing would be helpful in understanding the thoughts of the author. Additionally, it is unclear whether Watson was speaking to the nurse's responsibilities, or to the client's responsibilities in some interactions, or to both.

Simplicity

Watson draws on a number of disciplines in formulating her theory. The reader must have an understanding of a variety of subject matters in order to understand the theory as it is presented. Therefore this theory is not considered simple.

Generality

The scope of the framework encompasses all aspects of the health-illness continuum. In addition, the theory addresses aspects of preventing illness and experiencing a peaceful death, thereby increasing its generality.

Empirical Precision

Although the framework is difficult to study empirically, Watson draws heavily on widely accepted work from other disciplines. With this solid foundation, her views are strengthened.

Derivable Consequences

Considerable testing still needs to be undertaken, but Watson's theory can provide many useful and important concepts for the delivery of nursing care. Many of these concepts are not commonly stressed in traditional nursing education, that is, use of the self, client-identified needs, the caring process, and others. Using this theory could lead to the development of a new dimension of the nurse's role.

REFERENCES

1. Betz, B.J., & Whitehorn, J.C. (1956). *The relationship of the therapist to the outcome of therapy in schizophrenia.* Psychiatric Research Reports #5. Research techniques in schizophrenia. Washington, D.C.: American Psychiatric Association.
2. Chinn, P.L., & Jacobs, M.K. (1983). *Theory and nursing: A systematic approach.* St. Louis: C.V. Mosby.
3. Leininger, M. (1979). Preface. In J. Watson, *Nursing: the philosophy and science of caring.* Boston: Little, Brown.

4. Rogers, C.R. (1961). *On becoming a person: A therapist's view of psychology.* Boston: Houghton Mifflin.
5. Seeman, J. (1954). Counselor judgments of therapeutic process and outcome. In C.R. Rogers, & R.F. Dymond (Eds.), *Psychotherapy and personality change.* Chicago: University of Chicago Press, pp. 272-299.
6. Watson, J. (1979). *Nursing: The philosophy and science of caring.* Boston: Little, Brown.
7. Watson, J. (1981, July). Nursing's scientific quest. *Nursing Outlook, 29:*413-416.
8. Watson, J. (1981). The lost art of nursing. *Nursing Forum, 20:*244-249.
9. Watson, J., et al. (1979). *A model of caring: An alternative health care model for nursing practice and research.* American Nurses' Association NP-59 3W 8179190, Clinical and Scientific Sessions, Div. of Practice, Kansas City, Mo., pp. 32-34.
10. Watson, J. (1984). Telephone interview.
11. Whitehorn, J.C., & Betz, B.M. (1954). A study of psychotherapeutic relationships between physicians and schizophrenic patients. *American Journal of Psychiatry, 111:*321-331.

BIBLIOGRAPHY
Primary Sources
Books

Watson, J. (1979). *Nursing: The philosophy and science of caring.* Boston: Little, Brown.
Watson, J. (1985). *Nursing: Human science and health care.* Norwalk, Conn.: Appleton-Century-Crofts.

Book Chapters

Watson, J., et al. (1979). *A model of caring: An alternative health care model for nursing practice and research.* (Publication No. NP-59 3M 8179190). Kansas City, Mo.: American Nurses' Association.
Watson, J. (1980). Self losses. In F.L. Bower, and M.S. Brown, (Eds.), *Nursing and the concept of loss.* New York: John Wiley & Sons.
Watson, J. (1981). Some issues related to a science of caring for nursing practice. In M. Leininger (Ed.), *Caring: An essential human need.* Thorofare, N.J.: Charles B. Slack, Inc.
Watson, J. (1983). Delivery and assurance of quality health care: A rights based foundation. In R. Luke, J. Krueger, and R. Madrow, (Eds.), *Orga-*

nization and change in health care quality assurance. Rockville, Md.: Aspen Systems.

Articles

Carozza, V., Congdon, J., & Watson, J. (1978, Nov.). An experimental educationally sponsored pilot internship program. *Journal of Nursing Education, 17:*14-20.
Watson, J. (1976, Jan.-Feb.). The quasi-rational element in conflict: A review of selected conflict literature. *Nursing Research, 25:*19-23.
Watson, J. (1976, Jan.-Feb.). Research and literature on children's responses to injections: Some general nursing implications. *Pediatric Nursing, 2:*7-8.
Watson, J. (1976, Nov.-Dec.). Research question and answer. Creative approach to researchable questions. *Nursing Research, 25:*439.
Watson, J. (1978, May-June). Conceptual systems of undergraduate nursing students as compared with university students at large and practicing nurses. *Nursing Research, 27:*151-155.
Watson, J. (1980, Spring). Response to review of Watson's book. *Western Journal of Nursing Research, 2:*514-515.
Watson, J. (1981, Spring). Conceptual systems of students, practitioners. *Western Journal of Nursing Research, 3:*172-192.
Watson, J. (1981, Spring). Response to "Conceptual systems of students, practitioners." *Western Journal of Nursing Research, 3:*197-198.
Watson, J. (1981, Aug.). Professional identity crisis: Is nursing finally growing up? *American Journal of Nursing, 81:*1488-1490.
Watson, J. (1981, July). Nursing's scientific quest. *Nursing Outlook, 29:*413-416.
Watson, J. (1982, Aug.). Traditional vs. tertiary ideological shifts in nursing education. *Australian Nurses' Journal, 12:*46-64.
Watson, J. (1983, Fall). The IDIR model for faculty research with students. *Western Journal of Nursing Research, 5:*301-312.
Watson, J., & Carozza, V. (1978, Nov.). An experimental educationally sponsored pilot internship program. *Journal of Nursing Education, 17:*14-20.

Book Review

Watson, J. (1977, July-Aug.). Review of J.W. Ganong & W.L. Ganong, *Help with the nursing audit: A management guide. Journal of Nursing Administration, 7:*12.

Secondary Sources
Book Reviews

Watson, J. (1979). *Nursing: The philosophy and science of caring.*
*Nursing Outlook, 28:*45, January 1980.
*Western Journal of Nursing Research, 2:*417-418, Winter 1980.

Other Sources

Betz, B.J., & Whitehorn, J.C. (1956). *The relationship of the therapist to the outcome of therapy in schizophrenia.* Psychiatric Research Reports #5. Research techniques in schizophrenia. Washington, D.C.: American Psychiatric Association.

Chinn, P.L., & Jacobs, M.K. (1983). *Theory and nursing: A systematic approach.* St. Louis: C.V. Mosby.

Leininger, M. (1979). Preface. In J. Watson, *Nursing: The philosophy and science of caring.* Boston: Little, Brown.

Reynolds, P.D. (1971). *A primer in theory construction.* Indianapolis: Bobbs-Merrill.

Rogers, C.R. (1961). *On becoming a person: A therapist's view of psychology.* Boston: Houghton Mifflin.

Stevens, B.J. (1979). *Nursing theory: Analysis, application, evaluation.* Boston: Little, Brown.

Whitehorn, J.C., & Betz, B.M. (1954). A study of psychotherapeutic relationships between physicians and schizophrenic patients. *American Journal of Psychiatry, 111:*321-331.

Yalom, I.G. (1975). *The theory, knowledge, and practice of group psychotherapy* (2nd. ed.). New York: Basic Books.

Rosemarie Rizzo Parse

15

Man-Living-Health

Larry P. Schumacher

CREDENTIALS AND BACKGROUND OF THE THEORIST

Rosemarie Rizzo Parse is one of nursing's most recent theorists. Although her model, *Man-Living-Health,* was published in 1981, she had expressed ideas about the model 8 years earlier in another book, *Nursing Fundamentals.* Parse received her Master's degree in nursing and a doctorate of philosophy from the University of Pittsburgh. She has held various positions in both nursing service and education. She is a

The author wishes to express appreciation to Dr. Rose Jackson for her consultation, and to Dr. Rosemarie Rizzo Parse for editing the chapter.

Professor of Nursing at Hunter College Graduate Nursing Division, New York, and a consultant in nursing education and service. She is also engaged in research to validate her model and is developing the practice and research methodologies consistent with Man-Living-Health. Research related to Man-Living-Health is published in *Nursing Research: Qualitative Methods.* Parse is married and resides in Pittsburgh.

THEORETICAL SOURCES

In developing Man-Living-Health, Parse drew from the work of Martha E. Rogers and from the existential-phenomenologists, primarily

Jean Paul Sartre, Maurice Merleau-Ponty, and Martin Heidegger. Parse emphasized the importance of building on existing theory to provide a strong foundation for theory development and a link to the past necessary for the creation of scientific knowledge. Parse defines nursing theory as "a system of interrelated concepts describing unitary man's interrelating with the environment while cocreating health."[2:13] Parse synthesizes the principles, tenets, and concepts of these previous theorists to build the assumptions of Man-Living-Health. The principles, concepts, and theoretical structures of Man-Living-Health arise from these assumptions.

Parse uses Rogers' major principles and concepts to build her theory. The principles of helicy, complementarity, and reasonancy and the corresponding concepts of energy field, openness, pattern and organization, and four dimensionality are used by Parse to develop the assumptions supporting Man-Living-Health. (The work of Rogers is presented in Chapter 28. The reader is encouraged to review these principles and concepts before reading this chapter.)

Parse borrows from the existential-phenomenologists the tenets of intentionality and human subjectivity and the corresponding concepts of coconstitution, coexistence, and situated freedom. "Intentionality posits that man is by nature an intentional being. This means that in being human man is open, knows, and is present to the world. . . . Human subjectivity posits that conscious man by nature is no-thing, but rather a unity of being and non-being."[4:18-19] The concept of coconstitution "refers to the idea that the meaning emerging in any situation is related to the particular constituents of that situation."[4:20] Coexistence, the second concept of the existential-phenomenological perspective, means "man is not alone in any dimension of becoming. Man, an emerging being, is in the world with others; indeed, even the act of coming into the world is through others."[4:20] The final existential-phe-

nomenological concept Parse uses is situated freedom. Situated freedom means that "reflectively and pre-reflectively, one participates in choosing the situations in which one finds oneself as well as one's attitude toward the situations."[4:21] The assumptions of Man-Living-Health, then, are synthesized from the works of Rogers, Heidegger, Sartre, and Merleau-Ponty.

USE OF EMPIRICAL EVIDENCE

Research related to the theories Parse has used to build Man-Living-Health is not identified in Man-Living-Health. Research on Rogers' Unitary Man theory is evolving. Empirical evidence from Parse's lived experience with nursing cocreated the origin of Man-Living-Health.[4:xiii]

MAJOR CONCEPTS AND DEFINITIONS

Parse builds Man-Living-Health from nine assumptions that have now been synthesized into three assumptions, and three principles are derived from them. Each principle addresses three concepts of Man-Living-Health. The first principle is, "Structuring meaning multidimensionally is cocreating reality through the languaging of valuing and imaging."[4:42] It includes the concepts of imaging, valuing, and languaging. "*Imaging* . . . is the cocreating of reality that, by its very nature, structures the meaning of an experience. . . . Imaging reality, that is, making concrete the meaning of multidimensional experience, then incarnates the simultaneity of the explicit-implicit knowing."[4:42,44] *Valuing*, consistent with L.E. Raths and colleagues, involves identifying potential beliefs, choosing from among them, and then consistently acting on the chosen belief. *Languaging* is a person's method of expressing valued images. Languaging encompasses all modes of presentation of self, including speech and movement—tone, syntax, silence, gaze, and posture. An individual's way of languaging reflects his or her cultural heritage.[4:45-50]

The second principle is, "Cocreating rhythmical patterns of relating is living the paradoxical unity of revealing-concealing and enabling-limiting while connecting-separating."[4:50] It includes the concepts of revealing-concealing, enabling-limiting, and connecting-separating. The concept of *revealing-concealing* deals with self-disclosure and is based on the idea that a person reveals-conceals simultaneously, gaining self-knowledge through this rhythmical pattern of relating.[2:52-53] *Enabling-limiting* posits that man is enabled and limited simultaneously in situations. "In this choosing, man enables self to move in one direction and limits movements in another."[4:53] The final concept of cocreating rhythmical patterns is *connecting-separating*. This concept "can be recognized as man is connecting with one phenomenon and simultaneously separating from others."[4:53-54] Parse[4:54] describes this concept further when she states that, "in separating from one phenomenon and dwelling with another, a person integrates thought, becomes more complex, and seeks new unions."

The final principle of Man-Living-Health is, "contranscending with the possibles is powering unique ways of originating in the process of transforming."[4:55] *Cotranscending* deals with environment going beyond the "what is" to the "what is not-yet." The concepts central to this principle are powering, originating, and transforming. "*Powering* is a process of man-environment energy interchange, recognized in the continuous affirming of self in light of the possibility of non-being."[2:57] Central to *powering* is the rhythm of pushing-resisting, which leads to tension and sometimes conflict. When tension or conflict presents itself, a person is faced with new possibles to choose from in movement toward the not-yet. *Originating* is Man's own creating of unique, distinct ways of living. Man originates in mutual energy interchange with the environment. "To distinguish oneself is to choose a unique way of living the paradoxical unity of conformity-nonconformity and certainty-uncertainty all at once."[2:60] *Transforming*

is man's constant movement toward greater diversity, through living with new ideas, and moving beyond the present. Parse calls transforming "the changing of change, coconstituting anew in a deliberate way."[2:62] Transforming is self-initiated and creative.

MAJOR ASSUMPTIONS

In building Man-Living-Health, Parse synthesizes the concepts of Rogers and the existential-phenomenologists to create nine assumptions. She identifies three of the underlying concepts used to form each assumption. Because Parse treats man, environment, and health as a construct, it is difficult to categorize her assumptions. To divide her assumptions into the categories of nursing, environment, man, and health would distort her intended meaning. Parse defines nursing as a scientific discipline, not as a concept coequal with man, environment, and health. Parse's assumptions are listed below, followed by summary discussions about nursing, man, environment, and health.

Man-Living-Health: Assumptions and Derivative Concepts*:

- Man is coexisting while coconstituting rhythmical patterns with the environment. [Concepts of coconstitution, coexistence, and pattern and organization.]
- Man is an open being, freely choosing meaning in situations and bearing responsibility for decisions. [Concepts of situated freedom, openness, and energy field.]
- Man is a living unity continuously coconstituting patterns of relating. [Concepts of energy field, coconstitution, pattern and organization.]
- Man is transcending multidimensionally with the possibles. [Concepts of four-dimensionality, situated freedom, and openness.]
- Health is an open process of becoming, ex-

---

*Reference 4:25,35,36.

perienced by people. [Concepts of openness, coconstitution, and situated freedom.]

- Health is a rhythmically coconstituting
  process of the man-environment interrelationship. [Concepts of coconstitution, pattern and organization, and four dimensionality.]
- Health is man's patterns of relating value
  priorities. [Concepts of patterns and organization, openness, and situated freedom.]
- Health is an intersubjective process of
  transcending with the possibles. [Concepts
  of coexistence, openness, and situated freedom.]
- Health is unitary man's negentropic unfolding. [Concepts of coexistence, energy
  field, and four dimensionality.]

These nine assumptions have been synthesized into three assumptions. The assumptions
underpinning Man-Living-Health are:

1. Man-Living-Health is freely choosing
   personal meaning in situations in the intersubjective process of relating value
   priorities.
2. Man-Living-Health is cocreating rhythmical patterns of relating in open interchange with the environment.
3. Man-Living-Health is cotranscending
   multidimensionally with the unfolding
   possibles.[5]

Nursing

By proposing that nursing is a human science,
Parse rejects the traditional natural science view
of nursing. Parse contends that nursing has par-
alleled medicine, a natural science, and that by
moving away from the medical model toward a
human science perspective nursing will take its
rightful place as a unique science. She believes,
"Nursing, rooted in human sciences, focuses on
Man as a living unity and Man's qualitative participation with health experiences."[4:4] In a
broad sense, Parse views nursing as an art and
science.

Nursing is not explicitly addressed as a con-

cept coequal to Man, Environment, and Health
by Parse in her listed assumptions because the
assumptions relating Man, Environment, and
Health underpin the science of nursing. In later
parts of the text she defines nursing's responsibility to society and nursing practice. Parse[4:81]
states, "The responsibility to society relative to
nursing practice is guiding the choosing of possibilities in the changing health process." Consistent with the family orientation evident in
the model, Parse[4:82] states, "Nursing practice is
directed toward illuminating and mobilizing
family interrelationships in light of the meaning
assigned to health and its possibilities as lan-
guaged in the cocreated patterns of relating."

In previous works, Parse discussed nursing
in greater depth. In *Nursing Fundamentals,* she
defines nursing as "a human science profession
primarily concerned with the care of unitary
man as he evolves from conception to death."[4:7]
In "Rights of Medical Patients," Parse[7] defines
nursing's role in health care more precisely than
in Man-Living-Health, as is to be expected in
the evaluation of thought that creates a theory.
In this article, she views the professionally educated nurse as the health care professional most
concerned with the client's total well-being. She
defines the nurse's role to include helping the
client make informed decisions about health
and as collaborating with the client to plan
nursing care, follow-up, and health maintenance. She asserts, in this article, that nursing's
contribution to health care be through expertise
in Man-Environment interrelations. In her previous works, Parse viewed nursing practice at
two levels, technical and professional. Her
opinion of the roles of the two levels is consistent with the American Nurses' Association
statement on level of entry into practice.

Person

Man is the central concept of Man-Living-
Health. Parse addresses man in all the assumptions and principles explicitly. Man is always
discussed in relation to environment. The Man-
Environment interrelationship is a focus of all

the assumptions. The most fundamental belief underlying Parse's work is man's participation in cocreation of health. Following the work of Rogers, Parse views man as a unitary, synergistic being, who is greater than and different from the sum of the parts.

Man is viewed as an open being, free to choose meaning in situations, and bound to accept responsibility for the outcomes of decisions. Man and environment are viewed as a construct Man-Environment together coconstituting situations. Parse believes Man is constantly moving toward greater diversity through coexistence with other humans and the environment. Man is identifiable by unique patterns of relating.[2;6:30]

Health

Parse views health as a process, rather than a state of well-being or the absence of disease. To view health on a continuum would contradict the philosophy of unitary man. Health is an experience perceived by man through the life cycle as man continuously grows through energy interchange with the environment toward greater complexity.* "Living health, then is an incarnation of man's choosing."[4:30] Thus, each individual's health reflects a choosing of lived values. These assumptions indicate man is responsible for personal health through prereflective and reflective choosing.

Environment

Man and environment are treated as a construct, Man-Environment. Man and environment are viewed as constantly moving toward greater diversity through energy interchange with each other. Environment is implicitly defined as all that man is not.[2;6:130]

THEORETICAL ASSERTIONS

Building from principles and concepts, Parse identifies three theoretical structures as state-

*Reference 2:30-33; 6:130.

ments to verify the interrelationships of the concepts. Research using qualitative methods has verified Man-Living-Health. Six completed research studies are published in *Nursing Research: Qualitative Methods.* Parse believes that the qualitative research methods are appropriately borrowed from other disciplines to verify Man-Living-Health until an appropriate research method is carved out for the study of Man-Living-Health, which is being done now. Parse incorporates three concepts into each theoretical structure (Figure 15-1). The theoretical structures are:

1. Powering is a way of revealing and concealing imaging.
2. Originating is a manifestation of enabling and limiting valuing.
3. Transforming unfolds in the languaging of connecting and separating.[2:68]

Parse identifies lived experiences that might be studied to verify the relationships that may exist. If the reader is interested in seeing an example, consult Parse's text *Man-Living-Health.* Also refer to *Nursing Research: Qualitative Methods.*

LOGICAL FORM

Through a deductive approach, Parse builds Man-Living-Health from Rogers' Unitary Man theory and from existential phenomenology. Complying with the rules of logic, Parse builds her assumptions, principles, and concepts. Each assumption addresses three of the underlying concepts. Each principle groups three of her concepts. Each theoretical structure uses three concepts, one from each principle.

ACCEPTANCE BY THE NURSING COMMUNITY
Practice

Man-Living-Health, unlike more established models of nursing, has not been used extensively in the practice setting. The work is rela-

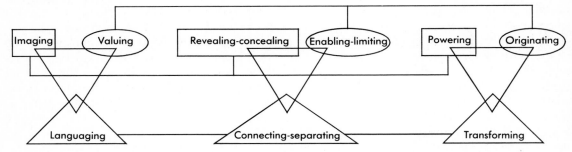

Principle 1: Structuring meaning multidimensionally is cocreating reality through the languaging of valuing and imaging.

Principle 2: Cocreating rhythmical patterns of relating is living the paradoxical unity of revealing-concealing and enabling-limiting while connecting-separating.

Principle 3: Cotranscending with the possibles is powering unique ways of originating in the process of transforming.

Relationship of the concepts in the squares:	*Powering* is a way of *revealing and concealing imaging.*
Relationship of the concepts in the ovals:	*Originating* is a manifestation of *enabling and limiting valuing.*
Relationship of the concepts in the triangles:	*Transforming* unfolds in the *languaging of connecting and separating.*

Figure 15-1. Relationship of principles, concepts, and theoretical structures of Man-Living-Health.

Used with permission from Parse, R.R. (1981). *Man-Living-Health: A theory of nursing.* New York: John Wiley & Sons, p. 69.

tively new and, as Parse indicates, the work is aimed at master's and doctoral nursing students and faculty. Since the model has not yet been integrated into curricula at the baccalaureate level, recent graduates have not been exposed to the model enough to use it in practice. Accounts of the model's use in practice have not yet appeared in the nursing literature, but papers have been presented in the United States and Canada reflecting the testing of the theory in practice.[1,2]

Education

Baccalaureate nursing education is the basis of professional entry into practice and is the appropriate level for the introduction to nursing theory. As previously stated, Parse has designed this model primarily for master's and doctoral students and faculty with the idea that these groups will conduct research to validate the model and use it for curriculum development.

Parse presents a sample master's nursing curriculum in family health nursing incorporating the principles, concepts, and theoretical structures of Man-Living-Health in the components of the curriculum. This process-oriented curriculum is outlined in great detail, including course descriptions and course sequencing, in her text. Consistent with the philosophical origins of this model, two courses in nursing theory are included in the curriculum. For students lacking a strong background in philosophy, a suitable course in philosophy might prove very beneficial. At this time there are no programs using Parse's model as basis for curriculum design.

Research

Parse invites empirical verification of her model. She has outlined three theoretical structures to be studied in relation to this model. Parse states the model has been verified by descriptive methodologies, consistent with the belief system espoused by this model. The model is in evolution, and empirical testing in research and practice of the relationships are leading to revision of the model. With further development and a research methodology designed particularly for Man-Living-Health, this model has potential to explain and describe lived experiences.

FURTHER DEVELOPMENT

This model will be further developed through testing of relationships in practice and research. The abstract concepts of this model are difficult to understand. If nursing continues to build theory from these origins, suitable education in the area of philosophy is necessary as a foundation.

The testing of relationships will lead to refinement of the concepts, identification of existing relationships, and perhaps higher levels of theory development. Curricula based on this model will educate nurses who will use it in practice settings. The usefulness of this model in practice will be recognized through nursing's ability to give guidance to clients and their families in the changing health process.

CRITIQUE

Man-Living-Health is a very complex, abstract conceptual model. The concepts and relationships presented in Parse's work have been empirically verified in research. Thus, the work fits the definition of a formal model that is a theory.

Simplicity

The major concepts are defined, but in highly abstract and philosophical terms, as all concepts in theories should be. The numerous quotations frequently complicate an understanding of the concepts. Some concepts, such as valuing, imaging, and languaging, are easy to understand. However, other concepts, such as powering with the underlying rhythm of push-resisting and originating with the underlying rhythms of conformity-nonconformity and certainty-uncertainty, are more complex and diffi-

cult to understand. The examples given in the text are simple and understandable, perhaps too simple to convey the complexity inherent in this model. The principles and theoretical structures identified by Parse outline clearly the relationships she perceives to exist.

This model has potential for description, but does not explain, predict, or control. Nursing is identified as a scientific discipline. The related terminology of existential-phenomenological thought is not present in the vocabulary of most nurses, making it easy for one to become lost in the rhetoric.

Generality

The framework of this model is broad in scope and could be applicable for families in change or crisis. The model deals with the discipline of nursing and does not focus on nursing as a concept equal to health and Man-Environment. Because the model purports to describe and not predict or control, its generalizability is limited. The model does not address biological dissonance or any other particular attribute of man. This is consistent with the assumptions. Parse addresses man individually in the concepts and points to man's responsibility for choosing lived values. Thus it is applicable to all settings.

Empirical Precision

The concepts in this model are defined in a highly abstract manner and are denotative. Although the concepts are highly theoretical and philosophical, in reality they are potentially observable through the application of knowledge and expertise of prepared nurses. Parse's model stimulates thinking regarding debatable issues applicable to nursing practice.

Derivable Consequences

Parse presents a model based in the human sciences, in contrast to most nursing models, which parallel the medical model. With increased consumer awareness and emphasis in society on health promotion and the quality of life, Parse's emphasis upon man's participation in health experiences and accepting responsibility for health is timely. Parse clearly outlines her intentions for the model in education and research, but because of the complex vocabulary and deep philosophical origins, it may be some time before the model moves from the academic setting to the practice setting.

The model deals with humanity at all times, but does not explicitly address the caring concept central to nursing. Because the model itself centers on man's health, it is specific to nursing.

REFERENCES

1. Magan, S. (1983, Oct. 15; 1984, Jan. 28; 1985, Aug. 22-23). *Mobilizing energies in the structuring of meaning of changing health patterns.* Unpublished paper presented at Nursing Science Symposium, Pittsburgh, Penn.; Dayton, Ohio; Nurse Theorist Conference, Edmunton, Alberta, Canada.
2. Magan, S. (1984, Sept. 22). *Shifting rhythms in changing health patterns.* Unpublished paper presented at Nursing Science Symposium, Pittsburgh, Penn.
3. Parse, R.R. (1981). Caring from a human science perspective. In M.M. Leininger, *Caring: An essential human need.* Thorofare, N.J.: Charles B. Slack, Inc.
4. Parse, R.R. (1981). *Man-Living-Health: A theory of nursing.* New York: John Wiley & Sons.
5. Parse, R.R. (1978). Rights of medical patients. In C. Fisher, *Client participation in human services.* New Brunswick: N.J.: Transaction.
6. Parse, R.R. (1974). *Nursing fundamentals.* Flushing, N.Y.: Medical Examination.
7. Parse, R.R., Coyne, A.B., & Smith, M.J. (1985). *Nursing research: Qualitative methods.* Bowie, Md.: Robert J. Brady.

BIBLIOGRAPHY
Primary Sources
Books

Parse, R.R. (1974). *Nursing fundamentals.* Flushing, N.Y.: Medical Examination.
Parse, R.R. (1981). *Man-Living-Health: A theory of nursing.* New York: John Wiley & Sons.
Parse, R.R., Coyne, A.B., & Smith, M.J. (1985). *Nursing research: Qualitative methods.* Bowie, Md.: Robert J. Brady.

Book Chapters

Parse, R.R. (1978). Rights of medical patients. In C. Fisher, *Client participation in human services.* New Brunswick, N.J.: Transaction.
Parse, R.R. (1981). Caring from a human science perspective. In M.M. Leininger (Ed.), *Caring: An essential human need.* Thorofare, N.J.: Charles B. Slack, Inc.

Articles

Parse, R.R. (1967, Aug.). The advantages of the ADN program. *Journal of Nursing Education, 6:*15.

Secondary Sources
Book Reviews

Parse, R.R. (1975). *Nursing fundamentals.* *Australian Nurses Journal, 5:*37, August, 1975.
Parse, R.R. (1982). *Man-Living-Health: A theory of nursing.* *Western Journal of Nursing Research, 5:*105-106, Winter 1982.

Books

Chinn, P.L., & Jacobs, M.K. (1983). *Theory and nursing: A systematic approach.* St. Louis: C.V. Mosby.

Book Chapters

Winkler, S.J. (1983). Parse's theory of nursing. In J.J. Fitzpatrick & A.L. Whall, *Conceptual models of nursing: Analysis and application* Bowie, Md.: Robert J. Brady.

Unpublished Papers

Magan, S. (1983, Oct. 15; 1984, Jan. 28; 1985, Aug. 22-23). *Mobilizing energies in the structuring of meaning of changing health patterns.* Presented at Nursing Science Symposium, Pittsburgh, Penn.; Dayton, Ohio; Nurse Theorist Conference, Edmunton, Alberta, Canada.
Magan, S. (1984, Sept. 22). *Shifting rhythms in changing health patterns.* Presented at Nursing Science Symposium, Pittsburgh, Penn.

Other Sources

Heidegger, M. (1962). *Being and time.* New York: Harper & Row.
Heidegger, M. (1972). *On time and being.* New York: Harper & Row.

Merleau-Ponty, M. (1963). *The structure of behavior.* Boston: Beacon Press.

Merleau-Ponty, M. (1973). *The prose of the world.* Evanston, Ill.: Northwestern University Press.

Merleau-Ponty, M. (1974). *Phenomenology of perception.* New York: Humanities Press.

Rogers, M.E. (1961). *Educational revolution in nursing.* New York: Macmillan.

Rogers, M.E. (1970). *An introduction to the theoretical basis of nursing.* Philadelphia: F.A. Davis.

Sartre, J.P. (1964). *Nausea.* New York: New Dimensions.

Sartre, J.P. (1966). *Being and nothing.* New York: Washington Square.

Stevens, B.J. (1984). *Nursing theory: Analysis, application, evaluation.* Boston: Little, Brown.

UNIT III

Interpersonal Relationships

Hildegard E. Peplau

16

Psychodynamic Nursing

Elizabeth T. Carey, LyNette Rasmussen, Bryn Searcy, Nancy L. Stark

CREDENTIALS AND BACKGROUND OF THE THEORIST

Hildegard E. Peplau was born September 1, 1909, in Reading, Pennsylvania. She graduated from Pottstown, Pennsylvania, Hospital School of Nursing in 1931. She received a B.A. in interpersonal psychology from Bennington College, Vermont, in 1943, an M.A. in psychiatric nursing from Teachers College, Columbia, New York, in 1947, and an Ed.D. in curriculum development from Columbia in 1953.[2]

The authors wish to express appreciation to Hildegard E. Peplau for critiquing the chapter.

Peplau's professional and teaching experiences have been broad and varied. She was operating room supervisor at Pottstown Hospital, and later headed the staff of the Bennington infirmary while pursuing her undergraduate degree. She did clinical work at Bellevue and Chestnut Lodge psychiatric facilities and was in contact with renowned psychiatrists Freida Fromm-Riechman and Harry Stack Sullivan. A member of the Army Nurse Corps during World War II, she worked in a neuropsychiatric hospital in London.

After obtaining her master's degree at Columbia, she was invited to develop and teach in the graduate program in psychiatric nursing. She remained on the faculty 5 years. In 1954

Peplau went to Rutgers, where she developed and chaired the graduate psychiatric nursing program until her retirement in 1974.[10]

Peplau's contribution to nursing and the specialty of psychiatric nursing has been enormous, beginning in 1952 with her book *Interpersonal Relations in Nursing*. Throughout the 1950s and 1960s she conducted workshops, "abundantly sharing her knowledge and clinical skills . . . [and] encouraging nurses to use their competence . . . in a continuous, experiential and educative process."[25;31:123] She analyzed verbatim notes of sessions with medical and psychiatric patients to develop numerous lectures, articles, and workshops. She has maintained a part-time private practice since 1960 and has given many lectures throughout the United States, Canada, Africa, and South America. During the 1970s William E. Field, Jr., took copious notes on the numerous lectures Peplau delivered to psychiatric nurses. He published them for his mentor in *The Psychotherapy of Hildegard E. Peplau*.

In 1969 Peplau became executive director of the American Nurses' Association. She served as president of the ANA from 1970-1972, and as second vice-president from 1972-1974.[28] She has also served as director of the New Jersey State Nurses' Association; a member of the Expert Advisory Council of WHO; the National Nurse Consultant to the Surgeon General of the Air Force; and a nursing consultant to the United States Public Health Services, the National Institute of Mental Health, and various foreign countries.[2] She chaired the editorial board of *Perspectives in Psychiatric Care* when the journal was founded and served as chief advisor of *Nursing 74*.

Peplau's archives are deposited in the Arthur and Elizabeth Schlesinger Library on the History of Women in America, Radcliffe College, Cambridge, Massachusetts.

THEORETICAL SOURCES

The nature of science in nursing refers to the "body of verified knowledge found within the discipline of nursing . . . [that is] mainly knowledge from the biological and behavioral sciences."[1:35] The "synthesis, reorganization, or extension of concepts drawn from the basic and applied sciences, which in their reformation tend to become new concepts," has led to the growth of nursing science.[14:292] Thus, the evolution of Peplau's theory of interpersonal relations resulted.

Peplau used knowledge borrowed from behavioral science and what can be termed the *psychological model*. Borrowing from the psychological model "enabled the nurse to begin to move away from a disease orientation to one whereby the psychologic meaning of events, feelings, and behaviors could be explored and incorporated into nursing interventions. It gave nurses an opportunity to teach patients how to experience their feelings and to explore with clients how to bear their feelings."[27:6] The conceptual framework of interpersonal relations seeks to develop the nurse's skill in using these concepts. Harry Stack Sullivan,[34] Percival Symonds,[35] Abraham Maslow,[17] and Neal Elgar Miller[18] are some of the major sources Peplau used in developing her conceptual framework. Some of the therapeutic conceptions devised by these theorists arose directly from the works of Freud[7] and Fromm.[8]

Peplau was committed to incorporating established knowledge into her conceptual framework, thus developing a theory-based nursing model. Peplau integrated theories into her model at a time when nursing theory development was relatively new.

USE OF EMPIRICAL EVIDENCE

Theories available when Peplau developed her theory described behavior within the prospectives of psychoanalytic theory, the principles of social learning, the concept of human motivation, and the concept of personality development. Peplau combined the various ideas of Maslow, Sullivan, Miller, and Symonds. These theories were initiated by the genius of Freud, Fromm, and Pavlov.[21]

Freud's hypotheses have been a rich source of research study. He emphasized the importance of motivation, conflict, and the role of the family in early childhood, and discovered the significance of the unconscious. Extensive testing of Freudian principles has been done, and his influence on later theorists' hypotheses is obvious.

Maslow's theory of human motivation is well known, and a great deal of sound research has followed its publication. Maslow[17:371] states, "The present theory must be considered to be a suggested program for future research and must stand or fall, not so much on facts available or evidence presented, as upon research yet to be done."

Miller's work focused on personality theory, adjustment mechanisms, psychotherapy, and principles of social learning. Pavlov's stimulus-response model influenced Miller's principles of social learning. Most of Miller's work consisted of developing hypotheses, the basis for research, rather than proving principles. Miller based his hypotheses on experimental studies.

Sullivan was a pioneer in the field of modern psychiatry. A comprehensive evaluation of Sullivan's work regarding personality development and interpersonal relations was written by Patrick Mullahy in 1945. Sullivan's theoretical positions in *Conceptions of Modern Psychiatry* were tested by the Washington School of Psychiatry, leading to further refinement of his theoretical positions.

MAJOR CONCEPTS AND DEFINITIONS

PSYCHODYNAMIC NURSING. Peplau defines psychodynamic nursing because her model evolves through this type of nursing. "Psychodynamic nursing is being able to understand one's own behavior to help others identify felt difficulties, and to apply principles of human relations to the problems that arise at all levels of experience."[22:xiii]

Peplau develops the model by describing the structural concepts of the interpersonal process,

which are the phases of the nurse-patient relationship, and further defines the role of nurses within the relationship. She holds this to be basic to psychodynamic nursing.

NURSE-PATIENT RELATIONSHIP. Peplau describes four phases of the nurse-patient relationship. Although separate, they overlap and occur over the time of the relationship.

Orientation. During the orientation phase, the individual has a "felt need" and seeks professional assistance. The nurse helps the patient recognize and understand his problem and determine his need for help.[22:18-30]

Identification. The patient identifies with those who can help him (relatedness). The nurse permits exploration of feelings to aid the patient in undergoing illness as an experience that reorients feelings and strengthens positive forces in the personality and provides needed satisfaction.[22:30-37]

Exploitation. During the exploitation phase the patient attempts to derive full value from what is offered him through the relationship. New goals to be achieved through personal effort can be projected, and power shifts from the nurse to the patient as the patient delays gratification to achieve the newly formed goals.[22:37-39]

Resolution. Old goals are gradually put aside and new goals adopted. This is a process in which the patient frees himself from identification with the nurse.[22:39-41]

NURSE-PATIENT RELATIONSHIPS. Peplau[22] describes six different nursing roles that emerge in the various phases of the nurse-patient relationship (Figure 16-1).

Role of the stranger. The first role is the role of the stranger. Peplau states that because the nurse and patient are strangers to each other, the patient should be treated with ordinary

Figure 16-1. Overlapping phases in nurse-patient relationships.
Used with permission from Peplau, H.E. (1952). *Interpersonal relations in nursing.* New York: G.P. Putnam & Sons, p. 21.

courtesy. In other words, the nurse should not prejudge the patient, but accept him as he is. During this nonpersonal phase, the nurse should treat the patient as emotionally able, unless evidence indicates otherwise. This coincides with the identification phase.[22:44-47]

Role of resource person. In the role of the resource person, the nurse provides specific answers to questions, especially health information, and interprets to the patient the treatment or medical plan of care. These questions often arise within the context of a larger problem. The nurse determines what type of response is appropriate for constructive learning, either straightforward factual answers or providing counseling.[22:47-48]

Teaching role. The teaching role is a combination of all roles and "always proceeds from what the patient knows and . . . develops around his interest in wanting and ability to use . . . information."[22:48]

Peplau[24] expands on the role of teacher in later writings. She separates teaching into two categories: *instructional,* which consists largely of giving information and is the form explained in educational literature, and *experiential,* which

is "using the experience of the learner as a basis from which learning products are developed."[24:98] The products of learning are generalizations and appraisals the patient makes about his experiences. This concept of learning used in the teaching role overlaps with the nurse counselor role, because the concept of learning is carried out through psychotherapeutic techniques.[24]

Leadership role. The leadership role involves the democratic process. The nurse helps the patient meet the tasks at hand through a relationship of cooperation and active participation.[22:49-51]

Surrogate role. The patient casts the nurse in the surrogate role. The nurse's attitudes and behaviors create *feeling tones* in the patient that reactivate feelings generated in a prior relationship. The nurse's function is to assist the patient in recognizing similarities between herself and the person recalled by the patient. She then helps the patient see the differences in her role and that of the recalled person. In this phase, both patient and nurse define areas of dependence, independence, and finally interdependence.[22:51-61]

Counseling role. Peplau believes the counseling role has the greatest emphasis in psychiatric nursing.[25] Counseling functions in the nurse-patient relationship by the way nurses respond to patient demands. Peplau[22:64] says the purpose of interpersonal techniques is to help "the patient remember and understand fully what is happening to him in the present situation, so that the experience can be integrated rather than dissociated from other experiences in life" (Figure 16-2).

PSYCHOBIOLOGICAL EXPERIENCES. Peplau describes four psychobiological experiences: needs, frustration, conflict, and anxiety. These experiences provide energy that is transformed into some form of action. Peplau uses nonnurs-

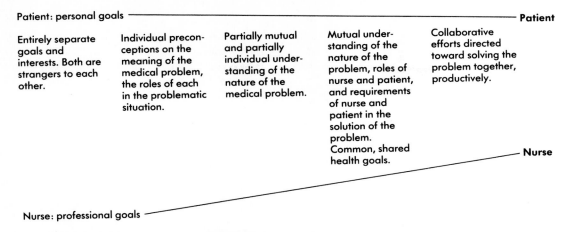

Figure 16-2. Continuum showing changing aspects of nurse-patient relations.
Used with permission from Peplau, H.E. (1952). *Interpersonal relations in nursing*. New York: G.P. Putnam & Sons, p. 10.

ing theoretical concepts to identify and explain these experiences that compel destructive or constructive responses from nurses and patients. This understanding provides a basis for goal formation and nursing interventions.[22]

MAJOR ASSUMPTIONS

Peplau[22:xii] identifies two explicit assumptions:

1. The kind of person the nurse becomes makes a substantial difference in what each patient will learn as he receives nursing care.
2. Fostering personality development toward maturity is a function of nursing and nursing education. Nursing uses principles and methods that guide the process toward resolution of interpersonal problems.

One implicit assumption was, "The nursing profession has legal responsibility for the effective use of nursing and for its consequences to patients."[22:6]

Nursing

Nursing is described as "a significant, therapeutic, interpersonal process. It functions coopera-

tively with other human processes that make health possible for individuals in communities." When professional health teams offer health services, nurses participate in the organization of conditions that facilitate natural ongoing tendencies in human organisms. "Nursing is an educative instrument, a maturing force that aims to promote forward movement of personality in the direction of creative, constructive, productive, personal, and community living."[22:16]

Person

Peplau defines person in terms of man. Man is an organism that lives in an unstable equilibrium.[22:82]

Health

Peplau defines health as "a word symbol that implies forward movement of personality and other ongoing human processes in the direction of creative, constructive, productive, personal, and community living."[22:12]

Environment

Peplau[22:163] implicitly defines the environment in terms of "existing forces outside the organism and in the context of culture," from which mores, customs, and beliefs are acquired. "However, general conditions that are likely to lead to health always include the interpersonal process."[22:14]

THEORETICAL ASSERTIONS

Peplau makes theoretical relationships throughout her book. In summarizing these relationships, Peplau addresses the patient-nurse relationship, the patient and his awareness of feelings, and the nurse and her awareness of feelings. She presents nursing as a maturing educative force that uses the experiential learning method for both patient and nurse (Figure 16-3).

LOGICAL FORM

The process Peplau uses is an inductive approach to theory building. Empirical generalizations are inductively established. "Induction is a type of relationship in which . . . one observes empirical events and generalizes from specific events to all similar events."[13:7] According to Peplau,[26:36] "Nursing situations provide a field of observations from which unique nurs-

ing concepts can be derived and used for the improvement of the professional's work." The selected concepts Peplau uses are organized into a larger component, forming relationships that are logical and complete. The relationships describe behaviors that occur in the nurse-patient interaction.

ACCEPTANCE BY THE NURSING COMMUNITY
Practice

Grace Sills[31:123] recalls Peplau brought "a new perspective, a new approach, a theoretically based foundation for nursing practice for therapeutic work with patients." She states, "Peplau's work is responsible for a second order change in the nursing culture."[31:123] Peplau's ideas provided a design for the practice of psychiatric nursing with explication of the design in usable form.

Some of Peplau's ideas were not accepted in the early years, such as the concept of experiential learning for the patient and students.[31] In a panel discussion on psychotherapeutic strategies Mertz, Mereness, and Mellow disagreed with Peplau on the methodology of psychotherapeutic functions and the role of nurse as

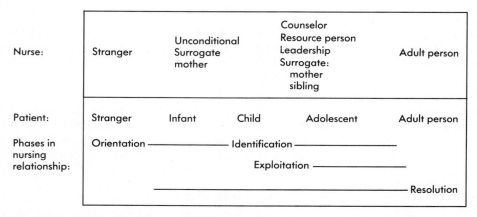

Figure 16-3. Phases and changing roles in nurse-patient relationships.
Used with permission from Peplau, H.E. (1952). *Interpersonal relations in nursing*. New York: G.P. Putnam & Sons, p. 54.

surrogate.[29] Later criticisms of Peplau's model indicate the lack of development of social systems that would broaden the knowledge base for understanding the patient's problem.

Peplau[22] used the interpersonal and intrapersonal theories of Sullivan and Freud as the theoretical base for her model and did not take into consideration interrelationships between man and society. These concepts were later developed in general systems theory by Ludwig von Bertalanffy.[2] However, systems theory was included in the curriculum of the Rutgers graduate program in psychiatric nursing. In 1968 Peplau began the first workshop on family therapy under a grant from NIMH to the University of New Mexico.

Education

Peplau's book, *Interpersonal Relations in Nursing,* was specifically written as an aid to graduate nurses and nursing students.

There are few early critiques of Peplau's model in the literature. Her model was designed and published in 1952, 1957, and 1962 with a particular emphasis in psychiatric nursing. The specialty journals in psychiatric nursing did not begin publication until 1963, 11 years after her model was first published. However, psychiatric nursing authors did write textbooks. Smoyak and Rouslin state that after 1952 no psychiatric nursing text could ignore Peplau's work. Peplau's impact was reflected in books in the 1950s and 1960s, such as G. Burton's *Personal, Impersonal, and Interpersonal Relations* (1959), Burd and Marshall's *Some Clinical Approaches to Psychiatric Nursing* (1963), Hofling and Leininger's *Basic Psychiatric Concepts in Nursing* (1960), and Orlando's *The Dynamic Nurse-Patient Relationship* (1961), to name but a few. Most comments on Peplau and her work were written 25 or more years after her published model.

Research

Sills[30] states that Peplau's work influenced the direction of clinical work and studies. Initial efforts to use research as a tool to develop a body of nursing knowledge were uneven in quality and quantity, and often did not explicitly recognize underlying assumptions. Early research followed the assumption that patient problems were within-the-person phenomena, and were explored in nurse-patient relationship studies. This followed Peplau's conceptual model. Since the 1960s, research has shifted to "within-the-social-system" point of view, as studies have examined broader sets of relationships.

For more than 30 years Peplau's model has formed the basis for numerous applications of research methods. M.D. Thomas, J.M. Baker, and N.J. Estes[36] used Peplau's concept of anxiety as a means to constructively resolve angry feelings through experiential learning within the nurse-patient relationship. D. Hays[11] described a study teaching the concept of anxiety that is predominantly based on Peplau's concept of anxiety and used her conceptual model. Hays was a Rutgers graduate student in psychiatric nursing and was a student of Peplau's. This study is one example of Peplau's influence on new nursing leaders with graduate education in the field of psychiatric nursing. M. Topf and B. Dambacher[37] interpret the findings in their study using Peplau's role of the nurse as a stranger. A. Garrett, D. Manuel, and C. Vincent[9] cite Peplau's concept of anxiety for their operational definition of stress and its relationship to learning. In a study by F.E. Spring and H. Turk,[33] the authors develop a behavior scale using Peplau's conceptual framework and her assumption that therapeutic behavior in the nurse-patient relationship promotes experiential learning. The authors concluded that their behavior score was objective, reliable, and valid. D. Methven and R.M. Schlotfeldt,[19] who developed a tool to evaluate verbal responses, based their study on Peplau's assumption that therapeutic communication can be used to reduce or redirect anxiety.

Assumptions from Peplau's model continue to be used in current research. La Monica[15] devised an empathy instrument using Peplau's model (and work from other theorists) as a theoretical framework. She states, "The primary goal of nurses . . . is to provide services that assist in moving clients to their optimum health levels . . . and involves a helping relationship."[15:389]

The impact and significance of Peplau's conceptual model can be best described by Suzanne Lego in a thorough discussion of the history, trends, patterns, and assessment of published research that notes the direction of the one-to-one nurse-patient relationship. She states that ambiguity about the nurse-patient relationship

> abruptly ended in the literature as a result of Peplau's *Interpersonal Relations in Nursing* (1952). As she would continue to do for the next 22 years, Dr. Peplau pulled together loose, ambiguous data and put them into systematic, scientific terms that could be tested, applied, and integrated into the practice of psychiatric nursing.[16:68]

Lego states that most of the published literature describing the one-to-one nurse-patient relationship is based on theoretical concepts inspired principally by Peplau.

Peplau makes a significant contribution to the nursing community through the research done to evaluate, validate, and make more precise the Theory of Interpersonal Relations.

FURTHER DEVELOPMENT

As nursing broadens its scope, there appears to be a need for further development of Peplau's theory for use with the healthy patient, group, and community. Further development is also indicated for clients who are unable to effectively use their communication skills. Increased use of Peplau's theory in practice is needed. Continued research is needed to further refine the theory and to build on nursing's knowledge base.

CRITIQUE
Simplicity

The major focus of Peplau's theory, interpersonal relations between patient and nurse, is easily understood. The theory's basic assump-

tions and key concepts are defined. Of the assumptions Peplau listed, two are explicit and one is implicit. Peplau sequentially describes her four phases of the interpersonal process. The roles of the nurse and the four psychobiological experiences are clearly indicated. Her logic is based on inductive reasoning. Ideas are taken from observations of the specific and applied to the general. Peplau draws from other disciplines' theories. She is consistent with established theories and principles, such as those of Sullivan, Freud, and Maslow. Peplau deals with the relationships of the interpersonal process, nurse, patient, and psychobiological experiences. Each of these relationships is then developed, within the theory, in an understandable way. Thus, Peplau's theory can be described as meeting the evaluative quality of simplicity.

Generality

In meeting the criteria of generality, Peplau[22] states, "While clinical situations are stressed, any nurse can apply principles that are presented in any other interpersonal relationship in any other area of living." The one drawback to the theory's generality is an interpersonal relationship must exist. The theory is adaptable only to nursing settings where there can be communication between the patient and nurse. Its use is limited in working with the comatose, senile, and newborn patient. In such situations, the nurse-patient relationship is often one-sided. The nurse and patient cannot work together to become more knowledgeable, develop goals, and mature. Even Peplau[22:41] admits, "Understanding of the meaning of the experience to the patient is required in order for nursing to function as an educative, therapeutic, maturing force." Since Peplau's theory cannot be applied to all patients, the quality of generality is not met.

Empirical Precision

Peplau provides us with a theory based on reality. The relationship between the theory and empirical data allows for validation and verification of the theory by other scientists. The definitions described by Peplau are in a middle range on a connotative-denotative continuum. Peplau operationally defines the four phases of the interpersonal process, the nurse with regard to her roles, and the patient with regard to his state of dependence. According to Duffey and Mullencamp,[5:573] "Peplau relates behavior to theory by naming and categorizing, operationalizing definitions of behavior, thematic abstractions of interaction phenomena, and diagnosis of problems and principles guiding nursing interactions." Peplau's theory can be considered empirically precise. With further research and development the degree of precision will increase.

Derivable Consequences

In historical perspective, Peplau is one of the first theorists since Nightingale to present a theory for nursing. Therefore her work can be considered pioneering in the nursing field. "She provided nursing with a meaningful method of self-directed practice at a time when medicine dominated the health-care field."[6:44]

Peplau's work, thoughts, and ideas have touched many nurses, from students to practitioners. Although her book was published in 1952, more than three decades ago, it continues to provide direction for nursing practice, education, and research. Peplau's work has provided a significant contribution to nursing's knowledge base. The evaluative criteria of derivable consequences are unquestionably met.

REFERENCES

1. Andreoli, R.G., & Thompson, C.E. (1977, June). The nature of science in nursing. *Image 9*(2):32-37.
2. Belcher, J.R., & Fish, L.J. (1980). Hildegard E. Peplau. In Nursing Theories Conference Group, J.B. George, Chairperson, *Nursing theories: The base for professional nursing practice*. Englewood Cliffs, N.J.: Prentice-Hall.
3. Burd, S.F. (1963). The development of an operational definition using the process of learning as a guide. In S.F. Burd, & A. Marshall (Eds.), *Some clinical approaches to psychiatric nursing*. New York: Macmillan.
4. Burton, G. (1958). Personal, impersonal, and interpersonal relations. Cited by S.A. Smoyak, & S. Rouslin (Eds.) (1982), *A collection of classics in psychiatric nursing literature*. Thorofare, N.J.: Charles B. Slack.
5. Duffey, M., & Mullencamp, A.F. (1974, Sept.). A framework for theory analysis. *Nursing Outlook, 22*:570-574.
6. Fitzpatrick, J.J., & Whall, A.L. (1983). *Conceptual models of nursing, analysis and application*. Bowie, Md.: Robert J. Brady.
7. Freud, S. (1936). The problem of anxiety. In H.E. Peplau, (1952), *Interpersonal relations in nursing*. New York: G.B. Putnam's Sons.
8. Fromm, E. (1947). Man for himself. Cited by H.E. Peplau, (1952), *Interpersonal relations in nursing*. New York: G.B. Putnam's Sons.
9. Garrett, A., Manuel, D., & Vincent, C. (1976, Nov.). Stressful experiences identified by student nurses. *Journal of Nursing Education, 15*(6):9-21.
10. Gregg, D.E. (1978). Hildegard E. Peplau: Her contributions. *Psychiatry Care, 16*:118-121.
11. Hays, D. (1961, Spring). Teaching a concept of anxiety. *Nursing Research, 10*(2):108-113.
12. Hofling, C.K., & Leininger, M.M. (1960). Basic psychiatric concepts in nursing. Cited by S.A. Smoyak, & S. Rouslin (Eds.), (1982), *A collection of classics in psychiatric nursing literature*. Thorofare, N.J.: Charles B. Slack.
13. Jacox, A. (1974, Jan.-Feb.). Theory construction in nursing: An overview. *Nursing Research, 23*:4-12.
14. Johnson, D.E. (1959). The nature of a science of nursing. *Nursing Outlook, 7*:292.
15. LaMonica, E. (1981). Construct validity of an empathy instrument. *Research in Nursing and Health, 4*:389-400.
16. Lego, S. (1980). The one-to-one nurse-patient relationship. *Perspectives in Psychiatric Care, 18*(2):67-89. (Reprinted from *Psychiatric nursing 1946-1974: A report on the state of the art*. American Journal of Nursing Co.)
17. Maslow, A.H., & Mittleman, B. (1941). *Principles in abnormal psychology*. New York: Harper & Brothers.
18. Miller, N.E., & Dollard, J. (1941). *Social learning and initiation*. New Haven, Conn.: Yale University Press.

19. Methven, D., & Schlotfeldt, R.M. (1962, Spring). The social interaction inventory. *Nursing Research, 11*(2):83-88.
20. Orlando, I. (1961). The dynamic nurse-patient relationship. Cited by S.A. Smoyak, & S. Rousin (Eds.) (1982), *A collection of classics in psychiatric nursing literature.* Thorofare, N.J.: Charles B. Slack.
21. Pavlov, I. (1927). *Conditioned reflexes: An investigation of the physiological activity of the cerebral cortex.* London: Oxford University Press.
22. Peplau, H.E. (1952). *Interpersonal relations in nursing.* New York: G.P. Putnam's Sons.
23. Peplau, H.E. (1964). *Basic principles of patient counseling* (2nd ed.). Philadelphia: Smith, Kline, & French Laboratories.
24. Peplau, H.E. (1957). Therapeutic concepts. In S.A. Smoyak, & S. Rouslin, (Eds.), (1982), *A collection of classics in psychiatric nursing literature.* Thorofare, N.J.: Charles B. Slack. (Reprinted from National League of Nursing League Exchange No. 26: Aspects of psychiatric nursing.)
25. Peplau, H.E. (1962). Interpersonal techniques: The crux of psychiatric nursing. *American Journal of Nursing, 62*:629-633.
26. Peplau, H.E. (1969). Theory: The professional dimension. In C. Norris (Ed.), *Proceedings of the first nursing theory conference.* Kansas City, Kansas, University of Kansas Medical Center, Dept. of Nursing Education.
27. Phillips, J.R. (1977, Feb.). Nursing systems and nursing models. *Image, 9*(1):6.
28. Profile 1974, Feb. *Nursing 74, 4*:13.
29. Psychotherapeutic strategies (1968). Current concepts in psychiatric care: The implications for psychiatric nursing practice. Proceedings of the Institute on Psychiatric Nursing, cosponsored by Yale School of Nursing, Department of Psychiatric Nursing and the Community Mental Health Center Department of Nursing. In *Perspectives of Psychiatric Care, 6*(6):271-289.
30. Sills, G.M. (1977, May-June). Research in the field of psychiatric nursing 1952-1977. *Nursing Research, 28*(3):201-207.
31. Sills, G.M. (1978). Hildegard E. Peplau: Leader, practitioner, academician, scholar, and theorist. *Perspectives in Psychiatric Care, 16*(3):122-128.
32. Smoyak, S.A., & Rouslin, S. (Eds.) (1982). Introduction. *A collection of classics in psychiatric nursing literature.* Thorofare, N.J.: Charles B. Slack.
33. Spring, F.E., & Turk, H. (1962, Fall). A therapeutic behavior scale. *Nursing Research, 11*(4):214-218.
34. Sullivan, H.S. (1947). Conceptions of modern psychiatry. Cited by H.E. Peplau (1952), in *Interpersonal relations in nursing.* New York: G.P. Putnam's Sons.
35. Symonds, P. (1946). *The dynamics of human adjustments.* New York: Appleton-Century-Crofts.
36. Thomas, M.D., Baker, J.M., & Estes, N.J. (1970, Dec.). Anger: A tool for developing self-awareness. *American Journal of Nursing, 70*(12):2586-2590.
37. Topf, M., & Dambacher, B. (1979). Predominant source of interpersonal influence in relationships between psychiatric patients and nursing staff. *Research in Nursing and Health, 2*(1):35-43.
38. von Bertalanffy, L. (1968). *General systems theory: Foundations, development, applications.* New York: G. Braziller.

BIBLIOGRAPHY
Primary Sources
Books

Peplau, H.E. (1952). *Interpersonal relations in nursing.* New York: G.P. Putnam & Sons.
Peplau, H.E. (1964). *Basic principles of patient counseling* (2nd ed.). Philadelphia: Smith, Kline, & French Laboratories.

Book Chapters

Peplau, H.E. (1969). Theory: The professional dimension. In C. Norris, (Ed.), *Proceedings of the first nursing theory conference,* (March 21-28). University of Kansas Medical Center, Dept. of Nursing Education, Kansas City.

Articles

Peplau, H.E. (1942, Oct.). Health program at Bennington College. *Public Health Nursing, 34* (10):573-575, 581.
Peplau, H.E. (1947, May). Discussion: A democratic participation technique. *American Journal of Nursing, 47*(5):334-336.
Peplau, H.E. (1951, Dec.). Toward new concepts in nursing and nursing education. *American Journal of Nursing, 51*(12):722-724.

Peplau, H.E. (1952, Dec.). The psychiatric nurses' family group. *American Journal of Nursing,* 52(12):1475-1477.

Peplau, H.E. (1953, Feb.). The nursing team in psychiatric facilities. *Nursing Outlook,* 1(2):90-92.

Peplau, H.E. (1953, Oct.). Themes in nursing situations: Power. *American Journal of Nursing,* 53(10):1221-1223.

Peplau, H.E. (1953, Nov.). Themes in nursing situations: Safety. *American Journal of Nursing,* 53(11):1343-1346.

Peplau, H.E. (1955, Dec.). Loneliness. *American Journal of Nursing,* 55(12):1476-1481.

Peplau, H.E. (1956). Discussion. The League Exchange No. 18: *Psychology and psychiatric nursing research,* pp. 20-22.

Peplau, H.E. (1956, Spring). Present day trends in psychiatric nursing. *Neuropsychiatry,* 111(4):190-204.

Peplau, H.E. (1956, July 8). An undergraduate program in psychiatric nursing. *Nursing Outlook,* 4:400-410.

Peplau, H.E. (1957, July). What is experiential teaching? *American Journal of Nursing,* 57(7):884-886.

Peplau, H.E. (1958). Educating the nurse to function in psychiatric services. *Nursing Personnel for Mental Health Programs,* Southern Regional Educational Board, Atlanta, Ga., pp. 37-42.

Peplau, H.E. (1958, Sept.). Public health nurses promote mental health. *Public Health Reports,* 73(9):828.

Peplau, H.E. (1960). Talking with patients. *American Journal of Nursing,* 60:964-967.

Peplau, H.E. (1960, Jan.). Must laboring together be called teamwork? Problems in team treatment of adults in state mental hospitals. *American Journal of Orthopsychiatry,* 30:103-108.

Peplau, H.E. (1960, March). A personal responsibility: A discussion of anxiety in mental health. *Rutgers Alumni Monthly,* pp. 14-16.

Peplau, H.E. (1960, May). Anxiety in the mother-infant relationship. *Nursing World,* 134(5):33-34.

Peplau, H.E. (1962). The crux of psychiatric nursing. *American Journal of Nursing,* 62:50-54.

Peplau, H.E. (1963). An approach to research in psychiatric nursing. *Training for Clinical Research in Psychiatric-Mental Health Nursing.* The Catholic University of America, pp. 5-44.

Peplau, H.E. (1963, Oct.-Nov.). Interpersonal relations and the process of adaptations. *Nursing Science,* 1(4):272-279.

Peplau, H.E. (1964). Psychiatric nursing skills and the general hospital patient. *Nursing Forum, III,* (2):28-37.

Peplau, H.E. (1964, Nov.). Professional and social behavior: Some differences worth the notice of professional nurses. *Quarterly,* 50(4):23-33. (Published by the Columbia University-Presbyterian Hospital School of Nursing Alumni Association, New York.)

Peplau, H.E. (1965). The 91st day: A challenge to professional nursing. *Perspectives in Psychiatric Care, III*(2):20-24.

Peplau, H.E. (1965, April). The heart of nursing: Interpersonal relations. *Canadian Nurse,* 61(4):273-275.

Peplau, H.E. (1965, Aug.). Specialization in professional nursing. *Nursing Science,* 3(4):268-287.

Peplau, H.E. (1965, Nov.). The nurse in the community mental health program. *Nursing Outlook,* 13(11):68-70.

Peplau, H.E. (1966). Nurse-doctor relationships. *Nursing Forum,* 5(1):60-75.

Peplau, H.E. (1966). Nursing's two routes to doctoral degrees. *Nursing Forum,* 5(2):57-67.

Peplau, H.E. (1966, March-April). An interpretation of the ANA position. *NJSNA-News Letter,* 22(2):6-10.

Peplau, H.E. (1966, May-June). Trends in nursing and nursing education. *NJSNA-News Letter,* 22(3):17-27.

Peplau, H.E. (1967, Feb.). The work of psychiatric nurses. *Psychiatric Opinion,* 4(1):5-11.

Peplau, H.E. (1967, Nov.). Interpersonal relations and the work of the industrial nurse. *Industrial Nurse Journal,* 15(10):7-12.

Peplau, H.E. (1968). Psychotherapeutic strategies. *Perspectives in Psychiatric Care, VI*(6):264-289.

Peplau, H.E. (1969). Professional closeness as a special kind of involvement with a patient, client, or family group. *Nursing Forum,* 8(4):342-360.

Peplau, H.E. (1969, Fall). The American Nurses' Association and nursing education. *Utah Nurse,* 20(3):6.

Peplau, H. (1970, Jan.) ANA's new executive director states her views. *American Journal of Nursing,* 70:84-88.

Peplau, H.E. (1970, Summer). Professional closeness as a special kind of involvement with a patient, client or family group. *Comprehensive Nurse Quarterly*, 5(3):66-81.

Peplau, H. (1970, Nov.-Dec.). Changed patterns of practice. *Washington State Journal of Nursing*, 42:4-6.

Peplau, H.E. (1970, Nov.-Dec.). Keynote address at the 68th annual convention of the New Jersey state nurses' association. *New Jersey Nurse*, 26:3-10.

Peplau, H.E. (1970, Dec.). ANA: Who needs it? *Nursing News*, 43:5-8.

Peplau, H.E. (1970, Dec.). What it means to be a professional nurse today. *Alabama Nurse*, 24:8-17.

Peplau, H.E. (1970, Dec.). The road ahead. *Maine Nurse*, 1(3):3-8.

Peplau, H.E. (1971, Jan.). ANA: Who needs it? *Nursing News*, 44(1):12-14.

Peplau, H.E. (1971). Dilemmas of organizing nurses. *Image*, 4:4-8.

Peplau, H.E. (1971, Spring). In support of nursing research. *Journal of the New York State Nurses' Association*, 2:5.

Peplau, H.E. (1971, Summer). Time of decision. *Nevada Nurses' Association Quarterly Newsletter*, pp. 1-3.

Peplau, H.E. (1971, July). Responsibility, authority, evaluation, and accountability of nursing in patient care. *Michigan Nurse*, 44:5-7.

Peplau, H.E. (1971, Sept.). The task ahead. *American Journal of Nursing*, 71:1800-1802.

Peplau, H. (1971, Nov.). The now nurse in nursing: Some problems of diversity. *Oklahoma Nurse*, 46:1.

Peplau, H.E. (1971, Nov.). What it means to be a professional nurse in today's society. *Kansas Nurse*, 46:1-3.

Peplau, H.E. (1971, Winter). Communication in crisis intervention. *Psychiatric Forum*, 2:1-7.

Peplau, H.E. (1971, Winter). Where do we go from here? *Pelican News*, 27:14-16.

Peplau, H.E. (1972, Spring). The nurse's role in health care delivery systems. *Pelican News*, 28:12-14.

Peplau, H.E. (1972, May). The independence of nursing. *Imprint*, 9:11.

Peplau, H.E. (1972, June). The president challenges nurses in address to delegates. *Kansas Nurse*, pp. 2-4.

Peplau, H.E. (1972, Nov.-Dec.) Some issues and developments that should be of concern to nurses. *New Jersey State Nurses' Association News*, 2:14-16.

Peplau, H.E. (1973, July). Meeting the challenge. *Mississippi RN*, 35:1-6.

Peplau, H.E. (1974). Creativity and commitment in nursing, *Image* 6:3-5.

Peplau, H.E. (1974). Is health care a right? Affirmative response. *Image*, 7:4-10.

Peplau, H.E. (1974, Jan.). Nurses: Collaborate or isolate. *Pennsylvania Nurse*, 29:2-5.

Peplau, H.E. (1974, Autumn). Talking with patients. *Comprehensive Nursing Quarterly*, 9(3):30-39.

Peplau, H.E. (1975, March-April). An open letter to a new graduate. *Nursing Digest*, 3:36-37.

Peplau, H.E. (1975, Oct.). Interview with Dr. Peplau: Future of nursing. *Japanese Journal of Nursing*, 39(10:1046-1050.

Peplau, H.E. (1975, Oct.). Midlife crisis. *American Journal of Nursing*, 75:1761-1765.

Peplau, H.E., et al. (1976, Aug.). What future for nursing? *AORN*, 24: 217-235.

Peplau, H.E. (1977, March-April). The changing view of nursing. *International Nursing Review*, 24:43-45.

Peplau, H.E. (1978, March-April). Psychiatric nursing: Role of nurses and psychiatric nurses. *International Nursing Review*, 25:41-47.

Peplau, H.E. (1980, April). New statement defines scope of practice. *American Nurse*, 12(4):1,8, 24.

Peplau, H. (1980, May-June). The psychiatric nurses: Accountable? to whom? for what? *Perspectives in Psychiatric Care*, 18:128-134.

Peplau, H.E. (1982, Aug.). Some reflections on earlier days in psychiatric nursing. *Journal of Psychosocial Nursing Mental Health Services*, 20:17-24.

Peplau, H.E. (1984, Jan.-Feb.). Internal versus external regulation, *New Jersey Nurse*, 14:12-14.

Peplau, H.E. (1985, Feb.). Is nursing self-regulatory power being eroded *American Journal of Nursing*, 85(2):140-143.

Chapters, Pamphlets, Proceedings, Reports.

Peplau, H.E. (1951). *Understanding ourselves*. Fifty-seventh annual report, National League for Nursing Education.

Peplau, H.E. (1952). *The responsibility of professional nursing in psychiatry*. Fifty-eighth annual report, National League for Nursing Education.

Peplau, H.E. (1954, Sept. 15). *Some problems of the psychiatric nursing team*. Second Annual Psychiatric Institute, New Jersey Neuropsychiatric Institute, Proceedings.

Peplau, H.E. (1956). *The yearbook of modern nursing.* New York: G.P. Putnam's Sons.

Peplau, H.E. (1958, June). Current concepts of psychiatric nursing care. *ANA Proceedings.*

Peplau, H.E. (1959). Principles of psychiatric nursing. In *American Handbook of Psychiatry* (Vol. II). New York: Basic Books.

Peplau, H.E. (1960). Ward atmosphere: Cliche or task? In *Nursing papers.* Illinois State Psychiatric Institute.

Peplau, H.E. (1962). Will automation change the nurse, nursing, or both? *Technical Innovations in Health Care: Nursing Implications* (Pamphlet 5). New York: American Nurses' Association.

Peplau, H.E. (1963). Counseling in nursing practice. In E. Harms, & P. Schreiber (Eds.), *Handbook of Counseling Techniques.* New York: Pergamon.

Peplau, H.E. (1963). Leadership responsibility in toleration of stress: The leader's role in helping staff to tolerate stress. In *Conferences on preparation for leadership in psychiatric nursing service.* Department of Nursing Education, Teachers College, Columbia University, New York.

Peplau, H.E. (1963, Dec. 2-3). A personal challenge for immediate action. In AHA Conference Group in Psychiatric Nursing Practice, National Institute, *Proceedings,* Kansas City.

Peplau, H.E. (1967). Psychiatric nursing. In A.M. Freedman and A.I. Kaplan (Eds.), *Comprehensive textbook of psychiatry.* New York: Williams and Wilkins.

Peplau, (1968). Operational definitions and nursing practice. In L.T. Zderad, & H.C. Belcher (Eds.), *Developing behavioral concepts in nursing.* SREB.

Peplau, H.E., & Smoyak, S. (1968, Nov. 14-16). *Pattern perpetuation and intellectual competencies in schizophrenia.* Paper presented at Conference on Schizophrenia: Current concepts and research. Waldorf Astoria, New York.

Peplau, H.E. (1969 March 20-21). *Theory: The professional dimension.* Presented at the Nursing Theory Conference, University of Kansas Medical Center, Kansas City.

Peplau, H.E. (1969). Pattern perpetuation in schizophrenia. In D. Sankar, *Schizophrenia: Current concepts and research.* Hicksville, N.Y.: PJD Publications.

Peplau, H.E. (1974). *Associate degree education for nursing: Current issues, 1974.* ANA and the professional nurse. Publication #23-1539. National League of Nursing, Dept. of Associate Degree Programs.

Thesis

Peplau, H.E. (1953). *An exploration of some process elements which restrict or facilitate instructor-student interaction in a classroom, Type B.* Doctoral Project, Teachers' College, Columbia University.

Forewords

Peplau, H.E. (1963). In S.F. Burd, & M.A. Marshall (Eds.), *Some clinical approaches to psychiatric nursing.* New York: MacMillan.

Peplau, H.E. (1963). In S. Armstrong, & S. Rouslin. *Group psychotherapy in nursing practice.* New York: Macmillan.

Editorial Statements, Letters, Reactions

Peplau, H.E. (1963, Sept.). Nursing has lost its way. *Journal RN, 25(9)*:103-105.

Peplau, H.E. (1963, Jan.-Feb.) On semantics. *Perspectives in Psychiatric Care, 1:*10-11.

Letter to Editor. (1962, March). *American Journal of Nursing, 62(3)*:16, 25, 26.

Reviews

Peplau, H.E. (1955, May). Review of *The psychiatric interview* by H.S. Sullivan. *American Journal of Nursing, 55(5)*:614.

Peplau, H.E. (1957, April). Review of *The foundation of human behavior* by T. Muller. *Mental Hygiene, 41(2)*:285-286.

Peplau, H.E. (1957, Oct.) Review of *Beyond laughter* by M. Grotjohn. *American Journal of Nursing, 57(10)*:1349-1450.

Peplau, H.E. (1963). Review of *The management of the anxious patient* by Ainslic Meares. *Perspectives in Psychiatric Care, II(1), 1964*:46-47.

Peplau, H.E. (1964). Review of *More for the mind: A study of psychiatric services in Canada. Perspectives in Psychiatric Care, 11(3)*:39-42.

Peplau, H.E. (1964, Fall). Review of *Attitudes of nursing students toward direct patient care* by Sr. L.M. Vaugh, *Journal of Nursing Research, 13(4)*:348-349.

Secondary Sources

American Nurses' Association new executive director states her views. (1970, Jan.). *American Journal of Nursing, 70*(1):84-88.

Belcher, J.R., & Fish, L.J. (1980). Hildegard E. Peplau. In Nursing Theories Conference Group, J.B. George, Chairperson, *Nursing theories: The base for professional practice*. Englewood Cliffs, N.J.: Prentice-Hall.

Burd, S.F. (1963). The development of an operational definition using the process of learning as a guide. In S.F. Burd, & A. Marshall, *Some clinical approaches to psychiatric nursing*. New York: MacMillan.

Burton, G. (1958). Personal, impersonal, and interpersonal relations. Cited by S.A. Smoyak, & S. Rouslin (Eds.), (1982), *A collection of classics in psychiatric nursing literature*. Thorofare, N.J.: Charles B. Slack.

Field, W.E., Jr. (Ed.). (1979). *The psychotherapy of Hildegard E. Peplau*. New Brunfels, Tex.: PSF Publications.

Fitzpatrick, J.J., & Whall, A.L. (1983). *Conceptual models of nursing: Analysis and Application*. Bowie, Md.: Robert J. Brady.

Chinn, P.L., & Jacobs, M.K. (1983). *Theory and nursing: A systematic approach*. St. Louis: C.V. Mosby.

Garrett, A., Manuel, D., & Vincent, C. (1976, Nov.). Stressful experiences identified by student nurses. *Journal of Nursing Education, 15*(6):9-21.

Gregg, D.E. (1978, May-June). Hildegard E. Peplau: Her contributions. *Perspective Psychiatric Care, 16*(3):118-121.

Hays, D. (1961, Spring). Teaching a concept of anxiety. *Nursing Research, 10*(2):108-113.

Hofling, C.K. & Leininger, M.M. (1960). Basic psychiatric concepts in nursing. Cited by S.A. Smoyak, & S. Rouslin (Eds.), (1982), *A collection of classics in psychiatric nursing literature*. Thorofare, N.J.: Charles B. Slack.

Iveson, J. (1982, November). A two-way process . . . theories in nursing practice . . . Peplau's nursing model. *Nursing Mirror, 155*(18):52.

Keda, A. (1970, Winter). From Henderson to Orlando to Wiedenback: Thoughts on completion of translation of *Basic Principles of Clinical Nursing*. *Comprehensive Nursing Quarterly, 5*(1):85-94.

LaMonica, E. (1981). Construct validity of an empathy instrument. *Research in Nursing and Health, 4*:389-400.

Lego, S. (1980). The one-to-one nurse-patient relationship. *Perspectives in Psychiatric Care, 18*(2):67-89. (Reprinted from *Psychiatric Nursing 1946-*

1974: A report on the State of the art, American Journal of Nursing Co.)

Marshall, J. (1963, March-April). Dr. Peplau's strong medicine for psychiatric nurses. *Smith, Kline & French Reporter, 7*:11-14.

McCarter, P. (1980, April). New statement defines scope of practice discussion with Dr. Lane and Dr. Peplau. *American Nurse, 12*(4):1, 8, 24.

Miller, N.E., & Dollard, J. (1941). *Social learning and imitiation*. New Haven, Conn.: Yale University Press.

Methven, D. & Schlotfeldt, R.M. (1962, Spring). The social interaction inventory. *Nursing Research, 11*(2):83-88.

Nursing Theories Conference Group, J.B. George, Chairperson. (1980). *Nursing theories: The base for professional nursing practice*. Englewood Cliffs, N.J.: Prentice-Hall, pp. 73-89.

Orlando, I. (1961). The dynamic nurse-patient relationship. Cited by S.A. Smoyak, & S. Roustin, (Eds.) (1982), *A collection of classics in psychiatric nursing literature*. Thorofare, N.J.: Charles B. Slack.

Osborne, O. (1984, Nov.). Intellectual traditions in psychiatric nursing. *Journal of Psychosocial Nursing, 22*(1):27-32.

Profile. (1974, Feb.). *Nursing 74, 4*:13.

Psychotherapeutic strategies. (1968). Current concepts in psychiatric care: The implications for psychiatric nursing practice. Proceedings of the Institute on Psychiatric Nursing, cosponsored by Yale School of Nursing, Department of Psychiatric Nursing and the Community Mental Health Center Department of Nursing. In *Perspectives of Psychiatric Care, 6*(6):271-289.

Sills, G.M. (1977, May-June). Research in the field of psychiatric nursing 1952-1977. *Nursing Research, 28*(3):201-207.

Sills, G.M. (1978). Hildegard E. Peplau: Leader, practitioner, academician, scholar, and theorist. *Perspectives in Psychiatric Care, 16*(3):122-128.

Smoyak, S.A., & Rouslin, S. (Eds.). (1982). Introduction. In *A collection of classics in psychiatric nursing literature*. Thorofare, N.J.: Charles B. Slack.

Spring, F.E., & Turk, H. (1962, Fall). A therapeutic behavior scale. *Nursing Research, 11*(4):214-218.

Thomas, M.D., Baker, J.M., & Estes, N.J. (1970, Dec.). Anger: A tool for developing self-awareness. *American Journal of Nursing, 70*(12):2586-2590.

Topf, M., & Dambacher, B. (1979). Predominant source of interpersonal influence in relationships between psychiatric patients and nursing staff. *Research in Nursing and Health, 2*(1):35-43.

Other Sources

Andreoli, R.G., & Thompson, C.E. (1977, June). The nature of science in nursing. *Image, 9*(2):32-37.

Duffey, M. & Mullencamp, A.F. (1974, Sept.). A framework for theory analysis. *Nursing Outlook, 22*:570-574.

Freud, S. (1936). The problem of anxiety. Cited by H.E. Peplau, (1952), *Interpersonal relations in nursing*. New York: G.B. Putnam's Sons.

Fromm, E. (1947). Man for himself. Cited by H.E. Peplau, (1952), *Interpersonal relations in nursing*. New York: G.B. Putnam's Sons.

Jacox, A. (1974, Jan.-Feb.). Theory construction in nursing: An overview. *Nursing Research, 23*:4-12.

Johnson, D.E. (1959). The nature of a science of nursing. *Nursing Outlook, 7*:272.

Maslow, A.H. (1943, July). A theory of human motivation. *Psychological Review, 50*:370-396.

Maslow, A.H., & Mittleman, B. (1941). *Principles in abnormal psychology*. New York: Harper & Brothers.

Miller, N.E., & Dollard, J. (1941). *Social learning and imitation*. New Haven, Conn.: Yale University Press.

Mullahy, P. (1948). *Oedipus: Myth and complex*. New York: Hermitage House.

Pavlov, I. (1927). *Conditioned reflexes: An investigation of the physiological activity of the cerebral cortex*. London: Oxford University Press.

Phillips, J.R. (1977, Feb.). Nursing systems and nursing models. *Image 9, (1)*:6.

Popper, K.R. (1963). *Conjectures and refutations: The growth of scientific knowledge*. New York: Basic Books.

Reynolds, P.D. (1971). *A primer in theory construction*. Indianapolis, Ind.: Bobbs-Merrill.

Solomon, A.P. (1943). Rehabilitation of patients with psychologically protracted convalescence. *Archives of Physical Therapy, 24*:270-273.

Sullivan, H.S. (1947). Concepts of modern psychiatry. Cited by H.E. Peplau (1952), *Interpersonal relations in nursing*. New York: G.B. Putnam's Sons.

Sullivan, H.S. (1948). *The meaning of anxiety in psychiatry and in life*. Washington, D.C.: William Alanson White Psychiatric Foundation.

Symonds, P. (1946). *The dynamics of human adjustment*. New York: Appleton-Century-Crofts.

von Bertalanffy, L. (1968). *General systems theory: Foundations, development, applications*. New York: Braziller.

Wertheimer, M. (1945). *Productive thinking*. New York: Harper & Brothers.

Joyce Travelbee
Human-to-Human Relationship Model

William H. Hobble, Theresa Lansinger

17

CREDENTIALS AND BACKGROUND OF THE THEORIST

Joyce Travelbee was a psychiatric nurse practitioner, educator, and writer. Born in 1926, she completed her basic nursing preparation in 1946 at Charity Hospital School of Nursing in New Orleans. She obtained a B.S.N. Ed. from Louisiana State University in 1956 and an M.S.N. from Yale in 1959. In the summer of 1973 Travelbee began a doctoral program in Florida, but was unable to complete the program because of her untimely death later that year.[1,2,7]

Travelbee began her career as a nursing educator in 1952 by teaching psychiatric nursing at DePaul Hospital Affiliate School, New Orleans, while working on her baccalaureate degree. She also taught psychiatric nursing at Charity Hospital School of Nursing, at Louisiana State University, at New York University in New York City, and at the University of Mississippi in Jackson. In 1970 she was named

Project Director at Hotel Dieu, School of Nursing in New Orleans. At the time of her death, Travelbee was the director of graduate education at Louisiana State University School of Nursing.[1,2,7]

Travelbee began publishing articles in nursing journals in 1963. Her first book, *Interpersonal Aspects of Nursing,* was published in 1966 and 1971. A second book, *Intervention in Psychiatric Nursing,* was published in 1969.

THEORETICAL SOURCES FOR THEORY DEVELOPMENT

Travelbee's experiences in her basic nursing education and initial practice in Catholic charity institutions greatly influenced the development of her theory. Travelbee believed the nursing care given patients in these institutions lacked compassion.[7] She felt nursing needed "a humanistic revolution—a return to focus on the 'caring' function of the nurse—in the caring for [and] the caring about ill persons."[9:2]

Travelbee was probably also influenced by Ida Jean Orlando, who was one of her instructors during her graduate studies at Yale. Orlando's model possesses some similarities to the model Travelbee proposes. Orlando[5,6] states, "The nurse is responsible for helping the pa-

The authors wish to express appreciation to Leigh DeNoon, Mary Ellen Doona, Joyce Lee, and Katharine Taylor for assistance with data collection. The authors have been unable to obtain a picture of Joyce Travelbee.

tient avoid and alleviate the distress of unmet needs." Orlando[5:8] also states the nurse and the patient are both people who interact with each other. The similarities between the two models are shown by Travelbee's assertion that the nurse and patient interact with each other and by her definition of the purpose of nursing. Travelbee[9:7] states the purpose of nursing is to assist "an individual, family, or community to prevent or cope with the experience of illness and suffering."

Travelbee also appears to have been influenced by Vicktor Frankl, a survivor of Auschwitz and other Nazi concentration camps. As a result of his experiences, Frankl[3:153] proposed the theory of Logotherapy, in which a patient "is actually confronted with and reoriented toward the meaning of his life." Travelbee[9:158] based the assumptions of her theory on the concepts of Logotherapy.

USE OF EMPIRICAL EVIDENCE

Katharine Taylor,[7] a former student and colleague of Travelbee, remembers Travelbee as a prolific reader whose office was often crammed with files of bibliography cards. Apparently, Travelbee's theory is based on the cumulation of her nursing experiences and her readings rather than the evidence of a particular research study.

MAJOR CONCEPTS AND DEFINITIONS

HUMAN BEING. "A human being is defined as a unique irreplaceable individual—a one-time-being in this world—like yet unlike any person who has ever lived or ever will live."[9:26]

PATIENT. The term *patient* is a stereotype useful for communicative economy. "Actually there are no patients. There are only individual human beings in need of the care, services, and assistance of other human beings, whom, it is believed, can render the assistance that is needed."[9:32]

NURSE. The nurse is also a human being. "The nurse possesses a body of specialized knowledge and the ability to use it for the purpose of assisting other human beings to prevent illness, regain health, find meaning in illness, or to maintain the highest maximal degree of health."[9:40]

ILLNESS. Illness is "a category and a classification."[9:49] Travelbee did not use the term illness as a definition of being unhealthy, but rather explored the human experience of illness. Travelbee defined illness by objective and subjective criteria. The objective criteria are determined by the outward effects of illness on the individual.[9:521] The subjective criteria refer to how a human being perceives himself as ill.[9:52]

SUFFERING. "Suffering is a feeling of displeasure which ranges from simple transitory mental, physical, or spiritual discomfort to extreme anguish, and to those phases beyond anguish, namely, the malignant phase of despairful 'not caring,' and the terminal phase of apathetic indifference."[9:62] Suffering can be placed on a continuum, such as the one in Figure 17-1.

PAIN. "Pain itself is not observable—only its effects are noted."[9:72] Pain is a lonely experience that is difficult to communicate fully to another individual.[9:72] The experience of pain is unique to each individual.

HOPE. "Hope is a mental state characterized by the desire to gain an end or accomplish a goal combined with some degree of expectation that what is desired or sought is attainable."[9:77] Hope is related to dependence on others, choice, wishing, trust and perserverence, and courage, and is future oriented.[9:78-80]

HOPELESSNESS. Hopelessness is being devoid of hope.[9:81]

Transitory feeling of displeasure	Extreme anguish	Malignant phase of despairful not caring	Terminal phase of apathetic indifference

Figure 17-1. Continuum of suffering. (Conceptualized by Theresa Lansinger, based on Joyce Travelbee's definition.)

COMMUNICATION. "Communication is a process which can enable the nurse to establish a human-to-human relationship and thereby fulfill the purpose of nursing, namely, to assist individuals and families to prevent and to cope with the experience of illness and suffering and, if necessary, to assist them to find meaning in these experiences."[9:93]

INTERACTION. "The term *interaction* refers to any contact during which two individuals have reciprocal influence on each other and communicate verbally and/or nonverbally."[9:120]

NURSE-PATIENT INTERACTION. "The term *nurse-patient interaction* refers to any contact between a nurse and an ill person and is characterized by the fact that both individuals perceive the other in a stereotyped manner."[9:120]

NURSING NEED. "A nursing need is any requirement of the ill person (or family) which can be met by the professional nurse practitioner, and which lies within the scope of the legal definition of nursing practice."[9:125]

THERAPEUTIC USE OF SELF. "The therapeutic use of self is the ability to use one's personality consciously and in full awareness in an attempt to establish relatedness and to structure nursing intervention."[9:19] It "requires self insight, self understanding, an understanding of the dynamics of human behavior, ability to interpret one's own behavior as well as the behavior of others, and the ability to intervene effectively in nursing situations."[9:19]

EMPATHY. "Empathy is a process wherein an individual is able to comprehend the psychological state of another."[9:43]

SYMPATHY. Sympathy implies a desire to help an individual undergoing stress.[8:68-69]

RAPPORT. "Rapport is a process, a happening, an experience, or series of experiences, undergone simultaneously by the nurse and the recipient of her care. It is composed of a cluster of interrelated thoughts and feelings, these thoughts, feelings and attitudes being transmitted, or communicated by one human being to another."[9:150]

HUMAN-TO-HUMAN RELATIONSHIP. "A human-to-human relationship is primarily an experience or series of experiences between a nurse and the recipient of her care. The major characteristic of these experiences is that the nursing needs of the individual (or family) are met."[9:123] "The human-to-human relationship, in nursing situations, is the means through which the purpose of nursing is accomplished."[9:119] The human-to-human relationship is established when the nurse and the recipient of her care attained a rapport after having progressed through the stages of the original encounter, emerging identities, empathy, and sympathy[9:119-120] (Figure 17-2).

MAJOR ASSUMPTIONS
Nursing

Travelbee[9:7] defines nursing as an "interpersonal process whereby the professional nurse

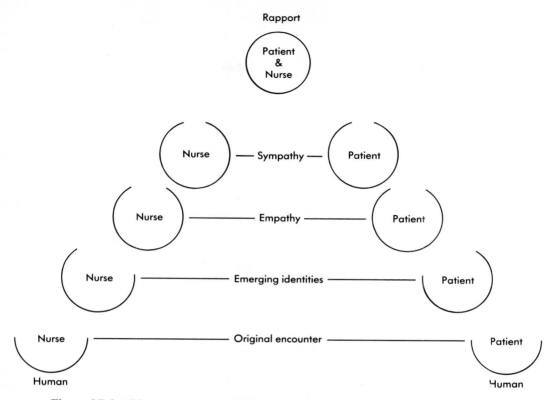

Figure 17-2. Human-to-human relationship. (Conceptualized by William Hobble and Theresa Lansinger, based on Joyce Travelbee's writings.)

practitioner assists an individual, family, or community to prevent or cope with the experience of illness and suffering and, if necessary, to find meaning in these experiences." Nursing is an interpersonal process since it is an experience that occurs between the nurse and an individual or group of individuals.[8:8]

Person

The term *person* is defined as a human being. Both the nurse and the patient are human beings. A human being is an unique, irreplaceable individual who is in the continuous process of becoming, evolving, and changing.[9:26-27]

Health

Travelbee defines health by the criteria of subjective and objective health. A person's subjective health status is how the individual perceives his health.[9:9] Objective health is "an absence of discernible disease, disability, or defect as measured by physical examination, laboratory tests, assessment by a spiritual director or psychological counselor."[9:10]

Environment

Travelbee does not explicitly define environment in the theory. She does define the human condition and life experiences encountered by all human beings as suffering, hope, pain, and illness. These human conditions can be equated to the environment.

THEORETICAL ASSERTIONS

"The purpose of nursing is achieved through the establishment of a human-to-human relationship."[9:16]

The quality and quantity of nursing care delivered to an ill human being is greatly influenced by the nurse's perception of the patient.[9:32]

The terms *patient* and *nurse* are stereotypes and only useful for communicative economy.

The roles of the nurse and patient must be transcended to establish a human-to-human relatedness.[9:33]

Illness and suffering "are spiritual encounters as well as emotional-physical experiences."[9:61]

The communication process enables "the nurse to establish a human-to-human relationship and thereby fulfill the purpose of nursing."[9:93]

"Individuals can be assisted to find meaning in the experience of illness and suffering. The meanings can enable the individual to cope with the problems engendered by these experiences."[9:158]

"The spiritual and ethical values of the nurse, or her philosophical beliefs about illness and suffering, will determine the extent to which she will be able to assist individuals and families to find meaning (or no meaning) in these difficult experiences."[9:158]

"It is the responsibility of the professional nurse practitioner to assist individuals and families to find meaning in illness and suffering (if this be necessary)."[9:158]

Human-to-human relationship

The human-to-human relationship model, shown in Figure 17-2, represents the interaction between the nurse and patient. The half circles at the point of the original encounter indicate the possibility of and need for develop-ing the encounter into a therapeutic relationship. As the interaction process progresses toward rapport, the circles join into one full circle—representing that the potential for a therapeutic relationship has been attained.

ORIGINAL ENCOUNTER. The original encounter is characterized by first impressions by the nurse of the ill person and by the ill person of the nurse. The nurse and ill person perceive each other in stereotyped roles.[9:131]

EMERGING IDENTITIES. The emerging identities phase is characterized by the nurse and ill person perceiving each other as unique individuals. The bond of a relationship is beginning to form.[9:132]

EMPATHY. The empathy phase is characterized by the ability to share in the other person's experience. The result of the empathic process is the ability to predict the behavior of the individual with whom one has empathized.[9:137] Travelbee believed two qualities that enhanced the empathy process were similarities of experience and the desire to understand another person.[9:138]

SYMPATHY. Sympathy goes beyond empathy and occurs when the nurse desires to alleviate the cause of the patient's illness or suffering. "When one sympathizes one is involved but not incapacitated by the involvement."[9:142] The nurse is to create helpful nursing action as a result of reaching the phase of sympathy. "This helpful nursing action requires a combination of the disciplined intellectual approach combined with the therapeutic use of self."[9:149]

RAPPORT. Rapport is characterized by nursing actions that alleviate an ill person's distress. The nurse and ill person are relating as human being to human being. The ill person exhibits both trust and confidence in the nurse. "A nurse is able to establish rapport because she possesses the necessary knowledge and skills required to assist ill persons, and because she is able to perceive, respond to, and appreciate the uniqueness of the ill human being."[9:155]

LOGICAL FORM

Travelbee's theory is inductive. She has used specific nursing situations to create general ideas. Travelbee appears to follow a logical form by first defining the labels in her theory, then listing the assumptions, and finally establishing specific nursing goals.

ACCEPTANCE BY THE NURSING COMMUNITY
Practice

Travelbee believed the condition of an individual exhibiting apathetic indifference is just as critical as that of an individual who is hemorrhaging. She felt both people need emergency resuscitative measures. But an examination of patient care given by nurses today indicates the patient's physical needs still hold top priority. The acceptance and use of nursing diagnosis does appear to focus nursing care more on the total needs of the patients as compared with 20 years ago when Travelbee published her theory. However, nursing has not yet reached the humanistic revolution Travelbee proposed.

Hospice is the one area of nursing practice where the philosophy closely adheres to the tenets of Travelbee's theory. The hospice nurse attempts to develop a rapport with the patient and his significant others. Most hospice nurses agree with Elisabeth Kübler-Ross[4:2] "that death does not have to be a catastrophic, destructive thing; indeed, it can be viewed as one of the most constructive, positive, and creative elements of culture and life." One hospice nurse believes the dying person must find meaning in his death before he can ever begin to accept the actuality of his death, just as his loved ones must find meaning in his death before they can complete the grieving process.[4]

Education

Nursing education appears to have identified the need to prepare nurses to address the emotional and spiritual needs of patients. The focus of nursing education has changed from the disease entity approach, that is, signs, symptoms, and nursing intervention, to a more holistic care approach. However, basic nursing programs do not seem to adequately prepare nurses to help individuals find meaning in illness and suffering as Travelbee proposed. Travelbee's second book, *Intervention in Psychiatric Nursing: Process in the One-to-One Relationship*, has been used in various nursing programs. But this book alone does not adequately prepare nurses to help individuals find meaning in illness and suffering. Nursing programs need to offer a much broader background in communication techniques, values clarification, and thanatology to adequately prepare nurses to fulfill the purpose of nursing stated in Travelbee's theory.

Research

Some aspects of the one-to-one relationship proposed by Travelbee have been quoted by several sources in research studies. However, there does not appear to be any major research generated by Travelbee's specific theory that could stimulate further development.

FURTHER DEVELOPMENT

The recent advent of diagnostic related groups (DRGs) is creating the need to produce the highest quality nursing care by the most economical method. Tools such as patient acuity systems have been devised to determine nursing staffing patterns in accordance with the nursing needs of patients. Although this type tool can account for the emotional needs of patients, emotional needs are not weighed as heavily as patients' physical needs. DRGs may shift the nursing focus back to solely meeting the patient's physical needs. If nurses are to prevent this, they must prove to health care administrators and health care consumers that the time taken by the nurse to meet a patient's emotional and spiritual needs is a valuable investment. Travelbee's theory could be used to provide the research data to justify this time investment. However, Travelbee's theory does not currently contain the empirical precision to support such research data. If it is to be more readily accepted, its major assumptions need to be assigned operational definitions. Once this is done, the theory could perhaps generate the data needed to facilitate further acceptance.

CRITIQUE
Simplicity

Travelbee's theory does not possess simplicity because there are many variables present. The theory is designed to help nurses appreciate not only the patient's humanness but also the nurse's humanness. To be human is to be unique; so the variables present in each phase of the human-to-human relationship will be numerous.

The definitions of terms used by Travelbee are often quite wordy. Travelbee also uses different terms for the same definition. She equates the terms rapport, human-to-human relationship, and human-to-human relatedness with the same definition. This leads to inconsistencies when labels are periodically substituted throughout the theory.

Generality

Travelbee's theory has a wide scope of application. It was primarily generated as a result of Travelbee's experience with psychiatric patients. However, the theory is not limited to use in psychiatric settings. It is applicable in all situations in which the nurse encounters ill persons in distress.

Empirical Precision

Travelbee's theory appears to have a low degree of empirical validity. Much of the lack of empirical validity can be traced to the lack of simplicity in the theory. The terms are given definitions, but these are often not operational definitions. The theory is difficult to validate with statistical data because of the lack of operational definitions.

Derivable Consequences

The usefulness of a theory is related to its ability to describe, explain, predict, and control phenomena. Travelbee's theory does explain some variables that may affect the establishment of a therapeutic relationship between nurse and patient. It also states the nurse should be able to predict the behavior of the ill person. But it lacks the ability to control phenomena of a therapeutic relationship. The lack of empirical precision also creates a lack of derivable consequences. Travelbee's theory focuses on the development of the attribute of caring. In this respect the theory can be useful, because caring is a major characteristic of the nursing profession.

REFERENCES

1. Doona, M.E. (1984, Oct.). Personal interview. (Nursing instructor, Boston College.)
2. Doona, M.E. (1984, Oct.). Telephone interview.
3. Frankl, V. (1963). *Man's search for meaning: An introduction to logotherapy.* New York: Washington Square Press.
4. Kübler-Ross, E. (1975). *Death: The final stage of growth.* Englewood Cliffs, N.J.: Prentice-Hall.
5. Orlando, I.J. (1961). *The dynamic nurse-patient relationship.* New York: G.P. Putnam.
6. Schoon, F. (1984, Oct.). Personal interview. (Hospice nurse.)
7. Taylor, K. (1984, Oct.). Telephone interview. (Former student and colleague of Joyce Travelbee.)
8. Travelbee, J. (1964, Jan.). What's wrong with sympathy? *American Journal of Nursing, 64:*68-71.
9. Travelbee, J. (1971). Interpersonal aspects of nursing. Philadelphia: F.A. Davis.

BIBLIOGRAPHY
Primary Sources
Books

Travelbee, J. (1966). *Interpersonal aspects of nursing.* Philadelphia: F.A. Davis.

Travelbee, J. (1969). *Intervention in psychiatric nursing: Process in the one-to-one relationship.* Philadelphia: F.A. Davis.

Travelbee, J. (1971). *Interpersonal aspects of nursing* (2nd ed.). Philadelphia: F.A. Davis.

Travelbee, J., & Doona, M.E. (1979). *Travelbee's intervention in psychiatric nursing* (2nd ed.). Philadelphia: F.A. Davis.

Articles

Travelbee, J. (1963, Feb.). Humor survives the test of time. *Nursing Outlook, 11*:128.

Travelbee, J. (1963, Feb.). What do we mean by rapport? *American Journal of Nursing, 63*:70-72.

Travelbee, J. (1964, Jan.). What's wrong with sympathy? *American Journal of Nursing, 64*:68-71.

Secondary Sources
Book Reviews

Travelbee, J. (1966). *Interpersonal aspects of nursing.*
Nursing Outlook, 14:77, June 1966.
American Journal of Nursing, 66:1504, July 1966.
Nursing Mirror, 122:438, August 5, 1966.
Supervisor Nurse, 2:44+, December 1971.
Nursing Outlook, 20:278, April 1972.
Journal of Nursing Administration, 3:14-15, January-February 1973.

Travelbee, J. (1969). *Intervention in psychiatric nursing: Process in the one-to-one relationship.*
American Journal of Nursing, 70:101-102, January 1970.
Nursing Outlook, 18:16, August 1970.
Nursing Mirror, 131:31, September 18, 1970.

Book Chapters

Chin, R. (1974). The utility of system models and development models for practitioners. In J. Riehl & C. Roy (Eds.), *Conceptual models for nursing practice.* New York: Appleton-Century-Crofts, pp. 46-53.

Meleis, A.I. (1985). Joyce Travelbee. In A.I. Meleis, *Theoretical nursing: Development and Progress.* Philadelphia: J.B. Lippincott, pp. 254-262.

Roy, C. (1974). Travelbee's developmental approach. In J.P. Riehl & C. Roy (Eds.), *Conceptual models for nursing practice.* New York: Appleton-Century-Crofts, pp. 267-268.

Thibodeau, J.A. (1983). An interaction model: The Travelbee model. In J.A. Thibodeau, *Nursing models: Analysis and evaluation.* Belmont, Calif.: Wadsworth, pp. 89-104.

Articles

Arnold, H.M. (1976). Working with schizophrenic patients: Guide to one-to-one relationships. *American Journal of Nursing, 76*:941-943.

Freihofer, P., & Felton, G. (1976). Nursing behaviors in bereavement. *Nursing Research, 25*:332-337.

Hinds, P.S. (1984). Introducing a definition of hope through the use of grounded theory methodology. *Journal of Advanced Nursing, 9*:357-362.

Koshi, P.T. (1976). Cultural diversity in nursing curricula. *Journal of Nursing Education, 15*:14-21.

Larson, P.A. (1977). Nurse perceptions of patient characteristics. *Nursing Research, 26*:416-421.

Limandri, B.J., & Boyle, D.W. (1978). Instilling hope. *American Journal of Nursing, 78*:78-80.

Morse, B.W., & Vandenberg, E. (1978). Interpersonal relationships in nursing practice, interdisciplinary approach. *Communication Education, 27*:158-163.

Schweer, S.F., & Dayani, E.C. (1973). Extended role of professional nursing: Patient education. *International Nursing Review, 20*:174+.

Sorgen, L.M. (1979). Student learning following an educational experience at an alcohol rehabilitation center in Saskatoon, Saskatchewan, Canada. *International Journal of Nursing Studies, 16*:41-50.

Spratlen, L.P. (1976). Introducing ethnic-cultural factors in models of nursing: Some mental health applications. *Journal of Nursing Education, 15*:23-29.

Stetler, C.B. (1977). Relationship of perceived empathy to nurses' communication. *Nursing Research, 26*:432-438.

Stoll, R.I. (1979). Guidelines for spiritual assessment. *American Journal of Nursing, 79*:1574-1577.

Wallston, K.A., & Wallston, B.S. (1975). Role-playing simulation approach toward studying nurses decisions to listen to patients. *Nursing Research, 24*:16-22.

Wallston, K.A., Wallston, B.S., & Devellis, B.M. (1976). Effect of a negative stereotype on nurse's attitudes toward an alcoholic patient. *Journal of Studies on Alcohol, 37*:659-665.

Correspondence

Doona, M.E. (1984, Oct. 19). Personal communication.

Interviews

Doona, M.E. (1984, Oct.). Telephone interview.
Taylor, K. (1984, Oct.). Telephone interview.

Other Sources

Barrett-Lennard, G.T. (1962). Dimensions of therapist responses as causal factors in therapeutic change. *Psychological Monographs, 76*:43. (Whole No. 562).
Cartwright, R.D., & Lerner, B. (1963). Empathy, need to change, and improvement with psychotherapy. *Journal of Consulting Psychology, 27*:138-144.
Chinsky, J.M., & Rappaport, J. (1970). Brief critique of the meaning and reliability of 'accurate empathy' ratings. *Psychological Bulletin, 73*:379-382.
Frankl, V. (1963). *Man's search for meaning: An introduction to logotherapy.* New York: Washington Square Press.
Kurtz, R.R., & Grummon, D.L. (1972). Different approaches to the measurement of therapist empathy and their relationship to therapy outcomes. *Journal of Consulting and Clinical Psychology, 30*:106-115.
May, R. (1953). *Man's search for himself.* New York: W.W. Norton.
McBride, M.A. (1967). Nursing approach, pain, and relief: An exploratory experiment. *Nursing Research, 16*(4):337-341.

Ida Jean Orlando (Pelletier)

18

Disciplined Professional Response Theory

Deborah I. Mills, Marcia K. Sauter

CREDENTIALS AND BACKGROUND OF THE THEORIST

Ida Jean Orlando was born August 12, 1926. In 1947 she received a diploma in nursing from New York Medical College, Flower Fifth Avenue Hospital School of Nursing in New York. She received a B.S. in Public Health Nursing from St. Johns University in Brooklyn, New York in 1951, and an M.A. in Mental Health Consultation from Columbia University Teachers College in New York in 1954. While pursuing her education, Orlando worked intermittently, and sometimes concurrently, as a staff nurse in obstetrical, medical, surgical, and emergency nursing services. She also worked as a supervisor in a general hospital. In addition, as an assistant director of nurses, she held responsibility for a general hospital's nursing service and responsibility for teaching several courses in the hospital's nursing school.

After receiving her master's in 1954 Orlando

The authors wish to acknowledge Ida Orlando Pelletier's review of the chapter and verification of this representation of her work.

went to the Yale School of Nursing in New Haven, Connecticut, for 8 years, where she was a Research Associate on a Federal Project Grant until 1958. The project focused on identifying factors influencing the integration of mental health principles in a basic nursing curriculum. Orlando carried out this project by observing and participating in student experiences with patients and medical, nursing, and instructional personnel throughout the basic curriculum. She recorded her observations for 3 years and then spent a fourth year analyzing the accumulated data. She reported her findings in 1958 in her first book, *The Dynamic Nurse-Patient Relationship: Function, Process and Principles of Professional Nursing Practice*. It was not published until 1961, but since then five foreign-language editions have appeared. The formulations in this book provided the foundation for Orlando's nursing theory.[21:243] During the next 4 years (1958-1961), as an associate professor and the director of the Graduate Program in Mental Health and Psychiatric Nursing, Orlando used her theory as the foundation of the program. She married Robert J. Pelletier and left Yale in 1961.

Orlando spent the years 1962-1972 as Clinical Nursing Consultant at McLean Hospital in Belmont, Massachusetts. From this position she studied the interaction of nurses with patients, other nurses, and other staff members and how these activities affected the process of the nurses' help to patients. Orlando convinced the hospital director that a training program for nurses was needed, whereupon McLean Hospital initiated one based on her theory. The nursing service of the hospital was reorganized as a result of this program.[25:45] Orlando subsequently applied for and received federal funding to evaluate training in the process discipline.

While at McLean Hospital, Orlando[26] published "The Patient's Predicament and Nursing Function" in a 1967 issue of *Psychiatric Opinion*. In 1972 she reported the 10 years of work at the hospital in her second book, *The Discipline and Teaching of Nursing Process: An Evaluative Study*.

Since 1972 Orlando has lectured, served as a consultant, and conducted about 60 workshops in her theory throughout the United States and Canada. She has served on the Board of the Harvard Community Health Plan in Boston, Massachusetts, since 1972 and on the Hospital Committee of the board since 1979.

Orlando's nursing theory emphasizes the reciprocal relationship between patient and nurse. Both are affected by what the other says and does. Orlando[23:133] may have facilitated the development of nurses as logical thinkers rather than conformers to the medical orders of a physician. She was one of the first nursing leaders to emphasize the elements of nursing process and the critical importance of the patient's participation during the nursing process.

Orlando[27] says that her search for facts in observing nursing situations influenced her most before the development of her theory and that she derived her theory from the conceptualization of those facts. Her overall goal was to find an organizing principle for professional nursing, that is, a distinct function.[24:viii] Orlando has made a major contribution to nursing theory and practice. Her conceptualizations fulfill the criteria of theory because she presents interrelated concepts that present a systematic view of nursing phenomena; she specifies relationships among the concepts; she explains what happens during the nursing process and why; she prescribes how nursing phenomena can be controlled; and she explains how the control leads to prediction of outcome. Although nursing writers such as Fitzpatrick and Whall[16:5] do not believe any current nursing model meets the level of specificity of theory described by Ellis, Orlando's theory has considerable merit in application to practice, education, and research.

THEORETICAL SOURCES

Orlando acknowledges no theoretical sources for the development of her theory. None of her publications includes a bibliography. In *The*

Discipline and Teaching of Nursing Process she referred only to her own publications and the dictionary.

USE OF EMPIRICAL EVIDENCE

Orlando synthesized facts from observations to develop her theory. She asserted that her theory was valid and applied it in her work with patients and nurses and the teaching of students. Orlando gathered a considerable amount of data before constructing her theory. She used a research process but did not follow research methodology for quantitative analysis.[13:59] However, her second book represents 10 years work and reports the results of a quantative research method to test her major formulations. She spent 3 years analyzing data gathered the previous 7 years while working at McLean Hospital.

MAJOR CONCEPTS AND DEFINITIONS

Orlando's theory[24:4] was derived from the systematic study of immediate nurse-patient situations. The major concepts in Orlando's theory include the patient's behavior and need for help, improvement in the patient's behavior, the nurses reaction and activity, and exploration by the nurse to correct or verify the nurse's perception of the patient's behavior. Orlando's concepts are bound to the immediate situation, but many are either operationally defined or have the potential for operational definition.[30:49-52]

PATIENT'S BEHAVIOR. The first concept is the patient's behavior. Orlando[25:10] assumed a patient may suffer helplessness while receiving medical care because he or she may not be in a position to control all that happens. She emphasizes that a patient can be anyone who suffers a sense of helplessness that requires the assistance of a nurse, even if this person actually receives no medical treatment or supervision.[25:13] However, Orlando's studies, and those of her students, were primarily limited to patients who were also under the medical treatment and supervision of a physician.

DISTRESS AND NEED FOR HELP. The concepts *need for help* and *distress* are closely tied to Orlando's categories of patient behavior. A need for help is situationally defined as a requirement of the patient which, if supplied, relieves or diminishes the immediate distress.[24:5] The nurse determines that the patient is in distress (has a need for help) by expressing and exploring her reactions to the patient's behavior with the patient.

IMPROVEMENT IN THE PATIENT'S IMMEDIATE BEHAVIOR. Improvement means change in the patient's behavior for the better after the immediate need for help is ascertained and met. Whether or not improvement occurs is observable in the patient's immediate verbal and nonverbal behavior when compared with the behavior exhibited when the process began. Thus improvement is the outcome of nursing action and provides the critieria for determining if the need for help has been met.

NURSE. Orlando[25:18-19] views the nurse, the nurse's activity, and the results of this activity, as "the basic operating unity of the nursing system." Orlando[25:12] views the professional nurse as one who provides "direct assistance to individuals in whatever setting they are found for the purpose of avoiding, relieving, diminishing, or curing the individual's sense of helplessness."

NURSE'S ACTION. Orlando defines nursing action as anything the nurse says or does. Within the nurse-patient situation the observation of behaviors, thoughts and feelings, and actions of each individual intermingle in a dynamic interaction.[25:25] The concept of nurse's action is not confined to the nurse-patient contact but also includes contacts between the nurse and other nurses and physicians. The nurse's action is discussed more fully in Theoretical Assertions.

EXPLORATION. The concept that has primary emphasis in Orlando's theory is the importance of exploration by the nurse and the patient of the nurse's thoughts and feelings related to and perceptions of the patient's behavior in order to obtain correction or verification. *Process discipline* is a term Orlando[25:29-31] used in formulating how this exploration should take place in order to comprehend the patient's experience and accurately determine his or her need for help. Process discipline is further examined in Theoretical Assertions.

MAJOR ASSUMPTIONS

Nearly all of the assumptions in Orlando's theory are implicit.

Nursing

The major assumption Orlando makes about nursing is it should be a distinct profession that functions autonomously. Although nursing has been historically aligned with medicine, and continues to have a close relationship with medicine, nursing and the practice of medicine are clearly separate professions.[25:8,12] These assumptions are reflected in Orlando's definition of the function of professional nursing. Orlando[25:7] emphasizes that inadequate patient care is "a generic manifestation of nursing's collective failure to fully articulate and exercise in its education and practice a distinct function." Another assumption Orlando[25:9] makes is that nurses should relieve physical or mental discomfort and should not add to the patient's distress. This assumption is evident in Orlando's concept of improvement in the patient's behavior as the intended outcome of nursing actions.

Person

Orlando assumes that persons behave verbally and nonverbally. Evidence of this assumption is found in Orlando's emphasis on behavior. Orlando assumes that persons are sometimes able to meet their own needs for help in some situations, but that persons become distressed when unable to do so. This is the basis for Orlando's assertion[24:22] that professional nurses should be concerned only with those persons who are unable to state the need for help clearly.

Health

Orlando[24:9] does not define health but assumes that freedom from mental or physical discomfort and feelings of adequacy and well-being contribute to health.[24:9]

Environment

Orlando does not define environment. She assumes that a nursing situation occurs when there is a nurse-patient contact and that both nurse and patient perceive, think and feel in the immediate environment.

THEORETICAL ASSERTIONS

Orlando[24:8] views the professional function of nursing as finding out and meeting the immediate needs for help of the patient. This function is fulfilled when the nurse ascertains and meets the patient's immediate needs for help. Consequently Orlando's theory focuses on how to produce improvment in the patient's behavior.

A person becomes a patient requiring nursing care when he or she has unmet needs for help that cannot be met independently because of physical limitations, a negative reaction to an environment, or experiences preventing the patient from communicating needs for help.[24:11] Orlando[24:10] asserts that these limitations on the patient's ability to meet his needs are most likely to occur while the patient is receiving medical care or supervision. Thus the restrictions Orlando has frequently placed on the concept of patient can be seen as a function of the impediments persons have in meeting their needs.

Patients experience distress or feelings of helplessness as a result of unmet needs for help.[24:61] Orlando[24:46-47] believes there is a positive correlation between the length of time the patient experiences the unmet needs and the degree of distress. Therefore immediacy is emphasized throughout her theory. In Orlando's view,[24:22] when persons are able to meet their own needs, they do not feel distress and do not require care from a professional nurse. For those persons who do have a need for help it is essential the nurse obtain correction or verification of the nurse's perceptions, thoughts, and feelings in order to determine whether the patient is in need of help.[24:29] It is the nurse's responsibility to see that "the patient's needs for help are met, either directly by her own activity or indirectly by calling in the help of others."[24:29]

Individuals in contact with each other go through an action process that involves observation of the other's behavior, the resulting thoughts and feelings about this observation and an action chosen by each individual in response to the reaction.[25:25] When the nurse acts, an action process transpires. This action process by the nurse in the nurse-patient contact is called nursing process.[25:29] The nursing process may be automatic or deliberative. Any behavior of the patient observed by the nurse must be viewed as a possible signal of distress, because it is possible for the patient to "react with distress to any aspect of an environment which was designed for therapeutic and helpful purposes."[24:17,40] Perception of patient behavior produces thoughts and feelings in the nurse. Orlando defines reaction as including perception, a physical stimulation of any one of a person's five senses; thought, an idea that occurs in an individual's mind; and feeling, a state of mind inclining a person toward or against a perception, thought, or feeling.[24:25] The nurse's reaction precipitates nursing actions.[24:61]

Asking the patient about the nurse's perception of the patient's behavior is more effective and less time consuming because the physical stimulus for perception has objective validity. Nursing actions that are not deliberative are au-

tomatic.[24:60] Automatic nursing actions are those having nothing to do with finding out and meeting patient's needs for help. Deliberative nursing activities are those designed to identify and meet the patient's immediate need for help and, therefore to fulfill the professional nursing function. Deliberative nursing actions require that the nurse seek validation or correction of her thoughts and feelings with the patient before she and the patient can know what nursing action will meet the need for help.[24:41]

In her second book Orlando renamed deliberative nursing activity a *process discipline* with three specific requirements. Application of the process discipline qualifies as a *disciplined professional response*.[25:29,31] Despite this change in terminology, Orlando provides a clear procedure for nurses to ascertain and meet a patient's needs for help. First, the nurse expresses to the patient any or all of the items contained in her reaction to the patient's behavior. Second, the nurse verbally states to the patient that the expressed item belongs to the nurse by use of the personal pronoun (an "I" message). Finally, the nurse asks about the item expressed, attempting to verify or correct her perceptions, thoughts, or feelings (reaction).[25:29-30]

The value of the process discipline is in determining whether the patient feels distressed and ascertaining what help is required to relieve the distress.[24:29] Without the investigation required by the process discipline the nurse does not have a reliable data base for action.[25:32] When the nurse responds automatically, the perceptions, thoughts, and feelings of each person are not available to the other. When the nurse uses the process discipline, the perceptions, thoughts, and feeling of the nurse are available to the patient and vice versa.[25:25-27] This latter response is viewed by Orlando[24:67] as a form of "continuous reflection as the nurse tries to understand the meaning to the patient of the behavior she observed and what he needs from her in order to be helped." The nurse evaluates her actions by comparing the patient's verbal and nonverbal behavior at the end of the contact with the behavior that was present when the process started.[24:68]

LOGICAL FORM

Orlando's theory is inductive. Orlando collected records of her observations of nurse-patient situations during a 3-year period. In analyzing this material, Orlando looked for "good" verses "bad" outcomes. Good nursing outcomes were defined as those that improved the patient's behavior. Bad nursing outcomes were defined as absence of improvement. Orlando concluded that the nurse's use of the process discipline was an effective means of achieving a good outcome. On this basis, Orlando synthesized her theory.[13:34]

Using Walker and Avant's criteria[34:125-128] for theory analysis, Orlando's theory is logically adequate. Because inductive argument can produce false conclusions even when the premises are true, Orlando's conclusions seem reasonable. The structure of relationships are clear and sufficiently precise; and it is possible to represent the relationships schematically. The relationships progress from existence and conditional statements to prediction and control. The predictions Orlando makes are acceptable to the nursing profession since improvement in patient care is always valuable. There are no logical fallacies within Orlando's theory because relationships are sufficiently developed.

ACCEPTANCE BY THE NURSING COMMUNITY
Practice

Orlando's theory is clearly applicable to nursing practice, yet little evidence of acceptance by the nursing community exists in the literature. Schmidt[31:72] reported using Orlando's theory as a basis for practice in 1972. Peitchinis[28] suggested that Orlando's deliberative approach reflected the elements of the therapeutic relationship, which include expression of empathy, warmth, and genuineness. She proposed that nursing practice based on Orlando's theory would increase the therapeutic effectiveness of nursing.[28:146] Henderson[19:119] wrote in 1978 that Orlando's insistence on validation was an important contribution to the practice of nursing. More recently, Schmieding[32] reported the advantages of adopting Orlando's theory throughout a department of nursing. Implementation of Orlando's theory produced several benefits. They included increased effectiveness in meeting patient needs; improvement in decision-making skills among staff nurses, particularly in determining what constituted nursing versus nonnursing activities; more effective conflict resolution among staff nurses and between staff and physicians; and a greater sense of identity and unity among staff.[32:761]

Orlando's nursing process is confined to every immediate nurse-patient contact. Observation of the patient's verbal and nonverbal behavior provides data for determining the patient's level of distress when the process discipline is used. The nurse then takes actions to meet the patient's need for help. Finally, the nurse investigates her newer observations to learn whether the action actually relieved the distress (evaluation). If the distress is not relieved, the process begins again.

Education

Orlando's theory is a conceptual framework for the process by which professional nursing should be practiced. Orlando's process recording has made a significant contribution to nursing education. Orlando[25:32-33] found that "training" in the process discipline was necessary in order for the nurse to be able to control the nursing process and achieve improvement in the patient's behavior. She therefore developed the process recording, a tool to facilitate self-evaluation of whether or not the process discipline was used. This "systematic repetitious examination and study of the nursing process" was designed to help students learn how to express their reactions to patients and to ask for correction or verification.[25:32-33] The process recording is an educational tool still used in nursing education.

Orlando[24:vii] wrote her first book "to offer the professional nursing student a theory of effective practice." Since 1961 numerous psychiatric nursing texts have included Orlando's theory. Orlando deserves credit for providing guidelines for the nurse to use in contacts with patients. Orlando's theory was instrumental in development of the interaction theory currently used in psychiatric nursing.[3:117]

Research

Orlando's theory has enjoyed considerable acceptance by the nursing profession in the area of research and has been applied to a variety of research settings. Many of the studies have provided empirical evidence that Orlando's theoretical assertions are valid. These are discussed under Empirical Precision.

Orlando's definition of the concept *need* was used by K. Dracup and C. Breu[9:213] in their study of the needs of grieving spouses, and by S. Hampe[18:114] in a similar study. Orlando's *deliberative nursing* has been designated the *experimental approach* in several studies to examine its effects on a patient's distress during admission and before surgery. B. Anderson, H. Mertz, and R. Leonard[1:151] found that deliberative nursing actions promoted stress reduction during admission. J. Wolfer and M. Visintainer[36:248] demonstrated this same result with children and their parents. R. Dumas and R. Johnson[11:140] determined that preoperative exploration with patients to determine the real source of distress permitted the nurse to take appropriate action to relieve the distress, and that lower distress before surgery correlated with fewer postoperative complications. Deliberative nursing was used as the experimental nursing action by Dumas and R. Leonard[12:12] in their study of postoperative vomiting. These studies using the deliberative nursing approach

can be considered both theory-testing and theory-generating. They have provided empirical support for Orlando's theory (theory-testing) and have produced new principles for practice, especially in the area of preoperative teaching (theory-generating).

FURTHER DEVELOPMENT

The process discipline needs to be taught and then implemented in a variety of settings. Orlando's study could be replicated to validate that the process discipline is directly related to effectiveness of a nursing system.

CRITIQUE
Clarity

Orlando's first book, *The Dynamic Nurse-Patient Relationship,* presented concepts clearly. The second book, *The Discipline and Teaching of Nursing Process,* redefined and renamed *deliberative nursing process* as *nursing process discipline.* Other changes in terminology related to the nursing process are confusing to the reader. Semantic clarity also suffers when the word "process" is included in several key terms. Clarity is further diminished because Orlando's writing style involves defining concepts minimally at first and then developing them throughout the book. Some terms are not fully developed, and readers do not get a distinct definition of many terms until the book is completed. Orlando's theory has several problems related to clarity and consistency, and the reader must be familiar with both books to evaluate her theory thoroughly.

Simplicity

Since Orlando deals with relatively few concepts and their relationships with each other, her theory would be considered simple. Her theory may also be viewed as simplistic because she is able to make some predictive statements as opposed to just description and explanation.

The simplicity of Orlando's theory has benefited research application.

Generality

Orlando discussed and illustrated nurse-patient contacts in which the patient is conscious, able to communicate, and in need of help. Although she did not focus on unconscious patients and groups, application of her theory to groups or unconscious patients is feasible. Actually, any other person could make use of the process discipline if educated properly. Therefore although Orlando's theory focuses on a limited number of situations, it could be adapted to other nursing situations and other professional fields.

Empirical Precision

Two thirds of Orlando's second book is a report of a research project designed to test the validity of her nursing formulations. A training program based on her formulations had been in progress for 3 years before the project began.[25:44] Nurses were trained to use the process discipline in nurse-patient contacts. Those nurses who became clinical nursing supervisors were trained to use the process discipline in their supervisory and other contacts as well. The following is a brief description of the research methodology.

The purpose of the project was to evaluate the effectiveness of the process discipline in the nurse's contacts at work and the effectiveness of the training program. But these evaluations could not take place before hypothetical measures for the process discipline and the effectiveness of the discipline were identified. A discipline variable was defined.[25:60] Effectiveness was determined by the presence or absence of a *helpful outcome,* as judged by two reliable outcome coders. The outcome coders compared the beginning behavior of the subject with the behavior at the end of the record.[25:76] Testing the relationship of the process discipline (in use) with the presence or absence of a helpful outcome in patient, staff, and supervisee contacts was also done. Evaluation of the training program was done by testing whether nurses increased their use of the process discipline after being trained.[25:63-66]

Two groups of nurses were included in the study. The control group consisted of "veterans"—previously trained supervisors and staff nurses. The experimental group consisted of "novices"—untrained supervisors and staff nurses. Transcripts were made of tape-recorded 10-minute periods (six for each subject) of novices' and veterans' contacts at work.

This report is extensive and detailed and may be difficult for those without a good understanding of statistics and research methodology to read and interpret. The complexity of the study probably contributed to the negative reviews it received. The study concludes that training in the nursing process discipline and its use achieves helpful outcomes in patient, supervisee, and staff contacts.

Although Orlando's work is difficult to understand, numerous studies by Orlando's first graduate students at Yale in the 1960s supported the validity of her theory.* Several that incorporated Orlando's deliberative nursing approach have already been mentioned in research application. Others, which specifically tested the usefulness of the deliberative approach, included: D. Pienschke,‡ who found that nursing intervention was more effective under conditions of open disclosure because patients' needs were perceived more accurately; M. Bochnak,[5:191-192] who found that a deliberative nursing process was more effective in relieving patients' pain; M. Dye,[14:194] who controlled for staff-patient ratios and amount of nursing time and still demonstrated that deliberative nursing actions met patient needs effectively; and J. Cameron,[6:192] who revealed that deliberative nursing actions led to the most consistent effective results in verifying patient needs.

*References 1, 5, 6, 10, 11, 12, 13, 14, 15.
‡Reference 29:484-489.

Orlando asserts that patient distress stems from reaction to the environment that the patient cannot control alone. Dye provided empirical evidence for this assertion in her study on clarifying patient needs. She found patients experienced distress more as a reaction to the hospital setting than to their illness.[13:59]

Orlando also asserts patient distress stems from misinterpretation by the nurse of the patient's experience or from the patient's initial inability to clearly communicate the need for help. Both necessitate use of the process discipline. Two studies, one by R. Elder and the other by N. Gowan and M. Morris provided support for this assertion. Both studies demonstrated that although patients frequently did not express their needs clearly, deliberative nursing actions alleviated the problem.*

Derivable Consequences

Orlando's theory is potentially beneficial in achieving valued outcomes. Identifying the patient's needs for help and the nurse's ability to meet these needs are very important to nursing practice. The systematic study of what nurses say and do and the effect on the immediate behavior of the patient can aid nursing education. Incorporating validation into the nursing process as Orlando suggests would allow for maximum participation by the patient in his or her care. Allowing the patient greater participation could change the focus of "nursing" care plans to "patient" care plans. Care based on patient needs for help would result in more effective nursing and enhance patient recovery.

REFERENCES

1. Anderson, B., Mertz, H., & Leonard, R. (1965). Two experimental tests of a patient-centered admission process. *Nursing Research, 14*:151-156.
2. Andrews, C. (1983). Ida Orlando's model of nursing. In J. Fitzpatrick, & A. Whall, *Conceptual models of nursing: Analysis, and application.* Bowie, Md.: Robert J. Brady, pp. 47-65.
3. Artinian, B. (1983). Implementation of the intersystem patient-care model in clinical practice. *Journal of Advanced Nursing, 8*:117-124.
4. Baron, R.A., & Byrne, D. (1977). *Social psychology: Understanding human interaction.* Boston: Allyn & Bacon.
5. Bochnak, M. (1963). The effect of an automatic and deliberative process of nursing activity on the relief of patients' pain: A clinical experiment. *Abstract in Nursing Research, 12*:191-192.
6. Cameron, J. (1963). An exploratory study of the verbal responses of the nurses in 20 nurse-patient interactions. *Abstract in Nursing Research, 12*:292.
7. Chaska, N. (1978). *The nursing profession: Views through the mist.* New York: McGraw-Hill.
8. Chinn, P., & Jacobs, M. (1983). *Theory and nursing: A systematic approach.* St. Louis: C.V. Mosby.
9. Dracup, K., & Breu, C. (1978). Using nursing research findings to meet the needs of grieving spouses. *Nursing Research, 27*:212-216.
10. Dumas, R. (1963). Psychological preparation for surgery. *American Journal of Nursing, 63*: 52-55.
11. Dumas, R., & Johnson, B. (1972). Research in nursing practice: A review of five clinical experiments. *International Journal of Nursing Studies, 9*:137-149.
12. Dumas, R., & Leonard, R. (1963). The effect of nursing on the incidence of postoperative vomiting. *Nursing Research, 12*:12-15.
13. Dye, M. (1963). Clarifying patients' communications. *American Journal of Nursing, 63*:56-59.
14. Dye, M. (1963). A descriptive study of conditions conducive to an effective process of nursing activity. *Abstract in Nursing Research, 12*:194.
15. Elder, R. (1963). What is the patient saying? *Nursing Forum, 11*:25-37.
16. Fitzpatrick, J., & Whall, A. (1983). *Conceptual models of nursing: Analysis, and application.* Bowie, Md.: Robert J. Brady.
17. Gowan, N., & Morris, M. (1964). Nurses' responses to expressed patient needs. *Nursing Research, 13*:68-71.
18. Hampe, S. (1975). Needs of the grieving spouse

---

*References 15:29-36; 17:70.

in a hospital setting. *Nursing Research, 24*:113-120.

19. Henderson, V. (1978). The concept of nursing. *Journal of Advanced Nursing, 3*:113-130.

20. Larson, P., Sr. (1977). Nurse perceptions of patient characteristics. *Nursing Research, 26*:416-421.

21. McCann-Flynn, J., & Heffron, B. (1984). *Nursing: From concept to practice*. Bowie, Md.: Robert J. Brady.

22. Murray, R., & Huelskoetter, M. (1983). *Psychiatric-mental health nursing: Giving emotional care*. Englewood Cliffs, N.J.: Prentice-Hall.

23. Nursing Theories Conference Group, J.B. George, Chairperson. (1980). *Nursing theories: The base for professional practice*. Englewood Cliffs, N.J.: Prentice-Hall.

24. Orlando, I. (1961). *The dynamic nurse-patient relationship*. New York: G.P. Putnam's Sons.

25. Orlando, I. (1972). *The discipline and teaching of nursing process*. New York: G.P. Putnam's Sons.

26. Pelletier, I.O. (1967). The patient's predicament and nursing function. *Psychiatric Opinion, 4*:25-30.

27. Pelletier, I. (1984). Personal correspondence.

28. Peitchinis, L. (1972). Therapeutic effectiveness of counseling by nursing personnel. *Nursing Research, 21*:138-147.

29. Pienschke, D., Sr. (1973). Guardedness or openness on the cancer unit. *Nursing Research, 22*:484-490.

30. Reynolds, P. (1971). *A primer in theory construction*. Indianapolis: Bobbs-Merrill.

31. Schmidt, J. (1972). Availability: A concept of nursing practice. *American Journal of Nursing, 72*:1086-1089.

32. Schmieding, N. (1984). Putting Orlando's theory into practice. *American Journal of Nursing, 84*:759-761.

33. Stevens, B. (1971). Analysis of structured forms used in nursing curricula. *Nursing Research, 20*:388-397.

34. Walker, L., & Avant, K. (1983). *Strategies for theory construction in nursing*. Norwalk, Conn.: Appleton-Century-Crofts.

35. Wilson, H., & Kneisel, C. (1983). *Psychiatric nursing*. Reading, Mass.: Addison Wesley.

36. Wolfer, J., & Visintainer, M. (1975). Pediatric surgical patients' and parents' stress responses and adjustment. *Nursing Research, 24*:244-255.

BIBLIOGRAPHY
Primary Sources
Books

Orlando, I. (1961). *The dynamic nurse-patient relationship*. New York: G.P. Putnam's Sons.

Orlando, I. (1972). *The discipline and teaching of nursing process*. New York: G.P. Putnam's Sons.

Book Chapters

Orlando, I. (1962). Function, process and principle of professional nursing practice. In *Integration of mental health concepts in the human relations professions*. New York: Bank Street College of Education.

Articles

Pelletier, I.O. (1967). The patient's predicament and nursing function. *Psychiatric Opinion, 4*:25-30.

Correspondence

Pelletier, I.O. (1984). Personal correspondence.
Pelletier, I.O. (1985). Personal correspondence.

Interviews

Pelletier, I.O. (1984). Telephone interviews.
Pelletier, I.O. (1985). Telephone interviews.

Secondary Sources
Book Reviews

Orlando, I. (1961). *The dynamic nurse-patient relationship*.
    AAINJ, 10:41, March, 1962.
    Nursing Outlook, 10:221, April 1962.
    Catholic Nurse, 10:54, June 1962.
    Journal of Psychiatric Nursing, 1:65, January 1963.

Orlando, I. (1972). *The discipline and teaching of nursing process*.
    Nursing Research, 22:10, January-February, 1973.
    Supervisor Nurse, 4:48-49, February, 1973.
    American Journal of Nursing, 73:926, May 1973.
    Nursing Outlook, 21:432, July 1973.
    Journal of Nursing Administration, 4:12, January-February 1974.

Dissertation

Schmieding, N. (1983). *A description and analysis of the directive process used by directors of nursing, supervisors, and head nurses in problematic situations based on Orlando's theory of nursing experience*. Doctoral dissertation. Boston: Boston University.

Books

Beck, C.M., Rawlins, R., & Williams, S. (1984). *Mental health: Psychiatric nursing.* St. Louis: C.V. Mosby.

Carter, F. (1981). *Psychosocial nursing.* New York: Macmillan.

Chaska, N. (1978). *The nursing profession: Views through the mist.* New York: McGraw-Hill.

Chinn, P.L., & Jacobs, M.K. (1983). *Theory and nursing: A systematic approach.* St. Louis: C.V. Mosby.

Fitzpatrick, J., & Whall, A. (1983). *Conceptual models of nursing practice: Analysis and application.* Bowie, Md.: Robert J. Brady.

Joel, L., & Collins, D. (1978). *Psychiatric nursing: Model and application.* New York: McGraw-Hill.

McCann-Flynn, J., & Heffron, B. (1984). *Nursing: From concept to practice.* Bowie, Md.: Robert J. Brady.

Murray, R., & Huelskoetter, M. (1983). *Psychiatric-mental health nursing: Giving emotional care.* Englewood Cliffs, N.J.: Prentice-Hall.

Nursing Theories Conference Group, J.B. George, Chairperson. (1980). *Nursing theories: The base for professional nursing practice.* Englewood Cliffs, N.J.: Prentice-Hall.

Stuart, G., & Sundeen, S. (1983). *Principles and practice of psychiatric nursing.* St. Louis: C.V. Mosby.

Wilson, H., & Kneisel, C. (1983). *Psychiatric nursing.* Reading, Mass.: Addison Wesley.

Book Chapters

Andrews, C. (1983). Ida Orlando's model of nursing. In J. Fitzpatrick, & A. Whall *Conceptual models of nursing: Analysis and application.* Bowie, Md.: Robert J. Brady.

Crane, M.D. (1980). Ida Jean Orlando. In Nursing Theories Conference Group, J.B. George, Chairperson, *Nursing theories: The base for professional nursing practice.* Englewood Cliffs, N.J: Prentice-Hall.

Meleis, A.I. (1985). Ida Orlando. In *Theoretical nursing: Development and progress.* Philadelphia: J.B. Lippincott.

Mertz, H. (1962). Nurse actions that reduce stress in patients. In *Emergency intervention by the nurse* (Monograph 1). New York: The American Nurses' Association.

Schmieding, N.J. (1983). An analysis of Orlando's theory based on Kuhn's theory of science. In P.L. Chinn, *Advances in nursing theory development.* Rockville, Md.: Aspen Systems.

Articles

Anderson, B., Mertz, H., & Leonard, R. (1965). Two experimental tests of a patient-centered admission process. *Nursing Research, 14*:151-156.

Artinian, B. (1983). Implementation of the intersystem patient-care model in clinical practice. *Journal of Advanced Nursing, 8*:117-124.

Beckstrand, J.A. (1980). A critique of several conceptions of practice model in nursing. *Research in Nursing and Health, 3*:69-79.

de la Cuesta, C. (1983). The nursing process: From development to implementation. *Journal of Advanced Nursing, 8*:365-371.

Diers, D. (1970). Faculty research development at Yale. *Nursing Research, 19*(1):64-71.

Dracup, K., & Breu, C. (1978). Using nursing research findings to meet the needs of grieving spouses. *Nursing Research, 27*:212-216.

Dumas, R. (1963). Psychological preparation for surgery. *American Journal of Nursing, 63*:52-55.

Dumas, R., & Johnson, B. (1972). Research in nursing practice: A review of five clinical experiments. *International Journal of Nursing Studies, 9*:137-149.

Dumas, R., & Leonard, R. (1963). The effect of nursing on the incidence of postoperative vomiting. *Nursing Research, 12*:12-15.

Dye, M. (1963). Clarifying patients' communications. *American Journal of Nursing, 63*:56-59.

Eisler, J., Wolfer, J., & Diers, D. (1972). Relationship between need for social approval and postoperative recovery and welfare. *Nursing Research, 21*:520-525.

Elder, R. (1963). What is the patient saying? *Nursing Forum, 11*:25-37.

Elms, R., & Leonard, R. (1966). Effects of nursing approaches during admission. *Nursing Research, 15*:39-48.

Gowan, N., & Morris, M. (1964). Nurses' responses to expressed patient needs. *Nursing Research, 13*:68-71.

Hampe, S. (1975). Needs of the grieving spouse in a hospital setting. *Nursing Research, 24*:113-120.

Henderson, V. (1978). The concept of nursing. *Journal of Advanced Nursing, 3*:113-130.

Larson, P., Sr. (1977). Nurse perceptions of patient characteristics. *Nursing Research, 26*:416-421.

Lipson, J., & Meleis, A.I. (1983, Dec.). Issues in health care of Middle-Eastern patients. *The Western Journal of Medicine, 139*:854-861.

McGilloway, F. (1980). The nursing process: A problem solving approach to patient care. *International Journal of Nursing Studies, 17*:79-80.

Peitchinis, L. (1972). Therapeutic effectiveness of counseling by nursing personnel. *Nursing Research, 21*:138-147.

Pienschke, D., Sr. (1973). Guardedness or openness on the cancer unit. *Nursing Research, 22*:484-490.

Powers, M., & Woldridge, P. (1982). Factors influencing knowledge, research, and compliance of hypertensive patients. *Research in Nursing and Health, 5*:171-182.

Rhymes, J. (1964). A description of nurse-patient interaction in effective nursing activity. *Nursing Research, 13*(4):365.

Schmidt, J. (1972). Availability: A concept of nursing practice. *American Journal of Nursing, 72*:1086-1089.

Schmieding, N. (1984). Putting Orlando's theory into practice. *American Journal of Nursing, 83*:759-761.

Silva, M. (1979). Effects of orientation information on spouses' anxieties and attitudes toward hospitalization and surgery. *Research in Nursing and Health, 2*:127-136.

Stevens, B. (1971). Analysis of structured forms used in nursing curricula. *Nursing Research, 20*:388-397.

Thibaudeau, M., & Reidy, M. (1977). Nursing makes a difference: A comparative study of the health behavior of mothers in three primary care agencies. *International Journal of Nursing Studies, 14*:97-107.

Tryon, P.A. (1963). An experiment of the effect of patients' participation in planning the administration of a nursing procedure. *Nursing Research, 12*:262-265.

Tryon, P.A., & Leonard, R.C. (1964). The effect of patients' participation on the outcome of a nursing procedure. *Nursing Forum, 3*(2):79-89.

Williamson, J. (1978). Methodologic dilemmas in tapping the concept of patient needs. *Nursing Research, 27*:172-177.

Wolfer, J., & Visintainer, M. (1975). Pediatric surgical patients' and parents' stress responses and adjustment. *Nursing Research, 24*:244-255.

Research Abstracts

Barron, M.A. (1966). The effects varied nursing approaches have on patients' complaints of pain. Abstract in *Nursing Research, 15*(1):90-91.

Bochnak, M. (1963). The effect of an automatic and deliberative process of nursing activity on the relief of patients' pain: A clinical experiment. Abstract in *Nursing Research, 12*:191-192.

Cameron, J. (1963). An exploratory study of the verbal responses of the nurses in 20 nurse-patient interactions. Abstract in *Nursing Research, 12*:192.

Diers, D.K. (1966). The nurse orientation system: A method for analyzing the nurse-patient interactions. Abstract in *Nursing Research, 15*(1):91.

Dye, M. (1963). A descriptive study of conditions conducive to an effective process of nursing activity. Abstract in *Nursing Research, 12*:194.

Faulkner, S. (1963). A descriptive study of needs communicated to the nurse by some mothers on a postpartum service. Abstract in *Nursing Research, 12*:26.

Fichelis, M. (1963). An exploratory study of labels nurses attach to patient behavior and their effect on nursing activities. Abstract in *Nursing Research, 12*:195.

Ernestine Wiedenbach

19

The Helping Art of Clinical Nursing

Marguerite Danko, Nancy E. Hunt, Judith E. Marich, Ann Marriner,
Cynthia A. McCreary, Margery Stuart

CREDENTIALS AND BACKGROUND OF THE THEORIST

Ernestine Wiedenbach's interest in nursing began with her childhood experiences with nurses. She greatly admired the private duty nurse who cared for her ailing grandmother and later enjoyed hearing accounts of nurses' roles in the hospital experiences of a young intern her sister was dating. Captivated by the

The authors wish to express appreciation to Catherine Martin, Janet Pezelle, and Nancy Preuss for their assistance with data collection and to Ernestine Wiedenbach for critiquing the chapter.

role of the nurse, Wiedenbach enrolled in the Johns Hopkins Hospital School of Nursing after graduating from Wellesley College with a bachelor's degree in liberal arts. After completing her study at Johns Hopkins, she held a variety of positions in hospitals and public health nursing agencies in New York. She also continued her education by attending evening classes at Teachers College, Columbia University, from which she received a master's degree and a Certificate in Public Health Nursing. During this period Hazel Corbin, director of the Maternity Center Association of New York, persuaded Wiedenbach to enroll in the Association's School for Nurse-Midwives. After completing

217

the program, Wiedenbach practiced as a nurse-midwife in the home delivery service of the Maternity Center Association.

In addition to her practice, she also developed her academic career. She taught an evening course in advanced maternity nursing at Teachers College, wrote several articles for professional publications, and wrote a textbook on clinical nursing. She was also active in professional nursing organizations. Then in 1952 she moved from New York to Connecticut, where she was subsequently appointed to the faculty of the Yale University School of Nursing. It was out of this vast practical experience and education that she developed her model.[7:1]

THEORETICAL SOURCES

At Yale, Wiedenbach's theory development benefited from her contact with fellow faculty members. Ida Orlando Pelletier stimulated Wiedenbach's understanding of the use of self and the effect a nurse's thoughts and feelings has on the outcome of her actions. In addition, Patricia James and William Dickhoff, who taught a course in nursing theory, reviewed the manuscript for Wiedenbach's book, *Clinical Nursing—A Helping Art*. In it they identified elements of a prescriptive theory, which Wiedenbach[7] developed more fully in *Meeting the Realities in Clinical Teaching*.

USE OF EMPIRICAL EVIDENCE

At present there is no specific research supporting Wiedenbach's work. Her model was developed on the basis of her years of experience in clinical practice and teaching.

MAJOR CONCEPTS AND DEFINITIONS

PATIENT. To understand Ernestine Wiedenbach's theory it is necessary to understand her concepts and how her definitions of common nursing terms may differ from or be similar to the current definitions of those words. She defines a patient as "any individual who is receiving help of some kind, be it care, instruction or advice, from a member of the health professions or from a worker in the field of health."[6:3] Thus, to be a patient, one does not necessarily have to be sick. Someone receiving preventive health care teaching would qualify as a patient.

NEED-FOR-HELP. Wiedenbach believed every individual experiences needs as a normal part of living. A need is anything the individual may require "to maintain or sustain himself comfortably or capably in his situation."[6:5] An attempt to meet the need is made by the intervention of help, which is "any measure or action that enables the individual to overcome whatever interferes with his ability to function capably in relation to his situation. . . . To be meaningful, help must be used by an individual and must succeed in enhancing or extending his capability."[6:5-6] Wiedenbach combines these two definitions into a more critical concept for her theory of a need-for-help.

A need-for-help is "any measure or action required and desired by the individual and which has potential for restoring or extending his ability to cope with the demands implicit in his situation."[6:6] It is crucial to the nursing profession that a need-for-help be based on the individual's perception of his own situation. If one does not perceive a need as a need-for-help, one may not take action to relieve or resolve it.

NURSE

The nurse is a functioning human being. As such she not only acts, but she thinks and feels as well. The thoughts she thinks and the feelings she feels as she goes about her nursing are important; they are intimately involved not only in what she does, but also in how she does it. They underlie every action that she takes, be it in the form of a spoken word, a written communication, a gesture, or a deed of any kind. For the nurse whose action is directed toward achievement of a specific purpose, thoughts and feelings have a disciplined role to play.[6:8]

PURPOSE

Purpose—that which the nurse wants to accomplish through what she does—is the overall goal toward which she is striving, and so is constant. It is her reason for being and for doing; it is the why of clinical nursing and transcends the immediate intent of her assignment or task by specifically directing her activities toward the "good" of her patient.[6:13]

PHILOSOPHY

Philosophy, an attitude toward life and reality that evolves from each nurse's beliefs and code of conduct, motivates the nurse to act, guides her thinking about what she is to do and influences her decisions. It stems from both her culture and subculture, and is an integral part of her. It is personal in character, unique to each nurse, and expressed in her way of nursing. Philosophy underlies purpose, and purpose reflects philosophy.[6:13]

PRACTICE

Overt action, directed by disciplined thoughts and feelings toward meeting the patient's need-for-help, constitutes the practice of clinical nursing. . . . It is goal-directed, deliberately carried out and patient-centered.[6:23]

Knowledge, judgment, and skills are three aspects of practice that are necessary to be effective.[6:25] Identification, ministration, and validation are three components of practice directly related to the patient's care. Coordination of resources is indirectly related to it.[6:31]

Knowledge

Knowledge encompasses all that has been perceived and grasped by the human mind; its scope and range are infinite. Knowledge may be acquired by the nurse, apart from judgment and skills, in a so-called ivory-tower setting. When acquired in this way, it has potentiality for use in directing, teaching, co-ordinating and planning care of the patient, but is not sufficient to meet his need-for-help. To be effective in meeting this need, such knowledge must be supplemented by opportunity for the nurse to function in a nurse-patient relationship with responsibility to exercise judgment and to implement skills for the benefit

of the patient. Knowledge may be factual, speculative, or practical.[6:25]

Factual knowledge. "Factual knowledge is something that may be accepted as existing or as being true."[6:25-26]

Speculative knowledge. "Speculative knowledge on the other hand, encompasses theories, general principles offered to explain phenomena, beliefs or concepts, and the content of such special subject areas as the natural sciences, the social sciences, and the humanities."[6:26]

Practical knowledge. "Practical knowledge is knowing how to apply factual or speculative knowledge to the situation at hand."[6:26]

Judgment

Judgment represents the nurse's potentiality for making sound decisions. Judgment grows out of a cognitive process which involves weighing facts—both general and particular—against personal values derived from ideals, principles and convictions. It also involves differentiating facts from assumptions, and relating them to cause and effect. Judgment is personal in character; it will be exercised by the nurse according to how clearly she envisions the purpose to be served, how available relevant knowledge is to her at the time, and how she reacts to prevailing circumstances such as time, setting, and individuals. Decisions resulting from the exercise of judgment will be sound or unsound according to whether or not the nurse has disciplined the functioning of her emotions and of her mind. Uncontrollable emotions can blot out knowledge as well as purpose. Unfounded assumptions can distort facts. Although whatever decision the nurse may make represents her best judgment at the moment of making it, the broader her knowledge and the more available it is to her, and the greater her clarity of purpose, the firmer will be the foundation on which her decisions rest.[6:27]

Skills

Skills represent the nurse's potentiality for achieving desired results. Skills comprise numerous and varied acts, characterized by harmony of movement, expression and intent, by precision, and by adroit use of self. These acts are always carried out with deliberation to achieve a specific purpose and are not goals in themselves. Deliberation and purpose, therefore, differentiate skills from nurses' actions, which, although they may be carried out with proficiency, are performed with the execution of the act as the end to be attained rather than the means by which it is reached.[6:27]

Skills may be classified as procedural or communication.

Procedural skills. "Procedural skills are potentialities for implementing procedures that the nurse may need to initiate and carry out in order to identify and meet her patients' need-for-help."[6:27-28]

Communication skills. "Communication skills are capacities for expression of thoughts and feelings that the nurse desires to convey to her patient and to others associated with his care. Both verbal and nonverbal expression may be used, singly or together, to deliver a message or to elicit a particular response."[6:28]

Identification. Identification involves individualization of the patient, his experiences, and recognition of the patient's perception of his condition.

> Activities in identification are directed toward ascertaining: (1) whether the patient has a need; (2) whether he recognizes that he has a need; (3) what is interfering with his ability to meet his need; and (4) whether the need represents a need-for-help, in other words, a need that the patient is unable to meet himself.[6:31-32]

Ministration. Ministration is providing the needed help. It requires the identification of the need-for-help and the acceptability of the help to the patient.[6:32]

Validation. "Validation is evidence that the patient's functional ability was restored as a result of the help given."[6:32]

Co-ordination. While striving for unity and continuity, the nurse co-ordinates all services provided to the patient so care will not be fragmented. Reporting, consulting, and conferring are functional elements of co-ordination.[6:33]

Reporting. "Reporting is the act of presenting information in written or oral form and is important in keeping others informed not only about the patient's health and social history, but also about his current condition, reaction, progress, care and plan of care."[6:33-34]

Consulting. "Consulting, the act of seeking information or of asking advice, is a means of gaining, from others, an opinion or suggestion that may help the nurse to broaden her understanding before deciding on a course of action."[6:34]

Conferring. "Conferring, the act of exchanging and comparing ideas, is most often initiated to review the patient's response to the care he has so far received, and to plan his future care."[6:35]

Art. Art is "the application of knowledge and skill to bring about desired results. . . . Art is individualized action. Nursing art, then, is carried out by the nurse in a one-to-one relationship with the patient, and constitutes the nurse's conscious responses to specifics in the patient's immediate situation."[6:36] Nursing art involves three operations: stimulus, preconception, and interpretation.[6:38-39] The nurse reacts based on those operations. "Her actions may be rational, reactionary, or deliberative."[6:40]

Stimulus. The helping process is triggered by a stimulus or the patient's presenting behavior.[6:38]

Preconception. Preconception is an expectation of what the patient may be like.

> This preconception is based on knowledge gained from a great variety of sources including the patient's chart, reports from other nurses, doctors or family members, what the nurse has read or heard

of patients in similar condition, her own experiences with patients in similar condition and, finally, her recollection of previous contacts with the patient.[6:38]

Interpretation. Interpretation is comparison of perception with expectation or hope. Perception is an interpretation of the stimulus and may misinterpret the patient's behavior.[6:39]

Rational action

Rational action is an overt act taken in response solely or mainly to the doer's immediate perception of another's action—verbal or nonverbal—or situation. In a nurse-patient relationship, the nurse's action would be called rational if she responds in a way guided by only her immediate perception of the patient's behavior—what he says, what he does, or how he appears.[6:40]

Reactionary action

Reactionary action, in contrast with rational action, is an overt act taken spontaneously in response to strong feelings the doer experiences when he compares his perception of another's behavior or situation with his expectation or hope about that behavior. In a nurse-patient relationship, the nurse's action is reactionary if it is taken solely or mainly in response to her reaction, to the feelings aroused in her by comparing what she perceived as the patient's behavior with what she hoped for or expected.[6:40]

Deliberative action

Deliberative action is in contrast with both rational action and reactionary action. A deliberative action is an overt act which, although not failing to take account of the doer's immediate perceptions and feeling-reactions is, nonetheless, not based solely on these perceptions or feelings. Rather, deliberative action is interaction, directed toward fulfillment of an explicit purpose and carried out with judgment and understanding of how the other means the behavior which he is manifesting either verbally or nonverbally. In a nurse-patient relationship, the nurse's action is deliberative if her overt action is based on the application—in the fulfillment of her nursing purpose—of principles of helping to gain

understanding of how the patient means the behavior he is manifesting.[6:41]

FRAMEWORK OF NURSING. Limits, supports, and research provide a broad framework in which clinical nursing functions. Limits, or boundaries, in a professional service give the individual guidelines to follow in practicing that profession. Professional limits are set by the profession's code; legal limits are those found in state laws and licensing requirements; local limits are set by the hospital, agency, or individual the nurse contracts to work for; and personal limits are self-imposed by the nurse herself.[6:63-73]

Supportive facilities for the practicing nurse are nursing administration, nursing education, and nursing organizations. Although these are rarely found at the patient's bedside or in the one-to-one relationship between the nurse and patient, they are nevertheless important to the nurse by maintaining standards of quality of nursing care for the profession.[6:73-80]

Wiedenbach recognized that nursing research had not received a great deal of emphasis from the profession in the past although more nursing research was beginning to occur. She acknowledged that such activity was essential to the growth of nursing and might even "prove to be crucial to the conservation of life and the promotion of health."[6:85]

MAJOR ASSUMPTIONS
Nursing

Nurses ascribe to an explicit philosophy. Basic to this philosophy of nursing are "(1) reverence for the gift of life; (2) respect for the dignity, worth, autonomy, and individuality of each human being; (3) resolution to act dynamically in relation to one's beliefs."[6:16] Wiedenbach identifies five essential attributes of a professional person. These characteristics are:

1. Clarity of purpose.
2. Mastery of skill and knowledge essential for fulfilling the purpose.

3. Ability to establish and sustain purposeful working relationships with others, both professional and nonprofessional individuals.
4. Interest in advancing knowledge in the area of interest and in creating new knowledge.
5. Dedication to furthering the goal of mankind rather than to self-aggrandizement.[6:2]

Person

Four explicit assumptions are stated in relation to human nature:

1. Each human being is endowed with unique potential to develop—within himself—resources which enable him to maintain and sustain himself.
2. The human being basically strives toward self-direction and relative independence and desires not only to make best use of his capabilities and potentialities but to fulfill his responsibilities.
3. Self-awareness and self-acceptance are essential to the individual's sense of integrity and self-worth.
4. Whatever the individual does represents his best judgment at the moment of his doing it.[6:17]

Health

The concept of health is neither defined nor discussed in Wiedenbach's model. The definitions of nursing, patient, and need-for-help, and the relationships among these concepts imply health-related concerns in the nurse-patient situation.

Environment

Wiedenbach does not specifically address the concept of environment. It is inferred that the environment may produce obstacles resulting in a need-for-help experienced by the person (Figure 19-1).

THEORETICAL ASSERTIONS

Identification of the patient's need-for-help involves four steps. First, the nurse uses her powers of observation to look and listen for consistencies and inconsistencies of the patient's behavior with her concept of comfort. Second, the nurse explores the meaning of the patient's behavior with him. Third, the nurse determines the cause of the patient's discomfort or incapability. Finally, the nurse determines if the patient can resolve his problem or if he has a need-for-help[6:52-57] (Figure 19-2).

Ministration of help needed involves the nurse making a plan to meet the needs and presenting it to the patient. If the patient concurs with the plan and accepts suggestions for implementing it, the nurse implements it and ministration of help needed occurs. If the patient does not concur with the plan or accept suggestions for implementation, the nurse needs to explore causes of the patient's nonacceptance. If the patient has an interfering problem, the nurse needs to explore the patient's ability to solve the problem. If the patient has a need-for-help, the nurse once again forms a plan to meet the need, presents the plan, and seeks patient concurrence with the plan and acceptance of suggestions for implementation[6:57,61] (Figure 19-3).

Validation that the need-for-help was met is important. The nurse perceives whether the patient's behavior is consistent with her concept of comfort and seeks clarification from the patient to determine if he believes his need-for-help was met. Then the nurse needs to take appropriate action based on the feedback.[6:57,62]

LOGICAL FORM

Wiedenbach developed this model through induction. The reasoning method in inductive logic begins with observation of specific instances, and then combines the specifics into a more generalized whole. The common features of the specific instances allow for grouping the specifics into a larger set of phenomena.[1:61] An analysis of clinical experiences (specific nursing situations) leads to the development and interrelationships of concepts for Wiedenbach's model.[4:79]

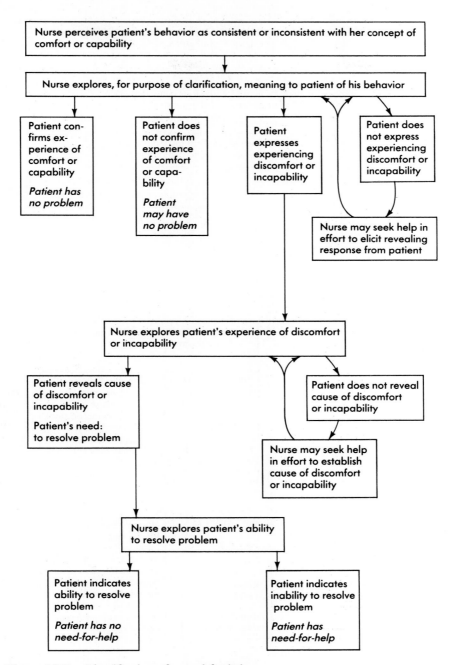

Figure 19-1.   Identification of a need-for-help.

Used with permission from Wiedenbach, E. (1964). *Clinical nursing: A helping art*. New York: Springer, p. 60.

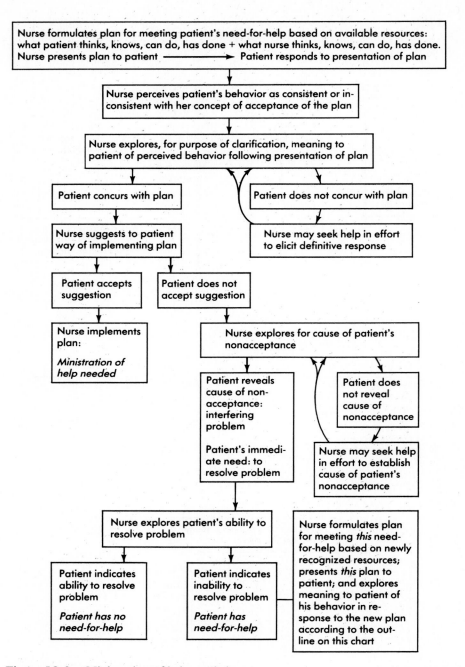

Figure 19-2. Ministration of help needed.

Used with permission from Wiedenbach, E. (1964). *Clinical nursing: A helping art.* New York: Springer, p. 61.

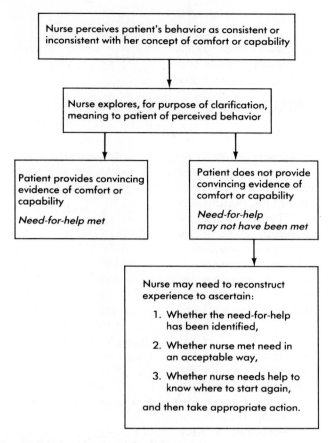

Figure 19-3. Validation that need for help was met.
Used with permission from Wiedenbach, E. (1964). *Clinical nursing: A helping art.* New York: Springer, p. 62.

Wiedenbach, Dickoff, and James[2] have identified four levels of theory development in a practice discipline. In order of increasing sophistication they are factor-isolating, factor-relating, situation-relating, and situation-producing. Wiedenbach[7] considers her work a situation-producing prescriptive theory.

ACCEPTANCE BY THE NURSING COMMUNITY
Practice

Today, nurses are applying Wiedenbach's concepts to their clinical practice more so than did

nurses in the 1950s and 1960s. According to Wiedenbach,[7:23] the practice of clinical nursing "is an overt action, directed by disciplined thoughts and feelings toward meeting the patient's need for help." Drawing from her many years of experience as a nurse midwife, she published "Childbirth as Mothers Say They Like It." In this article Wiedenbach noted that mothers wanted childbirth to be as natural as possible. In addition, mothers wanted instructions on childbirth, father participation, full participation in the labor and delivery process, and rooming-in with their infant in the postpartum periods.[5:417-421] But not until the 1970s were some or most of these needs for help met.

In the 1980s the health care industry is providing the supposedly unique concept of Family Centered Care, which Wiedenbach addressed some 20 years ago.

Education

Wiedenbach[6:75] proposed that nursing education serves the practice of nursing in four major ways:

1. It is responsible for the preparation of future practitioners of nursing;
2. It arranges for nursing students to gain experience in clinical areas of the hospital or in the homes of patients;
3. Its representatives may function in the clinical area and work closely with the staff; and
4. It offers educational opportunities to the nurse for special or advanced study.

Application of Wiedenbach's model to clinical practice requires the nurse to have a sound knowledge of the normal and pathological states, a thorough understanding of human psychology, competence in clinical skills and the ability to initiate and maintain therapeutic communication with patient and family. Also, the nurse must develop sound clinical judgment in decision making about patient care and be able to interpret the patient's behavior. These skills require a general education for nurses.

Today, many nursing schools are meeting this need for general education. Students are prepared with 2 years of courses in the humanities, biological science, and the social sciences, followed by 2 years in nursing science. This curriculum prepares a generalist in professional nursing and serves as the basis for graduate study.

Wiedenbach[6:78] saw graduate study as a means "for nurses to extend the personal limits of their practice and to realize, to a greater degree than before, their potentialities for creative and imaginative practice within the area of their responsibility in the total field of health." Today's focus on graduate education is much the same as Wiedenbach's. It is directed toward preparing advanced practitioners who are competent, self-directed, and concerned with the exploration of practice, issues, and problems of health care in a selected area of nursing.

Research

Before the development of Wiedenbach's model, nursing research focused more on the medical model than on a nursing model. But in Wiedenbach's model the focus of nursing research is to be related to the patient's response to the health care experience. Her model would support research designed to promote family relationships, to control factors responsible for disabling conditions, and to foster sound health care practices. Although not specifically based on Wiedenbach's model, numerous nursing research studies have been carried out in those areas. The results of those studies have been reported in nursing periodicals such as *Nursing Research*. Because of these nursing studies, nurses are better able to meet the patient's need for help.

FURTHER DEVELOPMENT

Wiedenbach is a pioneer in the writing of nursing theory. Her model of clinical nursing is one of the early attempts to systematically describe what it is that nurses do and what nursing is all about. It needs to be further developed by more clearly defining the concepts of health and environment. In addition, the component of nursing art needs to be identified in an operational way.

CRITIQUE

Wiedenbach's model evolved out of a desire to describe the practice of professional nursing. Her theory was influenced by Ida Orlando Pelletier and the philosophy of Dickoff and James, who were her colleagues at Yale University. Hers was one of the earlier nursing theories developed.

Clarity

Wiedenbach's model meets the criterion of clarity in that the concepts and definitions are clear, consistent, and intelligible.

Simplicity

There are too many relational statements for the theory to be classified as a simple theory. The concepts include the need-for-help, nursing practice, and nursing art. All of these concepts are interrelated, equal in importance, and have no meaning aside from their interaction.[5:76] Relationships between the major components can be linked, but it is difficult to diagram some of the concepts in the model. In addition, the concepts describe or explain phenomenon but do not predict.

Generality

The scope of the concepts of patient (person), nursing, and need-for-help are very broad and thus possess generality. However, the concept of need-for-help is based on the patient's recognition of his or her need for help. This concept is not applicable to the infant, comatose patient, or many other physiologically or psychologically incompetent persons. Also, the assumption that all nurses do not share a similar philosophy of nursing lessens the generality of the model.

Empirical Precision

Substantiation of a theory is accomplished through research, and thus the usefulness of the theory is determined. In Wiedenbach's model, the criterion is only partially met. The concepts of nursing practice and need-for-help are operationally defined and measurable. However, the concept of need-for-help is not always applicable. Also, within this theory is an attempt to operationally define nursing art. Therefore, it would be difficult to test this theory.

However, the potential exists for research to be done with this model. J. Fawcett believes three steps must be taken before the model can be tested. "First, the model must be formulated; second, a theory must be derived from the model; and third, operational definitions must be given to the concepts, and hypothesis derived."[3:26]

Derivable Consequences

Derivable consequences refer to the overall effect of the theory and its importance to nursing research, practice, and education. Wiedenbach's model fulfills the purpose for which it was developed: to describe professional practice. The theory focuses on nurse-patient interactions and regards the patient from a holistic point of view. Wiedenbach's work influenced the work of other early scholars, including Orlando and Peplau.

As one of the early nursing theorists, Wiedenbach made an important contribution to the nursing profession.

REFERENCES

1. Chinn, P.L., & Jacobs, M.K. (1983). *Theory and nursing: A systematic approach*. St. Louis: C.V. Mosby.
2. Dickoff, J.J., James, P.A., & Wiedenbach, E. (1968, Nov.-Dec.). Theory in a practice discipline: Practice-oriented theory. *Nursing Research, 17*:545-554.
3. Fawcett, J. (1984). *Analysis and evaluation of conceptual models of nursing*. Philadelphia: F.A. Davis.
4. Raleigh, E. (1983). Wiedenbach's model. In J. Fitzpatrick, & A. Whall, *Conceptual models of nursing analysis and application*. Bowie, Md.: Robert J. Brady.
5. Wiedenbach, E. (1949, Aug.). Childbirth as mothers say they like it. *Public Health Nursing, 5*:417-421.
6. Wiedenbach, E. (1964). *Clinical nursing: A helping art*. New York: Springer.
7. Wiedenbach, E. (1984, Spring). Written interview.

BIBLIOGRAPHY
Primary Sources
Books

Wiedenbach, E. (1958). *Family-centered nursing*. New York: G.P. Putnam's Sons.

Wiedenbach, E. (1964). *Clinical nursing: A helping art*. New York: Springer.

Wiedenbach, E. (1969). *Meeting the realities in clinical teaching*. New York: Springer.

Wiedenbach, E., & Falls, C.E. (1978). *Communication: Key to effective nursing*. New York: Tiresias.

Book Chapters

Wiedenbach, E. (1973). The nursing process in maternity nursing. In J.P. Clausen, et al., *Maternity nursing today*. New York: McGraw-Hill.

Articles

Dickoff, J.J., James, P.A., & Wiedenbach, E. (1968, Sept.-Oct.). Theory in a practice discipline I: Practice-oriented discipline. *Nursing Research, 17:* 415-435.

Dickoff, J.J., James, P.A., & Wiedenbach, E. (1968, Nov.-Dec.). Theory in a practice discipline II: Practice-oriented research. *Nursing Research, 17:*545-554.

Wiedenbach, E. (1940, Jan.). Toward educating 130 million people: A history of the nursing information bureau. *American Journal of Nursing, 40:*13-18.

Wiedenbach, E. (1949, Aug.). Childbirth as mothers say they like it. *Public Health Nursing, 5:*417-421.

Wiedenbach, E. (1960, May). Nurse-midwifery, purpose, practice, and opportunity. *Nursing Outlook, 8:*256.

Wiedenbach, E. (1963, Nov.). The helping art of nursing. *American Journal of Nursing, 63:*54-57.

Wiedenbach, E. (1965, Dec.). Family nurse practitioner for maternal and child care. *Nursing Outlook, 13:*50.

Wiedenbach, E. (1968, May). Genetics and the nurse. *Bulletin of the American College of Nurse Midwifery, 13:*8-13.

Wiedenbach, E. (1968, June). The nurse's role in family planning: A conceptual base for practice. *Nursing Clinics of North America, 3:*355-365.

Wiedenbach, E. (1970, May). Nurses' wisdom in nursing theory. *American Journal of Nursing, 70:*1057-1062.

Wiedenbach, E. (1970, Sept.-Oct.) Comment on beliefs and values: Basis for curriculum design. *Nursing Research, 19:*427.

Interviews

Wiedenbach, E. (1984, Spring). Written interview.

Wiedenbach, E. (1984, May 31). Telephone interview.

Secondary Sources
Book Reviews

Wiedenbach, E. (1958). *Family-centered maternity nursing.*
*Childbirth, 5:*229-230, November 1958.
*Nursing Outlook, 7:*193, April 1959.
*American Journal of Nursing, 59:*663, May 1959.
*Medical World News, 9:*82, January 19, 1968.
*Briefs, 32:*27, February 1968.
*Hospital Progress, 49:*98, July 1968.
*Nursing Outlook, 16:*71, August 1968.
*American Journal of Nursing, 68:*1758, August 1968.
*Obstetrics and Gynecology, 32:*446, September 1968.
*Nursing Journal of India, 60:*38, January 1969.

Wiedenbach, E. (1964). *Clinical nursing: A helping art.*
*Nursing Outlook, 12:*16, September 1964.
*Nursing Mirror, 119:*70, October 16, 1964.
*Journal of American Association of Nurse Anesthetists, 32:*401 +, December 1964.
*Canadian Nurse, 61:*83, February 1965.
*Catholic Nurse, 13:*34, June 1965.
*American Journal of Nursing, 65:*62, July 1965.

Wiedenbach, E. (1969). *Meeting the realities in clinical teaching.*
*Association of Operating Room Nurses, 10:*155. November 1969.

Wiedenbach, E., & Falls, C.E. (1978). *Communication: Key to effective nursing.*
*Occupational Health Nursing, 26:*54, July 1978.
*Supervisor Nurse, 9:*244, September 1978
*American Jorunal of Nursing, 78:*1976, November 1978
*California Nurse, 74:*28, March-April 1979.
*Nursing Times, 75:*588-589, April 5, 1979.

News Releases

Presentation of Hattie Hemschemeyer Award: 24th annual meeting of the American College of Nurse Midwives. *Journal of Nurse-Midwifery, 24:*35-36.

Books

Chinn, P.L., & Jacobs, M.K. (1983). *Theory and nursing: A systematic approach.* St. Louis: C.V. Mosby.

Fawcett, J. (1984). *Analysis and evaluation of conceptual models of nursing.* Philadelphia: F.A. Davis.

Yale University School of Nursing Index Staff. (1969) *Nursing studies index* (Vol. 4). Philadelphia: J.B. Lippincott.

Book Chapters

Bennett, A.M., & Foster, P.C. (1980). Ernestine Wiedenbach. In Nursing Theories Conference Group, J.B. George, Chairperson, *Nursing theories: The base for professional nursing practice.* Englewood Cliffs, N.J.: Prentice-Hall, pp. 138-149.

Meleis, A.I. (1985). Ernestine Wiedenbach. In A.I. Meleis, *Theoretical nursing: Development and progress.* Philadelphia: J.B. Lippincott, pp. 263-274.

Menke, E.M. (1983). Critical analysis of theory development in nursing. In N.L. Chaska (Ed.), *The nursing profession: A time to speak.* New York: McGraw-Hill, pp. 416-426.

Raleigh, E. (1983). Wiedenbach's model. In J. Fitzpatrick, & A. Whall, *Conceptual models of nursing analysis and application.* Bowie, Md.: Robert J. Brady, pp. 67-85.

Walker, L.O. (1983). Theory and research in the development of nursing as a discipline: Retrospect and prospect. In N.L. Chaska (Ed.), *The nursing profession: A time to speak.* New York: McGraw-Hill, pp. 406-415.

Articles

Barnard, K. (1981). Perinatal parental behavior: Nursing research and implications for newborn health—closing. *Birth Defects, 17:*285.

Roberts, J. (1981). Maternal positions in labor: Analysis in relation to comfort and efficiency. *Birth Defects, 17:*97.

Schmidt, W., & Valadian, I. (1964). A bookshelf on maternal-child health. *American Journal of Public Health, 54:*551.

Sheldon, R.S. (1974). Consolidation of hospital obstetric services. *Medical Clinics of North America, 58:*885.

Thompson, J.B. (1981). Nurse midwives and health promotion during pregnancy. *Birth Defects, 17:*29.

Wooden, H.E. (1965). Infection control in family-centered maternity care. *Obstetrics and Gynecology, 25:*232.

Other Sources

Eisler, J., Wolfer, J.A., & Diers, D. (1972). Relationship between the need for social approval and postoperative recovery welfare. *Nursing Research, 21*(5):520-525.

Larson, P.A. (1977). Nurse perception of client illness. *Nursing Research, 26*(6):416-421.

Leonard, R.C., Skipper, J.K., & Woolridge, P.J. (1967). Small sample field experiments for evaluating patient care. *Health Services Research, 2*(1):47-50.

Rickleman, B.L. (1971). Bio-psycho-social linguistics: A conceptual approach to nurse-patient interaction. *Nursing Research, 20*(5):398-403.

Shields, D. (1978). Nursing care in labor and patient satisfaction. A descriptive study. *Journal of Advances in Nursing, 3:*535-550.

Wolfer, J., & Visintainer, M. (1975). Pediatric surgical patients' and parents' stress responses and adjustment. *Nursing Research, 24*(4):244-255.

Imogene King

20

Theory of Goal Attainment

Mary Lee Ackermann, Sallie Anne Brink, Cathy Greenwell Jones,
Sandra L. Moody, Gwynn Lee Perlich, Beth Bruns Prusinski

CREDENTIALS AND BACKGROUND OF THE THEORIST

Imogene King earned a diploma in nursing from St. John's Hospital School of Nursing in St. Louis in 1945. She then worked as an office nurse, a school nurse, a staff nurse, and a private duty nurse to support herself while studying for a baccalaureate degree. In 1948 she received a Bachelor of Science in Nursing Education from St. Louis University. From

The authors wish to express appreciation to Dr. Imogene King for critiquing the chapter.

1947 to 1958 King worked as an instructor in medical-surgical nursing, then as an assistant director at St. John's Hospital School of Nursing. She went on to earn an M.S.N. in 1957 from St. Louis University, then a Doctor of Education degree from Teachers College, Columbia University, New York in 1961. King was awarded an honorary Ph.D. from Southern Illinois University in 1980.

From 1961 to 1966, King was an associate professor of nursing at Loyola University in Chicago, where she developed a master's degree program in nursing using a conceptual framework. During this time her book, *Toward a Theory for Nursing: General Concepts of Human Behavior,* was conceptualized, the literature reviewed, and a contract from a publishing company signed. Between 1966 and 1968 King served as Assistant Chief of Research Grants Branch, Division of Nursing in the Department of Health, Education, and Welfare. While she was in Washington, D.C., her article "A Conceptual Framework for Nursing" was published in *Nursing Research*. From 1968 to 1972 King was the director of the School of Nursing at The Ohio State University in Columbus. The manuscript for her book had been submitted to the publisher by the time she accepted this administrative position, and it was subsequently published in 1971. In *Toward a Theory for Nursing* King concludes, "A systematic representation of nursing is required ultimately for developing a science to accompany a century or more of art in the everyday world of nursing."[6:129]

King returned to Chicago in 1972 as a professor in the Loyola University graduate program. From 1978-1980 she also served as the Coordinator of Research in Clinical Nursing at the Loyola Medical Center, Department of Nursing. From 1972-1975 she was a member of the Defense Advisory Committee on Women in the Services for the Department of Defense. In 1980 King moved to Tampa, Florida, where she is currently a professor at the University of South Florida College of Nursing. The manuscript for her second book, *A Theory for Nursing: Systems, Concepts, Process,* was submitted to the publisher in June 1980 and published in 1981.

King is a member of the American Nurses' Association, the Florida Nurses' Association, and several honorary and professional societies. In addition to her books, she has authored several book chapters and multiple articles in professional journals. A third book, *Curriculum and Instruction in Nursing,* will be published in 1986.

THEORETICAL SOURCES

King[6:ix] states in the preface of *Toward a Theory for Nursing* that the book's purpose "is to propose a conceptual frame of reference for nursing . . . to be utilized . . . by students and teachers, and also by researchers and practitioners to identify and analyze events in specific nursing situations. The framework suggests that the essential characteristics of nursing are those properties that have persisted in spite of environmental changes." King[6:125] proposed that her first book was "a way of thinking about the real world of nursing" that it suggested "an approach for selecting concepts perceived to be fundamental for the practice of professional nursing," and that it showed "a process for developing concepts that symbolize experiences within the physical, psychological, and social environment in nursing." "A search of the literature in nursing and other behavioral science fields, discussion with colleagues, attendance at numerous conferences, inductive and deductive reasoning, and some critical thinking about the information gathered, lead me to formulate my own theoretical framework."[7:37] King[6:124] wrote in 1971 that although nurses were individuals and professionals, nursing was "not yet a science."

When King[12] was asked in a telephone interview, who influenced her work, she said the sources were "too numerous to mention." However, at a conference of nursing theorists she stated the Systems Theory from the behavioral sciences led to the development of her "dynamic interacting systems."[9] She identified in this system three distinct levels of operations: (1) individuals, (2) groups, and (3) society (Figure 20-1). King[4:10] states in her second book that "if the goal of nursing is concern for the health of individuals and the health care of groups, and if one accepts the premise that human beings are open systems interacting with the environment, then a conceptual framework for nursing must be organized to incorporate these ideas." King's concepts and definitions of those concepts were derived from many sources. E. Erikson, A.L. Gesell, Gibson, L. Hall, A.T. Jersild, J. Piaget, I. Orlando, H. Peplau, and H. Selye are just a few.

Figure 20-1. Dynamic interacting systems.

Used with permission from King, I.M. (1971). *Toward a Theory for Nursing*. New York: John Wiley & Sons. p. 20. Revised in I.M. King, *A theory for nursing: Systems concepts, process*. New York: John Wiley & Sons. p. 11.

USE OF EMPIRICAL EVIDENCE

King[11:11] defines theory as "a set of concepts, which, when defined, are interrelated and observable in the world of nursing practice." "Concepts are abstract ideas that give meaning to our sense perceptions, . . . mental images formed by generalizations from these particular impressions."[6:11-12] For King,[9] theory serves to "build scientific knowledge for nursing," and she has identified two methods for cultivating theory. First, a theory can be developed and then tested with research. But the procedure can also be reversed and enable research to initiate the development of theory. King[9] states, "It is my opinion that in today's world of building knowledge for a complex profession such as nursing, one must consider a composite of these two strategies."

Many research studies are cited in King's books, especially with regard to the development of the concepts relating to her theory, but only a few of those studies are briefly mentioned here. With regard to "perception" King examined studies by F.H. Allport, K.J. Kelley and K.R. Hammond, W.H. Ittleson and H. Cantril, and others. In her development of definitions for "space," R. Sommer and R. Ardrey's studies were used and B.B. Minkley's research was noted. For "time," D. Orem's work was acknowledged. In the examination of "communication," theories and models were presented and the studies of P. Watzlawick, J.H. Beavin, and D.D. Jackson; and D. Krieger were noted. Studies by J.F. Whiting, I. Orlando, and J. Bruner were examined for information on "interaction" and "transaction."[7] J. Dewey's theory of knowledge, which dealt with self-action, interaction, and transaction in knowing and the known, and A. Kuhn's work on transactions were also used.[13]

With regard to research, in 1975 King[7:9] noted, "Most studies have centered on technical aspects of patient care and of the health care systems rather than on patient aspects directly. . . . Few problems have been stated that begin with what the patient's condition demands or what the patient wants." In her 1981 book King[10:151-152] states, "Several theoretical formulations about interpersonal relations and nursing process have been described in nursing situations," citing studies by H. Peplau, I. Orlando, H. Yura and M. Walsh, and herself. However, "Few nursing studies have provided empirical data about nursing process phenomena related to human interaction."

King[10:152] notes that Orlando's study "supports the idea that nursing process is reciprocal" because goal identifications exists for nurses and patients. She adds that this study varies from others in that it "described the nurse-patient interaction process that leads to goal attainment."[10:153] King also discusses her own descriptive study, which tested goal attainment and operationally defined a concept of transaction as an integral component of the theory. A method of nonparticipant observation was used to collect information on nurse-patient interactions in a patient care hospital setting. Volunteer patients and graduate nursing students participated, and the students were specifically trained before the study. Multiple interactions were examined with both verbal and nonverbal communication activities recorded as raw data, including whether goals and the means to achieve them were explored and mutually agreed upon. The study provided a classification system useful in nurse-patient interactions.[10:150-156]

A systems approach is used in the development of the theory of goal attainment. King[10:4-10] notes that for about the last two decades, systems have been used to comprehend and respond to "changes and complexity in health care organizations." She adds, "Some scientists who have been studying systems have noted that the only way to study human beings interacting with the environment is to design a conceptual framework of interdependent variables and interrelated concepts."[10:10] In 1971 King[6:91] called the nursing act a process, stating, "The nursing process is a series of acts which connote action, reaction, interaction. Transaction follows when a reciprocal relationship is established by the nurse and patient" and both mutually set the goal to be achieved.

In her second book King[10:144] stated, "A theory of goal attainment was derived from the conceptual framework of interpersonal systems. The dyad, nurse and client, is one type of interpersonal system." In noting the intricate nature of nursing, King developed a conceptual framework consisting of an open system encompassing three parts. "An awareness of the complex dynamics of human behavior in nursing situations prompted the formulation of a conceptual framework that represents personal, interpersonal and social systems as the domain of nursing."[10:13]

Each of the three components uses human beings as the basic element because as individuals, human beings exchange matter, energy, and information with other individuals and the environment. Individuals exist within personal systems, and King provides an example of a "total system" as being a patient or a nurse. King[11-12,69] believes it is necessary to understand the concepts of perception, self, body image, growth and development, and time and space in order to comprehend human beings as persons. Interpersonal systems, or groups, are formed when two or more individuals interact, for example forming dyads (two people) or triads (three people). Families, when acting as small groups, would be considered in this area of the system. Comprehension of this system requires the concepts of role, interaction, communication, transaction, and stress.[10:10-11]

The final interacting system consists of groups with similar concerns or interests in a society, and is referred to as a social system. A religious, educational or health care system exists here. The influential behavior of a family on an individual's growth and development in the society is another example. Within the health care system the concepts of organization, power, authority, decision making and role are essential for comprehension of this dynamic.[10:11-12]

MAJOR CONCEPTS AND DEFINITIONS

"The major concepts in the theory of goal attainment are interaction, perception, communication, transaction, role, stress, growth and development, and time and space."[10:145]

INTERACTION. King[10:145] defines interaction as "a process of perception and communication between person and environment and between person and person, represented by verbal and nonverbal behaviors that are goal directed." Each individual in an interaction (nurse and client) "brings different knowledge, needs, goals, past experiences, and perceptions, which influence the interactions."[10:145]

PERCEPTION. Perception was defined as "each person's representation of reality."[10:146] According to King, this concept includes the import and transformation of energy, and processing, storing, and exporting information. "Perceptions are related to past experiences, concept of self, socioeconomic groups, biological inheritance, and educational background."[10:146]

COMMUNICATION. Communication was defined as "a process whereby information is given from one person to another either directly . . . or indirectly. . . . Communication is the information component of the interactions."[10:146] The exchange of verbal and nonverbal signs and symbols between nurse and client, or client and environment, is communication.[10:146-147]

TRANSACTION. "Transactions are defined as purposeful interactions that lead to goal attainment."[10:1] King goes on to subsequently expand the definition of transactions to include "observable behavior of human beings interacting with their environment . . . the valuation component of human interactions."[10:147]

ROLE. Role was defined as "a set of behaviors expected of persons occupying a position in a social system; rules that define rights and obligations in a position."[10:147] If expectations of a role differ, then role conflict and confusion exists. This may lead to decreased effectiveness of the nursing care provided.

STRESS. Stress is "a dynamic state whereby a human being interacts with the environment."[10:147] Stress "involves an exchange of energy and information between the person and the environment for regulation and control of stressors . . . an energy response of an individual to persons, objects, and events."[10:147] An increase in the stress of individuals interacting can narrow the perceptual field and decrease rationality. An increase in stress may also affect nursing care.

GROWTH AND DEVELOPMENT. King[10:148] defined growth and development as "continuous changes in individuals at the cellular, molecular, and behavioral levels of activities . . . conducive to helping individuals move toward maturity."

TIME. "Time is defined as a sequence of events moving onward to the future. . . . Time is a duration between one event and another as uniquely experienced by each human being."[10:148]

SPACE. "Space is defined as existing in all directions and is the same everywhere."[10:148] Space "is the immediate environment in which nurse and client interact."[10:149]

MAJOR ASSUMPTIONS

King's personal philosophy about human beings and life influenced her assumptions. Her conceptual framework and theory of goal attainment "are based on an overall assumption that the focus of nursing is human beings interacting with their environment leading to a state of health for individuals, which is an ability to function in social roles."[10:143]

Nursing

"Nursing is an observable behavior found in the health care systems in society."[6:125] The goal of nursing "is to help individuals maintain their health so they can function in their roles."[10:3-4] Nursing is viewed as an interpersonal process of action, reaction, interaction, and transaction. Perception of nurse and client also influences the interaction process.

Person

Specific assumptions relating to person follow:

> Individuals are social beings.
> Individuals are sentient beings.
> Individuals are rational beings.
> Individuals are perceiving beings.
> Individuals are controlling beings.
> Individuals are purposeful beings.
> Individuals are action-oriented beings.
> Individuals are time-oriented beings.[10:143]

King wrote, "Individuals have a right to knowledge about themselves, . . . a right to participate in decisions that influence their life, their health, and community service [and] . . . a right to accept or reject health care."[10:143]

Health

Health is viewed as a dynamic state in the life cycle; illness is an interference in the life cycle. Health implies continuous adaptation to stress "in the internal and external environment through optimum use of one's resources to achieve maximum potential for daily living."[10:5] "Health is the function of nurse, patient, physician, family and other interactions."[6:126]

Environment

King states, "An understanding of the ways that human beings interact with their environment to maintain health is essential for nurses."[10:2] Open system implies interaction occurs between the system and its environment, inferring that the environment is constantly changing. "Adjustments to life and health are influenced by [an] individual's interactions with environment. . . . Each human being perceives the world as a total person in making transactions with individuals and things in the environment."[10:141]

THEORETICAL ASSERTIONS

The propositions shown in the following box describe the relationships between King's concepts. Diagrams follow each proposition. When

the propositions are analyzed, 23 relationships are not specified, none are negative, and 22 are positive (Figure 20-2).

PROPOSITIONS

1. If perceptual accuracy (PA) is present in nurse-client interactions (I), transactions (T) will occur.

$$PA(I) \xrightarrow{+} T$$

2. If nurse and client make transactions (T), goals will be attained (GA).

$$T \xrightarrow{+} GA$$

3. If goals are attained (GA), satisfactions (S) will occur.

$$GA \xrightarrow{+} S$$

4. If goals are attained (GA), effective nursing care (NC_e) will occur.

$$GA \xrightarrow{+} NC_e$$

5. If transactions (T) are made in nurse-client interactions (I), growth and development (GD) will be enhanced.

$$(I)T \xrightarrow{+} GD$$

6. If role expectations and role performance as perceived by nurse and client are congruent (RCN), transactions (T) will occur.

$$RCN \xrightarrow{+} T$$

7. If role conflict (RC) is experienced by nurse and client or both, stress (ST) in nurse-client interactions (I) will occur.

$$RC(I) \xrightarrow{+} ST$$

8. If nurses with special knowledge and skills communicate (CM) appropriate information to clients, mutual goal setting (T) and goal attainment (GA) will occur. [Mutual goal setting is a step in transaction and thus has been diagrammed as transaction.]

$$CM \xrightarrow{+} T \xrightarrow{+} GA$$

From Austin, J.K., & Champion, V.L. (1983). King's theory for nursing: Explication and evaluation. In P.L. Chinn (Ed.), *Advances in nursing theory development*. Rockville, Md.: Aspen Systems. Used with permission by Aspen Systems Corporation.

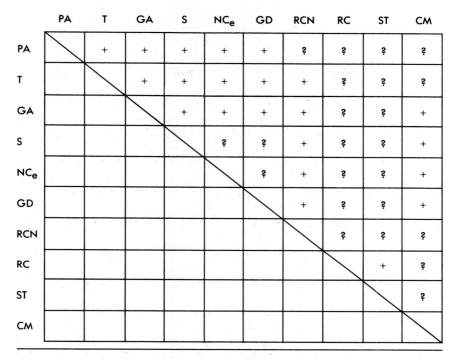

	PA	T	GA	S	NC$_e$	GD	RCN	RC	ST	CM
PA		+	+	+	+	+	?	?	?	?
T			+	+	+	+	+	?	?	?
GA				+	+	+	+	?	?	+
S					?	?	+	?	?	+
NC$_e$						?	+	?	?	+
GD							+	?	?	+
RCN								?	?	?
RC									+	?
ST										?
CM										

Figure 20-2. Relationship table. *PA,* perceptional accuracy; *T,* transactions; *GA,* goals attained; *S,* satisfactions; *NC$_e$,* effective nursing care; *GD,* growth and development; *RCN,* role congruency; *RC,* role conflict; *ST* stress; *CM,* communicate.

Used with permission from Austin J.K., & Austin V.L. (1983). King's theory for nursing: Explication and evaluation. In P.L. Chinn (Ed.), *Advances in nursing theory development.* Rockville, Md.: Aspen Systems. p. 58.

King's theory of goal attainment focuses on the interpersonal system and the interactions that take place between individuals, specifically in the nurse-client association, the dyadic phase. The relationships between King's major concepts that are important to this aspect of the interaction process can be explained through Figure 20-3. In this nursing process, each member of the dyad perceives the other and makes judgments; action results, and together these activities culminate in reaction. Interaction results, and if "perceptual accuracy" exists and any disturbances are conquered, transaction is the outcome. The system is open in order to permit feedback, because perception is potentially influenced by each phase of the activity.*

*References 6:90-93; 10:145-146.

As previously noted, King's descriptive study relating to the theory of goal attainment resulted in a means for analyzing interactions. This is presented in the box on p. 238.

King derived the following seven hypotheses from Goal Attainment Theory.

1. Perceptual accuracy in nurse-patient interactions increases mutual goal setting.
2. Communication increases mutual goal setting between nurses and patients and leads to satisfactions.
3. Satisfactions in nurses and patients increase goal attainment.
4. Goal attainment decreases stress and anxiety in nursing situations.
5. Goal attainment increases patient learning and coping ability in nursing situations.
6. Role conflict experienced by patients, nurses,

Figure 20-3. A process of human interactions.
Used with permission from King, I.M. (1971). *Toward a theory for nursing.* New York: John Wiley & Sons. p. 92.

or both, decreases transactions in nurse-patient interactions.

7. Congruence in role expectations and role performance increases transactions in nurse-patient interactions.[10:156]

Figure 20-4 combines some factors from the classification system and the process of human interaction. Both client and nurse perceive throughout the process; they communicate, thus creating action. Actions result in reactions, and, if there is no disturbance, goals may be set. At this point, means for goal achievement are explored and agreed upon, transactions are made, and goal attainment results.

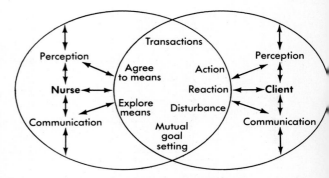

Figure 20-4. Schematic diagram of a theory of goal attainment.
Used with permission from King, I.M. (1981). *A theory for nursing.* New York: John Wiley & Sons. p. 157.

LOGICAL FORM

King[9] indicated at the second annual Nurse Educators' Conference in December 1978 that theory development is composed of inductive and deductive reasoning. She believes theory's primary purpose is to generate new knowledge through research.

King[8:36] wrote in 1975 that her "personal approach to synthesizing knowledge for nursing was to use data and information available from research in nursing and related fields and from my 25 years in active practice, teaching, and research. From all the knowledge available, a theoretical framework relevant for nursing was formulated." In this framework King placed four major concepts that centered

---

CLASSIFICATION SYSTEM OF NURSE-PATIENT INTERACTIONS THAT LEAD TO TRANSACTIONS

ELEMENTS IN INTERACTIONS

Action
Reaction
Disturbance
Mutual goal setting
Explore means to achieve goal
Agree on means to achieve goal
Transaction—goal achieved

Used with permission from King, I.M. (1981). *A theory for nursing.* New York: John Wiley & Sons. p. 156.

around man. She believed that man was an open system, but that energy exchange took place within and external to human organism, and that this led to behavioral responses. The four concepts were social systems, interpersonal relationships, perceptions, and health.[8:37] King proposed her theory of goal attainment in *A Theory for Nursing*. "This theory describes the nature of nurse-client interactions that lead to achievement of goals," she wrote.[8:142]

> Nurses purposefully interact with clients mutually to establish goals and to explore and agree on means to achieve goals. Mutual goal setting is based on nurses' assessment of client's concerns, problems, and disturbances in health, their perceptions of problems, and their sharing information to move toward goal attainment.[10:142-143]

In the 1981 publication there is less dichotomy between health and illness. Illness is referred to as an interference in the life cycle.[10:5] King also reformulated to provide a more open system relationship between person and environment. In the second book King[10] uses adjustment instead of adaptation, and the terms *person, human being,* and *individual* rather than man.

Although King's original framework was very abstract and dealt with "only a few elements of concrete situations."[6:128] She believed her four concepts were "relevant in every nursing situation."[6:128]

There was logical progression of development in the theory from 1971 to 1981. King derived her theory from the conceptual framework available in 1971. Her theory "organizes elements in the process of nurse-client interactions that result in outcomes, that is, goals attained."[10:143]

King[6:128] stated in her first book, "The discovery of knowledge must be disseminated continuously to the practitioners in such a way that they are able to use it in their practice. . . . Descriptive data collected systematically provide cues for generating hypotheses for research in human behavior in nursing situations." Dur-

ing the 1978 nursing theorist conference King[9] indicated that if nurses were taught this process they could begin to predict outcomes in nursing. "This theory should serve as a standard of practice related to nurse-patient interactions, and is in this sense a normative theory."[10:145]

ACCEPTANCE BY THE NURSING COMMUNITY
Practice

Although Goal Attainment Theory is relatively new to nursing, it appears to have been accepted for practice. Its relationship to practice is obvious because the profession of nursing is one that functions through interaction with individuals and groups within the environment. Before King's theory was published, Brown[2:469] stated, "This proposed intrasystems model provides an approach for stimulating continued learning, for establishing innovative foundations for nursing practice, and for generating inquiry through research." King[10:157] states, "Theory, because it is abstract, cannot be immediately applied to nursing practice or to concrete nursing education programs. When empirical referents are identified, defined, and described . . . theory is useful and can be applied in concrete situations."

King derived the Goal Oriented Nursing Record (GONR), based on L.L. Weed's Problem Oriented Medical Record (POMR), from Goal Attainment Theory. A method of collecting data, identifying problems and implementing and evaluating care, it has been used effectively in patient settings. King[11:12] states, "Nurses who have knowledge of the concepts of this theory of Goal Attainment are able to accurately perceive what is happening to patients and family members and are able to suggest approaches for coping with the situations." "The theory and the GONR are useful in practice as nurses have the ability to provide individualized plans and care while encouraging active participation from clients in the decision making phase."[11:11,17] The GONR is one approach to document effectiveness of nursing care.

Education

King's[12] conceptual framework was recently used at Ohio State University for curriculum design in the nursing program, and presently the graduate program at the University of Texas at Houston is doing the same. The Department of Medical-Surgical Nursing at Loyola University in Chicago is using portions of King's steps of nursing process at the graduate level. In 1980, Brown and Lee[2:468] noted that King's concepts were useful in developing a framework" for use in nursing education, nursing practice, and for generating hypotheses for research. . . . [It] provides a systematic means of viewing the nursing profession, organizing a body of knowledge for nursing, and clarifying nursing as a discipline." Shirley Steel used King's framework as the framework for her book, *Child Health and the Family.*

Research

"Research can be designed and conducted to implement this system in a hospital unit, in ambulatory care, in community nursing and home care. This information system can be designed for any patient population and for current and future computerization of records in health care systems."[10:17] In a telephone interview King[12] provided more examples of how her conceptual framework and her GONR are presently being or will soon be used in nursing practice and research. D. Polit and B. Hunger cite her theory in giving examples and discussing different aspects of the research process.

FURTHER DEVELOPMENT

Because this theory has been published only since 1981 there has been little time for digesting, testing, and evaluating. King[12] is preparing to initiate another research project, but is wait-

ing for the results of some studies by other researchers to be released. While maintaining her position as a professor at the University of South Florida, King serves as a consultant, and continues to expand her GONR in diverse situations. She states, "Any profession that has its primary mission in the delivery of social services requires continuous research to discover new knowledge that can be applied to improve practice. . . . The basis for the practice of nursing is knowledge; its activity is guarded by the intellect, and its intellectual application activity is applied in the practical realm."[6:112-113]

CRITIQUE
Simplicity

King's theory presents nine major concepts, thus making the theory complex. The concepts are easily understood, with the exception of some inconsistencies in the definitions of the concepts.

Some of the definitions of the basic concepts lack clarity. King's definition of stress lacks clarity because she states that stress has positive consequences and suggests that nurses should remove stressors from the hospital environment. She gives examples of the negative effects of stress on patients with sensory deprivation and sensory overload. The negative examples contradict the definition of stress.

King maintains that her definitions are clear and conceptually derived from the identified characteristics. She contends that the critics are stating examples of the use of knowledge of the concepts in nursing, but that the examples are not the definition of the concept. She thinks that most critics do not differentiate her definition from the stressors, and that they are different.[13]

Generality

King's theory has been criticized for having limited application in areas of nursing where patients are unable to competently interact with the nurse, such as working with comatose patients, newborns, and some psychiatric patients. Its use with groups has not been clarified.

King responds that 80% of communication is nonverbal. She says,

> Try observing a really good nurse interact with a baby or a child who has not yet learned the language. If you systematically recorded your observations, you would be able to analyze the behaviors and find many transactions at a nonverbal level. I have a beautiful example of that when I was working side by side with a graduate student in a neuro unit with a comatose patient. I was talking to the patient, explaining everything that was happening and showing the graduate student what I believe to be important in nursing care. When the patient regained consciousness a few days later, she asked the nurse in the unit to find that wonderful nurse who was the only one who explained what was happening to her. She wanted to thank her. I made transactions. I could observe her muscle movement. She was trying to help us as a physician poked a tube down her throat. A nurse midwife reports observing transactions between mothers and newborns. Psychiatric nurses have reported to me the value of my theory in their practice. So the need in nursing is to broaden nurses' knowledge of communication and that is what my theory is all about.[13]

King believes critics are assuming that a theory will address every person, event, and situation, which is impossible. She reminds critics that even Einstein's theory of relativity could not be tested completely until space travel made testing possible.[13]

Empirical Precision

King has gathered empirical data on the nurse-patient interaction process that leads to goal attainment. A descriptive study was conducted to test the goal attainment theory. From a sample of 17 patients, goals were attained in 12 cases (70% of the sample). If nursing students were taught the goal attainment theory, and if it were used in nursing practice, goal attainment could be measured along with the effectiveness of nursing care.

Because King's theory is relatively new, em-pirical testing is in the beginning stages, and it remains to be seen if relationships exist between the concepts. King is presently acting as a consultant to researchers testing hypotheses derived from her theory. She hopes researchers will continue to do more testing of the conceptual framework.[12]

Derivable Consequences

For a theory to be useful in nursing practice, it should focus on at least one aspect of the nursing process. King's theory focuses on the planning and implementation phases of the nursing process. The nurse-patient dyad interact, devise mutually agreed-on goals, explore means to achieve goals, transact, and attain goal achievement.

King maintains that her theory focuses on all aspects of the nursing process (APIE) but her process is not the same as the Yura and Walsh model. It requires human interaction. In her classes King compares her model, the Yura and Walsh nursing process model, the problem solving method, and the scientific method by identifying the elements of each of the four processes and their similarities. She believes one must assess to set mutual goals, plan to provide alternate means to achieve goals, and evaluate to determine if the goal was attained. King[13] says she is "the only one who has provided a theory that deals with choices, alternatives, participation of all individuals in decision making and specifically deals with outcomes of nursing care."

REFERENCES

1. Austin, J.K., & Champion, V.L. (1983). King theory for nursing: Explication and evaluation. In P. Chinn, *Advances in nursing theory development*. Rockville, Md.: Aspen Publications.
2. Brown, S.T., & Lee, B.T. (1980). Imogene King's conceptual framework: A proposed model for continuing nursing education. *Journal of Advanced Nursing*, 5(5):467-473.
3. Chinn, P.L., (1983). *Advances in nursing theory development*. Rockville, Md.: Aspen Systems.
4. Daubenmier, M.J., & King, I.M. (1973). Nurs-

ing process models: A systems approach. *Nursing Outlook, 21*:512-517.

5. Gonat, P.J. (1983). Imogene M. King: A theory for nursing. In J. Fitzpatrick, & A. Whall, *Conceptual models of nursing: Analysis and application.* Bowie, Md.: Robert J. Brady.

6. King, I.M. (1971). *Toward a theory for nursing: General concepts of human behavior.* New York: John Wiley & Sons.

7. King, I.M. (1975). Patient aspects. In L.J. Schumann, R.D. Spears, Jr., & J.P. Young (Eds.), *Operations research in health care: A critical analysis.* Baltimore: Johns Hopkins University Press.

8. King, I.M. (1975). A process for developing concepts for nursing through research. In P. Verhonick, *Nursing research.* Boston: Little, Brown.

9. King, I.M. (1978, Dec.). Speech presented at Second Annual Nurse Educators' Conference, New York. Audiotape available from Teach 'Em, Inc., Chicago.

10. King, I.M. (1981). *A theory for nursing: Systems, concepts, process.* New York: John Wiley & Sons.

11. King, I.M. (1984). Effectiveness of nursing care: Use of a goal oriented nursing record in end stage renal disease. *American Association of Nephrology Nurses and Technicians Journal, 11*(2):11-17, 60.

12. King, I.M. (1984). Telephone interview.

13. King, I.M. (1985). Personal correspondence.

14. Schwirian, P.M., & Kisker, K.L. (1977). Perceptions of health among baccalaureate nursing students. *Journal of Nursing Education, 16*:2-9.

BIBLIOGRAPHY
Primary Sources
Books

King, I.M. (1971). *Toward a theory for nursing: General concepts of human behavior.* New York: John Wiley & Sons.

King, I.M. (1981). *A theory for nursing: Systems, concepts, process.* New York: John Wiley & Sons.

Book Chapters

King, I.M. (1975). A process for developing concepts for nursing through research. In P.J. Verhonick (Ed.), *Nursing research* (Vol. I). Boston: Little, Brown.

King, I.M. (1975). Patient aspects. In L.J. Schuman,

R.D. Speas, Jr., & J.P. Young (Eds.), *Operations research in health care: A critical analysis.* Baltimore: The Johns Hopkins University Press.

King, I.M. (1976). The health care systems: Nursing intervention subsystem. In H.H. Werley, et al. (Eds.), *Health research: The systems approach.* New York: Springer.

King, I.M. (1983). King's theory of nursing. In I.W. Clements, & F.B. Roberts (Eds.), *Family health: A theoretical approach to nursing care.* New York: John Wiley & Sons.

King, I.M. (1984). A theory for nursing: King's conceptual model applied in community health nursing. In M.K. Asay, & C.C. Ossler (Eds.), *Proceedings of the Eighth Annual Community Health Nursing Conference: Conceptual models of nursing applications in community health nursing.* Chapel Hill: University of North Carolina.

Portions of Chapters

King, I.M. (1983). Analysis and application of King's theory of goal attainment. In The family coping with a medical illness. In I.W. Clements, & F.B. Roberts (Eds.), *Family health: A theoretical approach to nursing care.* New York: John Wiley & Sons.

Articles

Daubenmire, M.J., & King, I.M. (1973). Nursing process models: A systems approach. *Nursing Outlook, 21*(8):512-517.

King, I.M. (1964, Oct.). Nursing theory: Problems and prospects. *Nursing Science,* pp. 394-403.

King, I.M. (1968). A conceptual frame of reference for nursing. *Nursing Research, 17*(1):27-31.

King, I.M. (1970). A conceptual frame of reference for nursing. *Japanese Journal of Nursing Research, 3:* 199-204.

King, I.M. (1970). Planning for change. *Ohio Nurses Review, 45*:4-7.

King, I.M. (1978). U.S.A.: Loyola University of Chicago school of nursing. *Journal of Advanced Nursing, 3*(4):390.

King, I.M. (1984). Effectiveness of nursing care: Use of a goal-oriented nursing record in end-stage renal disease. *American Association of Nephrology Nurses and Technicians Journal, 11*(2):11-17:60.

King, I.M., & Tarsitano, B. (1982). The effect of structured and unstructured preop teaching: A replication. *Nursing Research, 31*(6):324-329.

NLN Publications

King, I.M. (1978). *How does the conceptual framework provide structure for the curriculum? Curriculum process for developing or revising baccalaureate nursing programs.* New York: NLN Publication 15-1700. pp. 23-34.

King, I.M. (1978). The "why" of theory development. In *Theory development: What, why, how?* New York: NLN Publication 15-1708. pp. 11-16.

Letters to the Editor

King, I.M. (1975). Reaction to "The patient rights advocate," by G.J. Annas, & J. Healey. *Journal of Nursing Administration, 5*(1):40-41.

Forewords

King, I.M. (1969). Symposium on neurologic and neurosurgical nursing. *Nursing Clinics of North America, 4*(2):199-200.

Audio Tapes

King, I.M. (1978, Dec. 4-6). *Nursing theory.* Nursing Resources, Inc., Wakefield, Mass.

King, I.M. (1978) *Second Annual Nurse Educators' Conference,* held in New York City. Audiotape available from Teach 'em, Inc. 160 E. Illinois Street, Chicago, IL 60611.

King, I.M. (1984, May). *Nurses' Theorist Conference* held at Edmonton, Alberta. Audio tapes available from Kennedy Recordings, R.R. 5, Edmonton, Alberta, T5P 487.

Personal Communication

King, I.M. (1984, Oct. 22). Telephone interview.

Presented Papers

King, I.M. (1980, April 21). *Theory development in nursing.* Paper presented at Georgia State University, Atlanta.

Secondary Sources
Book Reviews

King, I.M. (1971). *Toward a theory for nursing: General concepts of human behavior.*
Association of Operating Room Nurses' Journal, 1971, *14:*126.
*Canadian Nurse, 67:*40, 1971.
*Nursing Outlook, 19:*513, 1971.
*Nursing Research, 20:*462, 1971.

*American Journal of Nursing, 72:*1153, 1972.
*Journal of Nursing Administration, 2:*63, 1972.
*South African Nursing Journal, 40:*32, 1973.

King, I.M. (1981). *A theory for nursing: Systems, concepts, process.*
*American Association of Nurses and Nephrology Technicians Journal, 3:*39-40, 1981.
*Nursing Mirror, 154:*32, 1982.
*Nursing Outlook, 30:*414, 1982.
*Nursing Times, 78:*331, 1982.
*Research in Nursing and Health, 5:*166-167, September 1982.
*Today's OR Nurse, 4:*62, 1982.
*Western Journal of Nursing Research, 4:*103-104, 1982.
Australian Nurses Journal, 12(7):33-34, 1983.

Books

Bevis, E.O. (1982). *Curriculum building in nursing: A process.* St. Louis: C.V. Mosby.

Chaska, N.L. (Ed.). (1983). *The nursing profession: A time to speak.* New York: McGraw Hill.

Chinn, P.L. (Ed.). (1983). *Advances in nursing theory development.* Rockville, Md.: Aspen Systems.

Chinn, P.L., & Jacobs, M.K. (1983). *Theory and nursing: A systematic approach.* St. Louis: C.V. Mosby.

Fitzpatrick, J.J., & Whall, A.L. (1983). *Conceptual models of nursing: Analysis and application.* Bowie, Md.: Robert J. Brady.

Fitzpatrick, J.J., et al. (1982). *Nursing models and their psychiatric mental health applications,* Bowie, Md.: Robert J. Brady.

Kim, H.S. (1983). *The nature of theoretical thinking in nursing.* Norwalk, Conn.: Appleton-Century-Crofts.

Nursing Theories Conference Group, J.B. George, Chairperson. (1980). *Nursing theories: The base for professional nursing practice.* Englewood Cliffs, N.J.: Prentice-Hall.

Polit, D., & Hungler, B. (1983). *Nursing research: Principles and methods.* Philadelphia: J.B. Lippincott.

Steele, S., (1981). *Child health and the family: Nursing concepts and management.* New York: Masson.

Stevens, B.J. (1984). *Nursing theory: Analysis, application, evaluation* (2nd. ed.). Boston: Little, Brown.

Thibodeau, J.A. (1983). *Nursing models: Analysis and evaluation.* Monterey, Calif.: Wadsworth.

Walker, L.O., & Avant, K.C. (1983). *Strategies for theory construction in nursing*. Norwalk, Conn.: Appleton-Century-Crofts.

Who's Who in America (43rd. ed.) (1984). Chicago: Marquis.

Who's Who in the midwest. (1984). Chicago: Marquis.

Book Chapters

Austin, J.K., & Champion, V.L. (1983). King theory for nursing: Explication and evaluation. In P. Chinn, *Advances in nursing theory development*. Rockville, Md.: Aspen Publication. pp. 49-61.

Chinn, P.L., & Jacobs, M.K. (1983). Theory in nursing: A current overview. In *Theory and nursing: A systematic approach*. St. Louis: C.V. Mosby. pp. 190-191.

Fawcett, J. (1984). King's open systems model. In *Analysis and evaluation of conceptual models of nursing*. Philadelphia: F.A. Davis. pp. 83-113.

Fitzpatrick, J., et al. (1982). Nursing models. In *Nursing models and their psychiatric mental health application*. Bowie, Md.: Robert J. Brady. pp. 62-64.

George, J.B. (1980). Imogene M. King. In Nursing Theories Conference Group, J.B. George, Chairperson, *Nursing theories: The base for professional nursing practice*. Englewood Cliffs, N.J.: Prentice-Hall. pp. 184-198.

Gonot, P.J. (1983). Imogene M. King: A theory for nursing. In J. Fitzpatrick, & A. Whall, *Conceptual models of nursing: Analysis and application*. Bowie, Md.: Robert J. Brady. pp. 221-243.

Meleis, A.I. (1985). Imogene King. In *Theoretical nursing: Development and progress*. Philadelphia: J.B. Lippincott. pp. 230-237.

Thibodeau, J.A. (1983). History of the development of nursing models. In *Nursing models: Analysis and evaluation*. Monterey, Calif.: Wadsworth. pp. 37-38.

Articles

Brown, S.T., & Lee, B.T. (1980). Imogene King's conceptual framework: A proposed model for continuing nursing education. *Journal of Advanced Nursing*, 5(5):467-473.

Chance, K.S. (1982). Nursing models: A requisite for professional accountability. *Advances in Nursing Science*, 4(2):46-65.

Craig, S.L. (1980). Theory development and its relevance for nursing. *Journal of Advanced Nursing*, 5(4):349-355.

Daubenmier, M.J., & King, I.M. (1973). Nursing process models: A systems approach. *Nursing Outlook*, 21:512-517.

Gortner, S.R., & Nahm, H. (1977). An overview of nursing research in the U.S. *Nursing Research*, 26(1):10-33.

Jones, P.S. (1978, Nov.) An adaptation model for nursing practice. *American Journal of Nursing*, 78:1900-1906.

Luker, K.A. (1979). Measuring life satisfaction in an elderly female population. *Journal of Advanced Nursing*, 4(5):503-511.

McFarlane, E.A. (1980). Nursing theory: The comparison of four theoretical proposals. *Journal of Advanced Nursing*, 5(1):3-19.

Schwirian, P.M., & Kisker, K.L. (1977). Perceptions of health among baccalaureate nursing students. *Journal of Nursing Education*, 16(6):2-9.

Whall, A.L. (1980). Congruence between existing theories of family functioning and nursing theories. *Advances in Nursing Science*, 3(1):59-67.

Other Sources

Allport, F.H. (1955). *Theories of perception and the concept of structure*, New York: John Wiley & Sons.

Bruner, J.S., & Krech, W. (Eds.). (1968). *Perception and personality*. New York: Greenwood.

Bruner, J., Goodnow, J., & Austin, G. (1962). *A study in thinking*. New York: John Wiley & Sons.

Buber, M. (1958). *I and thou*. New York: Charles Scribner's Sons.

Churchman, C.W. (1968). *The systems approach*. New York: Dell.

Churchman, C.W., Ackoff, R., & Wilson, R. (1957). *Introduction to operations research*. New York: John Wiley & Sons.

Counte, M.A., & Christman, I.P. (1981). *Interpersonal behavior and health care*. Boulder, Colo: Westview.

Dewey, J., & Bentley, A.F. (1949). *Knowing and the known*. Westport, Conn.: Greenwood.

Dubin, R. (1978). *Theory building*. New York: Free Press.

Dubos, R. (1961). *Mirage of health*. New York: Doubleday.

Dubos, R. (1963). *The torch of life*. New York: Pocket Books.

Dubos, R. (1973). *Man adapting*. New Haven: Yale University Press.

Erikson, E. (1964). *Childhood and society*. New York: Norton.

Fawcett, J. (1978). The "what" of theory development. In *Theory development: What, why, how?* New York: NLN Publication 15-1708.

Feigl, H., & Brodbeck, M. (Eds.). (1953). *Readings in the philosophy of science*. New York: Appleton-Century-Crofts.

Freud, S. (1965). *New introductory lectures on psychoanalysis*. New York: W.W. Norton.

Gesell, A.L. (1946). *The child from five to ten*. New York: Harper & Sons.

Gesell, A.L. (1952). *Infant development*, New York: Harper & Row.

Hall, J.E., & Weaver, B.R. (1977). *Distributive nursing: A system approach to community health*. Philadelphia: J.B. Lippincott.

Ittleson, W.H., & Cantril, H. (1954). *Perception: A transactional approach*. Garden City, N.Y.: Doubleday.

Jersild, A.T. (1954). *Child psychology*. New York: Prentice Hall.

Jersild, A.T. (1963). *The psychology of adolescence*. London: Macmillan.

Kelley, K.J., & Hammond, K.R. (1964). An approach to the study of clinical inference. *Nursing Research, 13(4):*314-322.

Kerlinger, F. (1973). *Foundations of behavioral research* (2nd ed.). New York: Holt, Rinehart, & Winston.

Krieger, D. (1975, May). The therapeutic touch: The imprimatur of nursing. *American Journal of Nursing, 75:*784-787.

Knutson, A. (1965). *The individual, society, and health behavior*. New York: Russell Sage Foundation.

Kuhn, A. (1975). *Unified social science*. Homewood, Ill.: Dorsey Press.

Linton, R. (1936). *The study of man*. New York: Appleton-Century-Crofts.

Merton, R (1957). *Social theory and social structure*. New York: Macmillan.

Minckley, B.B. (1968, March). Space and place in patient care. *American Journal of nursing, 68:*510-516.

Nagel, E. (1961). *The structure of science*. New York: Harcourt Brace & World.

Orlando, I.J. (1961). *The dynamic nurse-patient relationship*. New York: G.P. Putnam's Sons.

Orlando, I.J. (1972). *The discipline and teaching of nursing process*. New York: G.P. Putnam's Sons.

Orem, D.E. (1971). *Nursing: Concepts of practice*. Scarborough, Ontario: McGraw-Hill.

Orem, D.E. (1979). *Concept formalization in nursing process and product*. Boston: Little, Brown.

Orme, D.E. (1969). *Time, experience and behavior*. New York: American Elsevier.

Parsons, T. (1951). *The social system*. New York: The Free Press.

Peplau, H. (1952). *Interpersonal relations in nursing*. New York: Putnam's.

Piaget, J. (1962). *Judgment and reasoning in the child*. New York: Humanities. (Reproduction of 1928 ed.).

Seyle, H. (1974). *Stress without distress*. Philadelphia: J.B. Lippincott.

Spiegel, J. (1971). *Transactions: The interplay between individual, family, and society*. New York: Science House.

Thibaut, J., & Jones, E. (1958). Interaction goals as bases of inference in interpersonal perception. In R. Tagiuri, & L. Petrullo (Eds.), *Persons, perception, and interpersonal behavior*. Palo Alto, Calif.: Stanford University Press.

von Bertalanffy, L. (1968). *General systems theory*. New York: Braziller.

Watzlawick, P., Beavin, J.H., & Jackson, D.D. (1967). *Pragmatics of human communication*. New York: Norton.

Weed, L.L. (1969). *Medical records, medical education, and patient care*. Cleveland: Case Western Reserve University Press.

Wiener, N. (1967). *The human use of human beings*. New York: Avon.

Whiting, J.F. (1955, Oct. 5). Q-sort: A technique for evaluating perceptions of interpersonal relationships. *Nursing Research, 4:*70-75.

Wilson, R.N. (1965). The social structure of a general hospital. In J. Skipper and R. Leonard (Eds.), *Social interaction and patient care*. Philadelphia: J.B. Lippincott.

Wooldridge, P.J., et al (1983). *Behavioral science and nursing theory*. St. Louis: C.V. Mosby.

Yura, H., & Walsh, M. (1978). *The nursing process*. New York: Appleton-Century-Crofts.

Joan Riehl Sisca

21

Symbolic Interactionism

Alta J.H. Gochnauer, Kathleen Millican Miller

CREDENTIALS AND BACKGROUND OF THE THEORIST

Although Joan Riehl was born in Davenport, Iowa, she spent most of her childhood and young adult life in a Chicago suburb. She attended the University of Illinois in Urbana and Chicago where she obtained her B.S.N. After graduation she worked as a clinical instructor, a supervisor, and an in-service director in Texas and in California before returning to college for her master's degree in nursing. After receiving her M.S.N. from UCLA, Riehl taught pediatric nursing at California State University for 3

years before joining the faculty at the University of California in Los Angeles. There she began teaching theoretical concepts and their application. Two major professional events resulted from this instruction. First, she began writing nursing textbooks on conceptual models to use for teaching graduate students, and she began to identify her own theoretical framework. Her interest resulted in doctoral study at UCLA in sociology, which afforded the opportunity to pursue the knowledge base needed to develop the particulars of her model. Symbolic interactionism is the foundation upon which this model is built. Role theory and self-concept are components of the theory. They constituted her dissertational investigation for her Ph.D., which she received in 1980.

The authors wish to express appreciation to Dr. Joan Riehl Sisca for critiquing the chapter.

Like many nurses who attend graduate school, Riehl worked part-time to maintain her clinical and research skills. The positions she held during this period included being a staff nurse in medical-surgical and psychiatric nursing and in the ICU-CCU, and being a supervisor in a gerontological hospital in Southern California. She also worked as a research assistant and coordinator in several research projects at the University of California at Los Angeles.

After graduation, Riehl moved to San Antonio, Texas. While there she taught sociology, psychiatric nursing, and mental health concepts as a lecturer in the Department of Social Science at the University of Texas and as an associate professor in the Division of Nursing at Incarnate Word College. She also served as a research evaluator on a government grant that examined numerous variables regarding the R.N. to B.S.N. student. When the three-year grant was completed, Riehl was named Chairperson of the Department of Nursing at the Harrisburg Area Community College in Harrisburg, Pennsylvania.

Riehl is a member of numerous professional organizations. They include the American Nurses' Association, the ANA Council of Nurse Researchers, Sigma Theta Tau, the American Sociological Association, and the American Association for the Advancement of Science.

THEORETICAL SOURCES

Riehl's theory is derived from symbolic interactionism (SI). In SI theory,

> interaction occurs between human beings who interpret or define each others' actions instead of merely reacting to them. The response is based on the meaning which the individual attaches to the action. Human interaction is mediated by the use of symbols, by interpretation, or by ascertaining the meaning of one another's action. This mediation is equivalent to inserting a process of interpretation between the stimulus and the response in the case of human behavior.[3:8]

Consequently, Riehl claims several theoretical sources from sociology and social psychology, including George Mead, Herbert Blumer, Arnold Rose, L. Edward Wells, Gerald Marwell, and Robert E.L. Faris.

EMPIRICAL EVIDENCE

During the past 50 years, the SI theory has been supported by numerous empirical studies. Many theoretical sources, including those mentioned above, have illustrated the utility of this theory and have contributed to further refinement and clarification of its components. Blumer[1:viii] eloquently states, "It is my conviction that an empirical science necessarily has to respect the nature of the empirical world that is its object of study. In my judgment symbolic interactionism shows that respect for the nature of human group life and conduct."

MAJOR CONCEPTS AND DEFINITIONS

Riehl's theory and model adapt four key concepts from the SI theory described by Blumer.[1:50] In addition, Riehl employs the "me" and "I" concepts developed by Mead. Last, she identifies role reversal and sick role as examples of the concept.

PEOPLE. "People, individually and collectively, are prepared to act on the basis of the meaning of the objects that comprise their world."[1:50] In the Riehl model, the term *people* includes the patient, the nurse, other health care professionals, and the patient's family and friends. Riehl[4:17] describes the nurse as one who knows her capabilities, is self-directed, and assumes more than one role in a given period.

ASSOCIATION. "The association of people is necessarily in the form of a process in which they are making indications to one another and interpreting each other's indications."[1:50] Riehl summarizes this as the defining process of role taking, a psychological concept instituted by Mead. Role taking occurs when an individual cognitively internalizes another person's perceptions of reality in varied situations.[4:352] Hence, the formative meanings of actions arise from this reciprocal interaction. The nurse-patient interface is an example of this interaction.

SOCIAL ACTS. "Social acts, whether individual or collective, are constructed through a process in which the actors note, interpret, and assess the situations confronting them."[1:50] Riehl[3:46] states, "Their interpretation of these situations influence their social acts toward each other." She expounds on the interpretive phase as described by Faris, in which a delayed response promotes clear thought, reduced frustration, and prospective learning.[4:354] This concept correlates to Riehl's method of process recordings, which allows the nurse to assess and respond more approximately to a patient's behavior.

INTERLINKAGES. "The complex interlinkages of acts that comprise organizations, institutions, division of labor, and networks of interdependency are moving and not static affairs."[1:50] From this concept Riehl derives that patient assessment is a dynamic process that often necessitates the use of several resources in meeting patient's needs, particularly in long-term care.

ME. Riehl defines *me* synonymously with a role taker in a given situation. In other words, the *me* learns and assumes the attitudes of others. This is a concept used in the development of one's behavior as well as a method of understanding another's actions.

I (SELF-CONCEPT). Riehl defines I, or self-concept, as the individual's total behavioral perceptions, reflecting the summation of roles. She states, "The self-concept refers to a global, relatively constant self-perception that an individual holds and it changes only gradually."[3:64]

ROLE REVERSAL. Role reversal is a potential consequence resulting during the interaction between nurse and patient. Riehl[4:355] defines role reversal as an inadvertent situation in which "the patient assumes the therapeutic role while the nurse becomes the recipient of the care." Rectification of this situation may require assistance from a third person.

SICK ROLE. Riehl[4:355] does not explicitly define sick role, but states there is a problem "when a patient is reluctant to part with the sick role." As with role reversal, this situation suggests the need of additional resources for the patient's rehabilitation.

MAJOR ASSUMPTIONS

Riehl relates Arnold Rose's generic and analytic assumptions to nursing and uses them in her derived theory. Rose divides his assumptions into two categories. The first, generic assumptions, deals with only the child. The second is the analytic assumptions, which focus on all ages of man other than the child.

Generic Assumptions

Rose cites the following four generic assumptions applicable to the SI theory.

1. "Society—a network of interacting individuals—with its culture—the related meanings and values by means of which individuals interact—precedes any existing individual."[4:353]
2. "The process by which socialization takes place can be thought of as occurring in three stages."[4:353] These stages are:
   a. "The infant is habituated to a certain sequence of behaviors and events through a psychogenic process such as trial and error."[4:353]

b. "When the habit is blocked, the image of the incomplete act arises in the infant's mind and he thus learns to differentiate the object . . . in that act by a symbol."[4:353]

c. "As the infant acquires a number of meanings he uses them to designate to others, and to himself, what he is thinking."[4:353]

3. "The individual is socialized into the general culture and also into various subcultures."[4:353]

4. "While some groups and personal meanings and values may be dropped and become lower on the reference-relationship scale, they are not lost or forgotten."[4:353]

Analytic Assumptions

The five analytic assumptions pertaining to the SI theory according to Rose follow.

1. "Man lives in a symbolic as well as in a physical environment and can be stimulated to act by symbols as well as by physical stimuli."[4:351]

2. "Through symbols, man has the capacity to stimulate others in ways other than those in which he himself is stimulated."[4:351] Riehl[4:351] states that role taking, a concept included under this assumption, is important in nursing.

3. "Through communication of symbols, man can learn huge numbers of meanings and values—and hence ways of acting—from other men."[4:351] Riehl summarizes that as a result of this assumption man's behavior is not learned through trial and error or through conditioning, but rather through symbolic communication.[4:351] "According to the SI theory, an individual's perception of how others evaluate him is more important in forming his self-concept than the actual evaluation that others hold."[3:12] Riehl[4:351] explains that it can be deduced from this assumption that "through the learning of a culture, or subculture, men are able to predict each other's behavior and gauge their own behavior accordingly."

4. "The symbols—and the meanings and values to which they refer—do not occur in isolated bits, but in large and complex clusters."[4:351] This assumption refers to man's role. As defined in the discussion of concepts, the "me" is the role-taker and the "I," or self-concept, is the perception of the person as a whole. "Since the 'me' is made up of the attitudes of others, these others can take this role and predict an individual's behavior in a given capacity."[3:351] Consequently, a person is able to gain insight into another's problem by taking the other's role, anticipating how he will act, and implementing a plan of action to help him accomplish his goal.[4:352]

5. "Thinking is the process by which possible symbolic solutions and other future courses of action are examined, assessed for their relative advantages and disadvantages in terms of the values of the individual, and chosen for action or rejected."[4:352] Riehl discusses two major points involving this assumption. First, the assumption encompasses the four steps of the nursing process: "nursing assessment, diagnosis, planned intervention, and evaluation of action."[4:352] Second, she points out, "Since meaning arises in the process of interaction between two persons, and individuals differ, even the most carefully thought out plan may go awry."[4:352]

THEORETICAL ASSERTIONS

Riehl has identified several theoretical assertions in her model. These include:

1. "The premise that social action is built up by the acting unit through the process of noting, interpreting, etc., implies how social action should be studied."[4:354] Riehl identifies the acting unit as the individual.

2. "According to Blumer (1969), in order to treat and analyze social action, one must observe the process by which it is constructed." Riehl[4:354] identifies "one" as the nurse, who must view the social action as the individual sees it.

3. "Since the self-concept is an integral part of this model, the nurse must continue to develop self-insight through self evaluation regarding his/her own actions to understand end results of interactions with others."[7,8]

4. "The goal of action is based upon a key factor of SI, which is taking the role of the others."[4:354] Riehl[4:354] identifies three methodological approaches the nurse uses to achieve this goal. The first approach, role taking, allows the nurse to understand why the patient does what he does. The second method entails interpretation of these actions. The third involves the use of process recordings. Riehl does not advocate recording all interactions, but she does recommend recordings be used until the nurse is able to respond effectively during on-the-spot interactions.

5. "It must be realized that it is not completely possible to take the role of the other, but genuine attempts to do so convey understanding of the other's position."[6,8]

6. "Three additional elements must be included to meet the requirements of an effective conceptual model for nursing, namely, the source of difficulty, the intervention, and the consequences."[4:354] Riehl[5,7] equates the source of difficulty with the nursing diagnosis, and the intervention with the plan of care arrived at after role taking, interpretation, and process recordings.

7. The eclipse shown in her model (Figure 21-1), "should never be complete, however, because maintaining a certain distance is essential for the preservation of the individuality of each person."[4:356] As

the nurse and patient gain knowledge and insight from their interactions, the circles in the model move toward each other and form an ecliptical image. However, Riehl[4,7] emphasizes that if the circles form a complete eclipse, objectivity and independence will be lost.

LOGICAL FORM

Riehl's derived theory uses deductive logic, because Riehl draws relationships between nursing and the SI theory. Her statements are consistent with Meads' concepts of role taking and self-concept. Her theoretical assertions deduced from Rose's assumptions demonstrate further consistency. This allows for easy identification of the interrelationships between the theoretical components, and thus enhances the generation of hypotheses for empirical testing.

ACCEPTANCE BY THE NURSING COMMUNITY
Practice

Riehl's theory has not been widely accepted in nursing practice, although some nursing literature describes its potential applicability. For example, it has been considered a middle range theory in nursing.[2:13] Middle range constitutes a relatively broad scope of phenomena, but its goals are not directed toward the global concerns of the discipline. Also, L.O. Walker and K. Avant[9:167] illustrate that Riehl's derivations of content and structure from the SI theory have "made sense in a nursing care setting."

As Figure 21-1 illustrates, Riehl views the nurse therapist and the patient as actively exchanging information and gleaning knowledge. This is accomplished through mutual role taking in conjunction with the nurse selecting and using known theoretical approaches. The unshaded areas of the model indicate active processes in the relationship, while the arrows represent the complex interdependencies of these

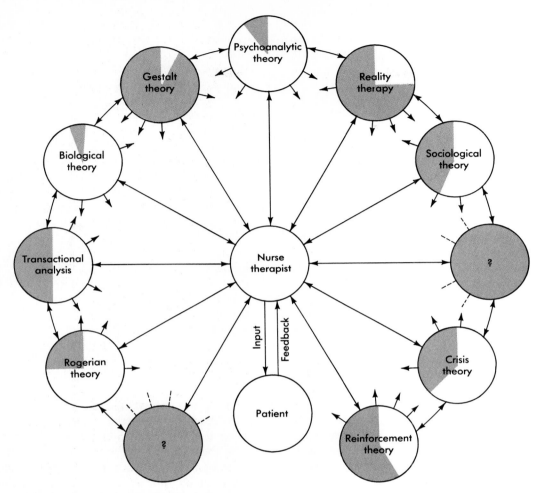

Figure 21-1. Schematic representation of model.
Used with permission from Preisner, J.M. (1980). A proposed model for the nurse therapist, In J.P. Riehl and C. Roy, *Conceptual models for nursing practice*. New York: Appleton-Century Crofts. p. 363.

elements, allowing for continual reassessment and evaluation.

Riehl's model provides a realistic approach for nursing practice in any situation where the focus is on role interaction in the nurse-patient relationship. Preisner demonstrates the applicability of Riehl's model in the psychiatric setting.[4:362-371] The nurse selects from multiple theories, therapies, and allied health disciplines in planning and implementing effective nursing interventions.

Wood demonstrates the use of role taking in a patient's hospital admission.[4:357-361] The nurse interprets the patient's response to the new environment and thereby helps the patient acquire the necessary perceptual changes or new roles in the health care system.

The nursing implications are evident, yet not restrictive to the interaction between the nurse and patient. The role interaction framework may also be effective in nurse-nurse relationships (nursing management, for example), nurse-physician dyads, nurse-patient-family triads, and other interactive situations. However, the model's emphasis remains on the nurse-patient relationship.

Education

The SI theory has long been prevalent among schools of sociology and psychology. Because the Riehl interaction model was introduced to the nursing discipline only recently, in 1980, it is uncertain whether any educational institutions have incorporated it into their nursing curriculum. As previously stated, Riehl[6,8] is in the process of implementing her model into theory and practice in the nursing curriculum at Harrisburg Area Community College in Pennsylvania. In addition, interaction models as a group, are moderately employed in B.S.N. programs.[4:396-398] Nursing is presently concerned with developing a distinct body of knowledge and delineating its professional role. Riehl's model, which focuses on the therapeutic processes in the nurse-patient relationship, will undoubtedly contribute to these goals.

Research

To date, no nursing research has been published involving the application and testing of Riehl's theory. Research relevant to her theory, although limited in scope, can be found in her own doctoral dissertation. This study examines autistic children's ability to role take as compared with their "normal" siblings. It implicates a positive correlation between the level of development of self-concept and the ability to role take.

The generation of implications for further research is inherent in empirical studies. Riehl makes several suggestions for further testing dealing specifically with autistic children, such as investigating their perceptions of their parent's treatment of them and simply increasing the sample size to study more variables in this population. Examples of other recommendations include applying this study to other handicapped children and developing more tools for measuring self-conception. Further

nursing research is essential for Riehl's theory to gain credibility, acceptance, and future application.

FURTHER DEVELOPMENT

Riehl has introduced an interesting and valuable model of SI to nursing. The theory is still in its early stages of development, but Riehl[5,6] is planning to include further development of her theory in future publications. She plans to incorporate the concepts of stress, decision making, and self-analysis into the theory and to better define the concepts of I, me, and process recordings.

More explicit definitions of many concepts in the current model, including SI itself are needed for in-depth descriptions in regard to the relationship statements between Blumer's concepts and nursing, and between Rose's assumptions and nursing. Furthermore, the theoretical assertions require refinement for lucidity and depth.

As a therapeutic nursing approach, Riehl's theory merits the involvement of the profession for progress in its development, understanding, and validation. Abundant potential for both nursing research and subsequent contributions to the theory seems to lie particularly in the psychiatric nurse setting. This testing may also generate new information. "Theory development is important to the growth of any discipline" and should be pursued.[4:3]

CRITIQUE
Complexity

The Riehl interaction model contains several key concepts and theoretical relationships; thus it is complex. With the future development of concepts and relationships, this level of complexity will increase.

Generality

Riehl's interaction mdoel is generalizable to the broad scope of nursing. However, in a situation with a nonresponsive comatose patient, this application may be limited to information and interpretations obtained from the patient's family and friends.

Empirical Precision

The derived concepts from Blumer and Mead have been defined explicitly and grounded in observable reality within their parent discipline. However, Riehl does not clarify all her concepts with denotative definitions and therefore obscures the means for accurate testability. For this reason, a high degree of empirical precision is not present.

Derivable Consequences

Riehl's interaction model employs the nursing process in implementing nursing care. Emphasis is on the nurse assessing and interpreting the patient's actions and then making predictions about the patient's behavior in order to plan interventions. Furthermore, the evaluation phase in the theory, regarding potential patient problems, presents important nursing implications. The theory's usefulness is evident not only in the delivery of nursing care, but also in delineating the nurse's professional role.

Summary

Riehl is in the beginning stages of development of her nursing theory, which is derived from SI. SI, as defined by Blumer, involves the interaction that transpires between people who "interpret or define each other's actions instead of just relating to them."[4:350] Riehl uses Rose's generic and analytic assumptions as her own. She identifies Blumer's concepts, the I and Me concepts of Mead, and the role reversal and sick role concepts in describing her model.

Using these assumptions and concepts, Riehl relates nursing to the SI theory. She believes that the nurse must view the actions of the individual as he seems them. By role playing, the nurse is able to understand why the patient does what he does, and is thus better able to identify the source of difficulty, or nursing diagnosis. Then, having interpreted the patient's action and studied the process recordings, the nurse is able to intervene with a plan of care. The plan of care involves helping the patient assume roles he has used in the past, or is currently using, to help him cope with his present illness. The evaluation process is then used to determine the success of this role taking. Riehl views this dynamic process as one that changes daily, requiring continuous assessment by both the nurse and the patient.

Although little has been done to test Riehl's theory within the science of nursing, the potential for research and contribution to nursing is there. Riehl plans to incorporate her model into the theory and practice in the nursing curriculum at Harrisburg Area Community College. As she continues to develop this theory, which she plans to expound upon in future publications, and as this theory is tested through research and practice, it may prove to be a valuable addition to the science of nursing.

REFERENCES

1. Blumer, H. (1969). *Symbolic interactionalism: Perspective and method.* Englewood Cliffs, N.J.: Prentice-Hall.
2. Kim, H.S. (1983). *The nature of theoretical thinking in nursing.* Norwalk, Conn.: Appleton-Century-Crofts.
3. Riehl, J.P. (1980). *The self-conception and role relationships of autistic children: A symbolic interactionist perspective.* Doctoral dissertation. Los Angeles: University of California, Department of Sociology.
4. Riehl, J.P., & Roy, C. (Eds.). (1980). *Conceptual models for nursing practice* (2nd ed.). New York: Appleton-Century-Crofts.
5. Riehl Sisca, J. (1984). Telephone interviews.
6. Riehl Sisca, J. (1985). Telephone interviews.
7. Riehl Sisca, J. (1984). Personal correspondence.
8. Riehl Sisca, J. (1985). Personal correspondence.
9. Walker, L.O., & Avant, K. (1983). *Strategies for theory construction in nursing.* Norwalk, Conn.: Appleton-Century-Crofts.

BIBLIOGRAPHY
Primary Sources
Books

Riehl, J.P., & McVay, J.W. (Eds.). (1973). *The clinical nurse specialist: Interpretations.* New York: Appleton-Century-Crofts.

Riehl, J.P., & Roy, C. (Eds.). (1974). *Conceptual models for nursing practice*. New York: Appleton-Century-Crofts.

Riehl, J.P., & Roy, C. (Eds.). (1980). *Conceptual models for nursing practice* (2nd ed.). New York: Appleton-Century-Crofts.

Book Chapters

Chrisman, M., & Riehl, J.P. (1974). The systems-developmental stress model. In J.P. Riehl, & C. Roy (Eds.), *Conceptual models for nursing practice*. New York: Appleton-Century-Crofts.

McVay, J.W., Riehl, J.P., & Chen, S. (1973). The clinical nurse specialist as perceived by the deans of baccalaureate and higher degree programs. In J.P. Riehl, & J.W. McVay (Eds.), *The clinical nurse specialist: Interpretations*. New York: Appleton-Century-Crofts.

Riehl, J.P. (1973). Role change and resistance: The baccalaureate student as practitioner. In J.P. Riehl, & J.W. McVay (Eds.), *The clinical nurse specialist: Interpretations*. New York: Appleton-Century-Crofts.

Riehl, J.P. (1974). Application of interaction theory. In J.P. Riehl, & C. Roy (Eds.), *Conceptual models for nursing practice*. New York: Appleton-Century-Crofts.

Riehl, J.P., & Roy, C. (1974). Conceptual models in nursing: Use of nursing models in education, research, and service. In J.P. Riehl, & C. Roy (Eds.), *Conceptual models for nursing practice*. New York: Appleton-Century-Crofts.

Riehl, J.P., & Roy, C. (1974). Discussion of a unified nursing model. In J.P. Riehl, & C. Roy (Eds.), *Conceptual models for nursing practice*. New York: Appleton-Century-Crofts.

Riehl, J.P., & Roy, C. (1974). The nature and history of models: Models related to theory: Use of models in other fields; and history of nursing models. In J.P. Riehl, & C. Roy (Eds.). *Conceptual models for nursing practice*. New York: Appleton-Century-Crofts.

Riehl, J.P., & Roy, C. (1974). Toward a unified nursing model. In J.P. Riehl, & C. Roy (Eds.), *Conceptual models for nursing practice*. New York: Appleton-Century-Crofts.

Riehl, J.P. & Roy, C. (1980). The nature of nursing models. In J.P. Riehl, & C. Roy (Eds.), *Conceptual models for nursing practice* (2nd ed.). New York: Appleton-Century-Crofts.

Riehl, J.P. (1980). Nursing models in current use. In J.P. Riehl, & C. Roy (Eds.), *Conceptual models for nursing practice* (2nd ed.). New York: Appleton-Century-Crofts.

Riehl, J.P. (1980). The Riehl interaction model. In J.P. Riehl, & C. Roy (Eds.), *Conceptual models for nursing practice* (2nd ed.). New York: Appleton-Century-Crofts.

Riehl, J.P., & Roy, C. (1980). A unified model of nursing. In J.P. Riehl, & C. Roy (Eds.), *Conceptual models for nursing practice* (2nd ed.). New York: Appleton-Century-Crofts.

Skolny, M.A., & Riehl, J.P. (1974). Hope: Solving patient and family problems by using a theoretical framework. In J.P. Riehl, & C. Roy (Eds.), *Conceptual models for nursing practice*. New York: Appleton-Century-Crofts.

Articles

Riehl, J.P. (1965). The effect of naturally occurring pain on the galvanic skin response and heart rate: A clinical study. *American Nurses' Association Regional Clinical Conference, 3*:16-23.

Riehl, J.P., & Chambers, J. (1976, July). Better salvage for the stroke victim. *Nursing, 6*:24-31.

Riehl Sisca, J. (1981, Aug.). Preparing to take the state board exams. *California Nurse, 77*:5.

Riehl Sisca, J. (1982). Nontraditional RN-BSN programs for ethnic minority students: A research paradigm. *Journal of Nursing Education, 21*(8):75.

Riehl Sisca, J., & Kerr, J. (1984). Passing the state board examination. *Journal of Nursing Education, 23*(8):358-360.

Professional Papers

Riehl, J.P. (1965). The effect of naturally occurring pain on the galvanic skin response and heart rate: A clinical study. Master's thesis. Los Angeles: University of California, Department of Nursing.

Riehl, J.P. (1980). The self-conception and role relationships of autistic children: A symbolic interactionist perspective. Doctoral dissertation. Los Angeles: University of California, Department of Sociology.

Secondary Sources
Book Reviews

Riehl, J.P., & McVay, J.W. (Eds.). (1973). *The clinical nurse specialist: Interpretations*.
The Canadian Nurse, 69:38, November 1973.

*Nursing Outlook, 21:*689-690, November 1973.
*Nursing Research, 23:*76-77, January-February 1974.
*American Journal of Nursing, 74:*960, May 1974.
*Hospitals, 48:*36, May 16, 1974.
*Nursing Mirror, 141:*72, October 2, 1975.
Riehl, J.P., & Roy, C. (Eds.). (1974). *Conceptual models for nursing practice.*
*The Canadian Nurse, 76:*48, December 1980.
Nursing Times, 77:825, May 7, 1981.
*Nursing Research, 30:*379, November-December 1981.
*American Journal of Nursing, 82:*696, April 1982.

Books

Chinn, P.L., & Jacobs, M.K. (1983). *Theory and nursing: A systematic approach.* St. Louis: C.V. Mosby.
Kim, H.S. (1983). *The nature of theoretical thinking in nursing.* Norwalk, Conn.: Appleton-Century-Crofts.
Walker, L.O., & Avant, K. (1983). *Strategies for theory construction in nursing.* Norwalk, Conn.: Appleton-Century-Crofts.

Book Chapters

Preisner, J.M. (1980). A proposed model for the nurse therapist. In J.P. Riehl, & C. Roy (Eds.), *Conceptual models for nursing practice* (2nd ed.). New York: Appleton-Century-Crofts. pp. 362-371.
Wood, M.J. (1980). Implementing the Riehl inter-action model in nursing administration. In J.P. Riehl, & C. Roy (Eds.), *Conceptual models for nursing practice* (2nd ed.). New York: Appleton-Century-Crofts. pp. 357-361.

Correspondence

Curriculum vitae of Joan Riehl Sisca revised November 1984.
Riehl Sisca, J. (1984, Nov. 2). Personal correspondence.
Riehl Sisca, J. (1985). Personal correspondence.

Interviews

Riehl Sisca, J. (1984, Oct. 10). Telephone interview.
Riehl Sisca, J. (1984, Oct. 17). Telephone interview.
Riehl Sisca, J. (1984, Nov. 30). Telephone interview.
Riehl Sisca, J. (1985). Telephone interview.

Other Sources

Blumer, H. (1969). *Symbolic interactionism: Perspective and method.* Englewood Cliffs, N.J.: Prentice-Hall.
Faris, R.E.L. (1964). *Handbook of modern sociology.* Chicago: Rand McNally.
Mead, G.H. (1934). *Mind, self, and society* (C.V. Morris, Ed.). Chicago: University of Chicago.
Rose, A.M. (1962). *Human behavior and social processes.* Boston: Houghton Mifflin.
Wells, L.E., & Marwell, G. (1976). *Self-esteem: Its conceptualization and measurement.* Beverly Hills: Sage Publications.

Helen C. Erickson, Evelyn M. Tomlin, Mary Ann P. Swain

22

Modeling and Role-Modeling

Jane A. Caldwell-Gwin, Connie Rae Jarlsberg, Judy McCormick, Kathryn W. Noone

CREDENTIALS AND BACKGROUND OF THE THEORISTS
Helen Erickson

Helen Erickson received a diploma from Saginaw General Hospital, Saginaw, Michigan, in 1957. Her degrees include a Bachelor of Science in Nursing in 1974, a Master of Science in Psychiatric Nursing in 1976, and a Doctor of Educational Psychology in 1984, all from the University of Michigan.

Erickson's professional experience began in the Emergency Room of the Midland Community Hospital in Midland, Texas, where she was the head nurse for 2 years. She then worked in Mt. Pleasant, Michigan, as night supervisor of nursing in the State Home for the Handicapped. She was then Director of Health Services at the Inter American University in San German Puerto Rico from 1960-1964. On her return to the United States, she worked as a staff nurse at both St. Joseph's and University Hospitals in Ann Arbor, Michigan. Erickson later served as a psychiatric nurse consultant to the Pediatric Nurse Practitioner Program at the University of Michigan. Her academic career began as a teaching assistant in the RN Studies program at the University of Michigan, where she later served as Chairperson of the Undergraduate Program and Interim Dean for Undergraduate Studies. Currently, she is an assistant professor of nursing. Erickson has also maintained an independent nursing practice since 1976.

Erickson is a member of the American Nurses' Association, American Nurses' Foundation, The Charter Club, American Public Health Association, Michigan Nurses' Association, National League for Nursing, and Sigma Theta Tau. She is actively researching the Modeling and Role-Modeling theory and has pre-

The authors wish to express appreciation to Dr. Helen C. Erickson, Evelyn M. Tomlin, and Dr. Mary Ann P. Swain for critiquing the chapter.

sented numerous seminars and papers on various aspects of the theory throughout Michigan and in Florida, Illinois, Minnesota, and Washington. She has served as a consultant in the implementation of the theory into clinical practice at the University of Michigan Medical Center in the surgical area and has consulted with faculty in various schools of nursing that have considered adopting the theory into their curriculum.

Erickson has been listed in *Who's Who Among University Students*. She received the Sigma Theta Tau Rho Chapter Award of Excellence in Nursing in 1980, the Amoco Foundation Good Teaching Award in 1982, and was accepted into ADARA, a university honor society, in 1982.

Evelyn Tomlin

Evelyn Tomlin's nursing education began in Southern California. She attended Pasadena City College, Los Angeles County General Hospital School of Nursing, and the University of Southern California where she received her Bachelor of Science in Nursing. She received a Master of Science in Psychiatric Nursing from the University of Michigan in 1976.

Tomlin's professional experiences are varied, beginning when she was a clinical instructor at Los Angeles County General Hospital School of Nursing in Surgical Nursing, Maternal and Premature Infant Nursing. She later lived in Kabul, Afghanistan, where she taught English at the Afghan Institute of Technology. In addition, she also served as school nurse and family nurse practitioner to the overseas American and European communities with which she was associated, a role that included attending more than 40 home deliveries with a Certified Nurse Midwife. After the establishment of medical services and hospital at the United States Embassy Hospital, Tomlin functioned as relief staff nurse at the Hospital. When she returned to the United States, she was employed by the Visiting Nurse Association as a staff nurse in Ann Arbor, Michigan. She then functioned as the coordinator and clinical instructor for student practical nurses. She has been a staff nurse in a coronary care unit and was briefly the head nurse of the Emergency Room at St. Joseph's Mercy Hospital in Ann Arbor. She has also been an assistant professor in the RN Studies Program at the University of Michigan School of Nursing. She has served as the mental health consultant to the Pediatric Nurse Practitioner Program at the University of Michigan. For 8 years she was Assistant Professor of Nursing in the fundamentals area at the University of Michigan.

Tomlin was among the first 12 nurses in the United States to be certified by the American Association of Critical Care Nurses. With several colleagues, she opened one of the first offices for independent nursing practice in Michigan. She continues to maintain her independent practice begun in 1976.

Tomlin is a member of the American Nurses' Association, the Michigan Nurses' Association, the American Association of Critical Care Nurses, Sigma Theta Tau Rho Chapter, the California Scholarship Federation, and the Philathian Society. She has presented programs incorporating a variety of nursing topics into the Modeling and Role-Modeling theory and paradigm with an emphasis on clinical applications.

Mary Ann Swain

Mary Ann Swain's educational background is in psychology. She received her Bachelor of Arts in psychology from DePauw University in Greencastle, Indiana, and her Master of Science and doctoral degrees from the University of Michigan, both in the field of psychology.

Swain has taught psychology research methods and statistics as a teaching assistant at DePauw University and later as a lecturer and an Associate Professor of Psychology in Nursing at the University of Michigan. She became Director of the Doctoral Program in Nursing in 1975 and served in that capacity for 1 year. She was Chairperson of Nursing Research from 1977-1982 and is currently Professor of Nursing Research at the University of Michigan.

Swain is a member of the American Psychological Association and an associate member of the Michigan Nurses' Association. She has developed and taught classes of psychology, research, and nursing research methods. She has collaborated with nurse researchers on various projects, including Health Promotion among Diabetics, and Influencing Compliance among Hypertensive Patients, and has worked with Erickson to develop a model for assessing potential adaptation to stress, which is significant to the Modeling and Role-Modeling theory.

Swain received the Alpha Lambda Delta, Psi Chi, Mortar Board, and Phi Beta Kappa awards while at DePauw University. In 1981, she was recognized by the Rho Chapter of Sigma Theta Tau for Contributions to Nursing.

THEORETICAL SOURCES

The theory, Modeling and Role-Modeling, uses psychological, cognitive, and biological theories as the theoretical base for the observations the theorists make regarding similarities and differences among individuals. The works of Abraham Maslow, Erik Erikson, Milton H. Erickson, Jean Piaget, George Engel, and Hans Selye are salient in the development of this theory.

Erickson, Tomlin, and Swain note a correspondence between their clinical observations and Abraham Maslow's growth principle and theory of human needs. "Maslow states that all people want to be the best they can possibly be; unmet basic needs interfere with holistic growth whereas satisfied needs promote growth."[6:45] The theorists believe that unmet basic needs can lead to initiation or aggravation of physical or mental illnesses.

The work of Erik Erikson describing the eight stages of psychosocial development provides another source of the development of this theory. Erikson's stages represent developmental tasks. As an individual resolves each task, strengths are gained that contribute to character and health. "The utility of Erikson's theory is the freedom we may take to view aspects of people's problems as uncomplicated tasks. This perspective provides a hopeful expectation for the individual's future since it connotes something still in progress."[6:62-63]

The cognitive developmental theory of Jean Piaget provides the basis for considering one of the ways individuals are alike: the development of thinking. The theorists believe that chronologically older individuals who do not develop the last stage of cognitive development, the formal operations stage, have encountered impediments in their learning process.[6:68]

The theorists identify object relations theory as important in the development of their concept of affiliated-individuation. The works of Winnicott, Klein, Mahler, and Bowlby have provided the vast majority of the literature related to this concept.[6:68] Object relations theory is a theory of attachment that progresses from an infant's attachment to its mother, to attachment to objects such as teddy bears and blankets in childhood, and finally to more abstract attachments in adulthood, such as an educational degree. According to the theorists, "research supports the notion that object attachment is vital for adaptive coping."[6:69]

The work of Selye and Engel provide the background theory for the beliefs the theorists hold regarding the stress response. Selye's theory is a biophysical one, whereas Engel's is psychosocial. The synthesis of these theories has led to the development of the Adaptive Potential Assessment Model (APAM) by Erickson, Tomlin, and Swain.

The final theoretical source for the development of Modeling and Role-Modeling are the psychiatric and hypnotic techniques of Milton H. Erickson. He urged Helen Erickson to "Model the client's world, understand it as they do, then role-model the picture the client has drawn—building a healthy world for them."[2]

USE OF EMPIRICAL EVIDENCE

The Adaptive Potential Assessment Model (Figures 22-1 and 22-2) has been tested by two of the theorists. Data from the study support the classification model. "This classification model distinguishes individuals in states of stress from those in nonstress states."[5:99] "While this study statistically supports the proposed classification model, the sample size prohibits generalizations. Replication with a larger sample . . . would provide the data necessary to further develop the adaptive potential model."[5:100-101]

With the exception of this study, there is little empirical evidence published to support the theory. However, studies are being conducted and manuscripts are under review; therefore, more empirical evidence will become available in the future.

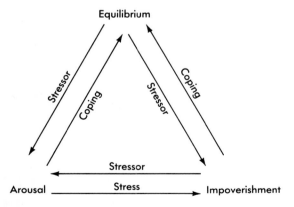

Figure 22-2. An illustration of the dynamic relationship among the states of the adaptive potential assessment model.

From Erickson, H.C., Tomlin, E.M., & Swain, M.A.P. *Modeling and role-modeling: A theory and paradigm for nursing.* © 1983. Reprinted with permission of Prentice-Hall, Englewood Cliffs, N.J. p. 82.

Figure 22-1. Adaptive potential assessment model.

From Erickson, H.C., Tomlin, E.M., & Swain, M.A.P. *Modeling and role-modeling: A theory and paradigm for nursing.* (1983) Reprinted with permission of Prentice-Hall, Englewood Cliffs, N.J. p. 81.

MAJOR CONCEPTS AND DEFINITIONS

The theory and paradigm modeling and role-modeling contains multiple concepts. These are defined as follows:

MODELING

The act of Modeling, then, is the process the nurse uses as she develops an image and understanding of the client's world—an image and understanding developed within the client's framework and from the client's perspective. . . . The art of Modeling is the development of a mirror image of the situation from the client's perspective. . . . The science of Modeling is the scientific aggregation and analysis of data collected about the client's model.[6:95]

"Modeling occurs as the nurse accepts and understands her client."[6:96]

ROLE-MODELING

The art of Role-Modeling occurs when the nurse plans and implements interventions that are unique for the client. The science of Role-Modeling occurs as the nurse plans interventions with respect to her theoretical base for the practice of nursing. . . . Role-Modeling is . . . the essence of nurturance. . . . Role-Modeling requires an unconditional acceptance of the person as the person is while gently encouraging and facilitating growth and development at the person's own pace and within the person's own model.[6:95]

"Role-Modeling starts the second the nurse moves from the analysis phase of the nursing process to the planning of nursing interventions."[6:96]

NURSING

Nursing is the holistic helping of persons with their self-care activities in relation to their health. This is an interactive, interpersonal process that nurtures strengths to enable development, release, and channeling of resources for coping with one's circumstances and environment. The goal is to achieve a state of perceived optimum health and contentment[6:49]

Nurturance

Nurturance fuses and integrates cognitive, physiological, and affective processes, with the aim of assisting a client to move toward holistic health. Nurturance implies that the nurse seeks to know and understand the client's personal model of his or her world and to appreciate its value and significance for that client from the client's perspective.[6:48]

Unconditional acceptance

Being accepted as a unique, worthwhile, important individual—with no strings attached—is imperative if the individual is to be facilitated in developing his or her own potential. The nurse's use of empathy helps the individual learn that the nurse accepts and respects him or her as is. The acceptance will facilitate the mobilization of resources needed as this individual strives for adaptive equilibrium.[6:49]

PERSON. People are alike because of their holism, lifetime growth and development, and their affiliated individuation. They are different because of their inherent endowment, adaptation, and self-care knowledge.

How are people alike

Holism. "Human beings are holistic persons who have multiple interacting subsystems. Permeating ill subsystems are the inherent bases. These include generic makeup and spiritual drive. Body, mind, emotion, and spirit are a total unit and they act together. They affect and control one another interactively. The interaction of the multiple subsystems and the inherent bases creates holism: Holism implies that the whole is greater than the sum of the parts."[6:44-45]

Basic needs. "All human beings have basic needs that can be satisfied, but only from within the framework of the individual."[1:58] "Basic needs are only met when the individual perceives that they are met."[6:57]

Lifetime development. Lifetime development evolves through psychological and cognitive stages.

Psychological stages. "Each stage represents a developmental task or decisive encounter resulting in a turning point, a moment of decision between alternative basic attitudes (for example, trust versus mistrust or autonomy versus shame and doubt). As a maturing individual negotiates or resolves each age-specific crisis or task, the individual gains enduring strengths and attitudes that contribute to the character and health of the individual's personality in his or her culture."[6:61]

Cognitive stages. "Consider how thinking develops rather than what happens in psychosocial or affective development. . . . Piaget believed that cognitive learning develops in a sequential manner and he has identified several periods in this process. Essentially, there are four periods: sensorimotor, preoperational, concrete operations, and formal operations."[6:63-64]

Affiliated-individuation. "Individuals have an instinctual need for affiliated-individuation. They need to be able to be dependent on support systems while simultaneously maintaining independence from these support systems. They need to feel a deep sense of both the 'I' and the 'we' states of being and to perceive freedom and acceptance in both states."[6:47]

How people are different

Inherent endowment. "Each individual is born with a set of genes that will to some extent predetermine appearance, growth, development, and responses to life events. . . . Clearly, both genetic makeup and inherited characteristics influence growth and development. They might influence how one perceives oneself and one's world. They make individuals different from one another, each unique in his or her own way."[6:74-75]

Adaptation. "Adaptation occurs as the individual responds to external and internal stressors in a health and growth-directed manner. Adaptation involves mobilizing internal and external coping resources. No subsystem is left in jeopardy when adaptation occurs."[6:47]

Mind body relationships. "We are all biophysical, psychosocial beings who want to develop our potential, that is, to be the best we can be."[6:70]

Self-care. Self-care involves the use of knowledge, resources, and action.

Self-care knowledge. "At some level a person knows what has made him or her sick, lessened his or her effectiveness, or interfered with his or her growth. The person also knows what will make him or her well, optimize his or her effectiveness or fulfillment (given circumstances), or promote his or her growth."[6:48]

Self-care resources. Self-care resources are "the internal resources, as well as additional resources, mobilized through self-care action that help gain, maintain, and promote as optimum level of holistic health."[6:254-255]

Self-care action. Self-care action is "the development and utilization of self-care knowledge and self-care resources."[6:254]

MAJOR ASSUMPTIONS
Nursing

"The nurse is a facilitator, not an effector. Our nurse-client relationship is an interactive, interpersonal process that aids the individual to identify, mobilize, and develop his or her own strengths."[6:48]

Person

A differentiation is made between patients and clients in this theory. A patient is given treatment and instruction; a client participates in his own care. "Our goal is for nurses to work with clients."[2:21] "A client is one who is considered to be a legitimate member of the decision-making team, who always has some control over the planned regimen, and who is incorporated into the planning and implementation of his or her own care as much as possible."[6:20]

Health

"Health is a state of physical, mental, and social well-being, not merely the absence of disease or infirmity. It connotes a state of dynamic equilibrium among the various subsystems [of a holistic person]."[6:46]

Environment

"Environment is not identified in the theory as an entity of its own. The theorists see environment in the social subsystems as the interaction between self and others both cultural and individual. Biophysical stressors are seen as part of the environment."[2]

THEORETICAL ASSERTIONS

The theoretical assertions of Modeling and Role-Modeling are based on the linkages between completion of developmental tasks and basic need satisfaction; between basic need satisfaction, object attachment and loss, and developmental tasks; and the relationship between the ability to mobilize coping resources and need satisfaction. Three generic theoretical assertions that constitute a number of theoretical linkages implied in the theory but less specifically delineated are:

1. "The degree to which developmental tasks are resolved is dependent on the degree to which human needs are satisfied."[6:87]
2. "The degree to which needs are satisfied by object attachment depends on the availability of those objects and the degree to which they provide comfort and security as opposed to threat and anxiety."[6:90]
3. "An individual's potential for mobilizing resources—the person's state of coping according to the APAM [Adaptive Potential Assessment Model]—is directly associated with the person's need satisfaction level."[6:91]

LOGICAL FORM

The theory, Modeling and Role-Modeling, is formulated by the use of retroductive thinking. The theorists go through all four levels of theory development and then recycle from inductive to deductive to inductive to deductive.[2] The theoretical sources were used to validate clinical observations. Clinical observations were tested in light of the theoretical bases. These sources were synthesized with their observations, which enabled Erickson, Tomlin, and Swain to develop a "multi-dimensional new whole the theory and paradigm—Modeling and Role-Modeling."[2]

The theorists label Modeling and Role-Modeling a theory and paradigm. This is a valid label because Modeling and Role-Modeling meets the five functions of a paradigm as identified by Merton,[7:70] who said paradigms "provide a compact arrangement of central concepts and their interrelations that are utilized for description and analysis." The theorists provide a clear presentation of their central concepts and build on the relationships as they described them. "Paradigms lessen the likelihood of inadvertently introducing hidden assumptions and concepts, for each new assumption and concept must be either logically derived from previous components or explicitly introduced into it."[7:71] Erickson, Tomlin, and Swain build on previous components as their paradigm is developed, each component being logically derived from clinical observations or based in theory. "Third, paradigms advance the cumulation of theoretical interpretation."[7:71] It appears the assumptions and concepts made by the theorists allow for interpretation in multiple clinical and research situations in which the concepts may be applied, thereby expanding the theory base of nursing. "Paradigms promote analysis rather than description of concrete details."[7:71] Modeling and Role-Modeling promotes analysis of significant concepts. The interrelationships among the concepts can also be empirically examined because they have broad applicability, and lend themselves to multiple research questions. "Fifth, paradigms make for codification of qualitative analysis in a way that approximates the logic if not the empirical rigor of quantitative analysis."[7:71] Erickson states that a qualitative approach has been used to form concepts. Based on that approach, scales were built using deductive logic to test those concepts.[2] The methods used will become available for replication of studies as they are published.

ACCEPTANCE BY THE NURSING COMMUNITY
Practice

Publication of the books *Modeling and Role-Modeling: A Theory and Paradigm for Nursing* and a chapter on Self-care in *Introduction to Person-Centered Nursing,* as well as publication of research studies based on the theory, have exposed practicing nurses to this theory. Currently, nurses on surgical units at the University of Michigan Medical Center are using the theory as the basis for their care.[2] They also collect data on their clients, using the tool developed by the theorists.[6:152]

The theorists have spoken prolifically on their theory and have held one-to-one consultations that exposed nurses from various practice and educational backgrounds to the theory. Nurses in critical care, mental health, and hospice are using the theory. Erickson[2] has noted that what seemed to be a revolutionary idea as recently as 7 to 8 years ago—"calling for the client to be the head of the Health Care Team"—is rapidly gaining acceptance, as is the notion that nurses can practice nursing independently. According to Erickson,[2] negative responses to the theory came from individuals who cannot accept the idea of "listening to the client first" or who do not take the concept of holism seriously.

Education

The theory is introduced into the curriculum in the sophomore year at the University of Michigan School of Nursing and is required for returning R.N. students as well. Faculty members at several nursing schools have contacted Erickson regarding the use of the theory in their curricula. She has recently assumed a position as Assistant Dean for Academic Programs and Associate Professor at the University of South Carolina College of Nursing, where she will work with masters and doctoral students in research and theory development related to modeling and role modeling. *Introduction to Person-Centered Nursing* with a chapter on "Self-care" by Tomlin is being used as a text in various nursing schools and is expanding exposure to theory concepts.

Research

The theorists identify multiple research projects that are tests of the theory. A study using Modeling and Role-Modeling with a more homogeneous population and expanding the work previously done with diabetics and hypertensive clients has been submitted for federal funding. Several doctoral students at the University of Michigan School of Nursing are pursuing various research questions based in the theory. A research study is under way at the University of Michigan Medical Center by three nurses who have hypothesized that length of hospital stay correlates with stages of development. They are using an updated version of the theorists' data collection tool and newly developed scales based on Erikson's and Piaget's theories, and are assessing the states of coping, which are predictors of length of stay.[2] Further development of the Adaptive Potential Assessment Model is currently under way.

FURTHER DEVELOPMENT

Currently, only a paucity of published data related to the theory exists. As stated above, research in progress at the University of Michigan will, when published, serve to support the theory and enhance its clinical applicability. Erickson[2] states, "Every part of it [the theory] needs further development. . . . There are a thousand research questions in that book. . . .

You can take any one statement we make and ask a research question about it. . . . Modeling and Role-Modeling has only begun."

EVALUATION OF THE THEORY
Clarity

Erickson, Tomlin, and Swain present their theory clearly. Definitions in the theory are denotative with the concepts explicitly defined. They use everyday language and offer many examples to illustrate their meaning. Their definitions and assumptions are consistent and there is a logical progression from assumptions to assertions.

Simplicity

The theory appears simple at first. However, on closer inspection, it becomes complex. It is based on biological and psychological theories and several of the theorists' own assumptions. The interactions among the major concepts, assumptions, and assertions add depth to the theory and increase its complexity.

Generality

Because its major assumptions that deal with developmental tasks, basic needs satisfaction, object attachment and loss, and adaptive potential are broad enough to be applicable in multiple diverse nursing situations, the theory is generalizable to all nursing and client situations. The theorists cite many examples of the applicability of their concepts, both in clinical practice and research. It may be argued that the theory lacks applicability in the pediatric or comatose population. But we believe the theory is applicable in these situations, although it may take some creativity on the part of the clinician to make those applications. Modeling and Role-Modeling is generalizable to all aspects of professional nursing practice.

Empirical Precision

Empirical precision is increased if the theory has operationally defined concepts, identifiable subconcepts, and denotative definitions. The major concepts, Modeling and Role-Modeling, are reality-based, which makes them more empirical than general. Definitions in the theory are denotative, making it possible to empirically test the concepts identified. The theorists provide an outline for collecting, analyzing, and synthesizing data, and guidelines for implementing their theory based on the client's model. These explicit guidelines increase the empirical precision of the theory by allowing any practitioner to test the theory using these tools.

Chinn and Jacobs[1:42] state, "Empirical precision is necessarily increased with research testing." Data reflecting research testing of the theory is not currently readily available; however, as has been stated, studies are ongoing. We believe Modeling and Role-Modeling will gain empirical precision when data become available for critical analysis. The theorists recognize the need for further research of their theory and encourage practicing nurses to do it.[2]

Derivable Consequences

The theory is limited by its relative newness. It simply has not been available long enough to determine the value of its outcomes. We believe the consequences of this theory will prove invaluable to the practice of professional nursing. The theory provides a framework for the autonomous practice of nursing separate from other disciplines, designed specifically to collaborate with the client. This theory recognizes the client as head of the health care team and helps the practitioner promote optimum functioning of the client within the client's model of the world. The nurse implementing this theory will role-model a healthier world for the client by developing interventions designed to meet need deficits, developmental needs, and resolve loss and grief. Anticipating what this theory, when implemented, may accomplish is exciting indeed. The theorists encourage nurses to develop a philosophy of practice, to examine clinical situations in light of existing theories, to collaborate with clients, to validate their observations, and to test those observations empirically; in essence, to practice professional nursing.

REFERENCES

1. Chinn, P.L., & Jacobs, M.K. (1983). *Theory and nursing: A systematic approach.* St. Louis: C.V. Mosby.
2. Erickson, H.C. (1984, Nov. 5). Telephone interview.
3. Erickson, H.C. (1984, Nov. 7). Telephone interview.
4. Erickson, H.C. (1984, Oct.). Curriculum vitae.
5. Erickson, H.C., & Swain, M.A. (1982). A model for assessing potential adaptation to stress. *Research in Nursing and Health, 5:*93-101.
6. Erickson, H.C. Tomlin, E.M., & Swain, M.A. (1983). *Modeling and role-modeling: A theory and paradigm for nursing.* Englewood Cliffs, N.J.: Prentice-Hall.
7. Merton, R.K. (1968). *Social theory and social structure.* New York: The Free Press.
8. Swain, M.A. (1984, Oct.). Curriculum vitae.
9. Tomlin, E.M. (1984, Oct.). Curriculum vitae.
10. Tomlin, E.M. (1982). Self-care. In J. Lindberg, M. Hunter, & A. Pruszewski, *Introduction to person-centered nursing.* Philadelphia: J.B. Lippincott.

BIBLIOGRAPHY
Primary Sources
Books

Erickson, H.C., Tomlin, E.M., & Swain, M.A. (1983). *Modeling and role-modeling: A theory and paradigm for nursing.* Englewood Cliffs, N.J.: Prentice-Hall.
Raush, H., et al. (1974). *Communication, conflicts, and marriage.* San Francisco: Jossey-Bass.

Book Chapters

Erickson, H.C. (1977). Communication in nursing. In *Professional nursing matrix: A workbook.* Ann Arbor, Mich.: Media Library, University of Michigan. pp. 1-150.
Tomlin, E.M. (1983). Self-care. In J. Lindberg, M. Hunter, & A. Kruszewski, *Introduction to person-centered nursing.* Philadelphia: J.P. Lippincott. pp. 51-60.

Articles

Erickson, H., & Swain, M.A. (1977). *The utilization of a nursing care model for treatment of essential hypertension. 56* Supp. III (1977, Oct.): 145. Circulation. (Abstract).
Erickson, H., & Swain, M.A. (1982, June). A model for assessing potential adaptation to stress. *Research in Nursing and Health, 5:*93-101.
Schulman, B.A., & Swain, M.A. (1980, Jan.). Active patient orientation. *Patient Counseling and Health Education, 2:*32-37.
Steckel, S., & Swain, M.A. (1977, Dec.). The use of written contracts to increase adherence. *Hospitals, 51:*81-84.
Swain, M.A., & Steckel, S. (1981, March). Influencing adherence among hypertensive. *Research in Nursing and Health, 4:*213-222.
Tomlin, E.M. (1953, Oct.). Los Angeles Program for Premature Infant Care (Section III). *Nursing Outlook, 1:*568-569.

Thesis

Erickson, H. (1976). *Identification of states of coping utilizing physiological and psychological data.* Master's thesis. The University of Michigan.

Dissertation

Erickson, H. (1984). *Self-care knowledge: Relationships among the concepts of support, hope, control, and satisfaction with daily life.* Doctoral dissertation, The University of Michigan.

Correspondence

Erickson, H.C. (1984, Oct.). Curriculum vitae.
Swain, M.A. (1984, Oct.). Curriculum vitae.
Tomlin, E.M. (1984, Oct.). Curriculum vitae.

Interviews

Erickson, H. (1984, Nov. 5). Telephone interview.
Erickson, H. (1984, Nov. 7). Telephone interview.

Secondary Sources
Book Reviews

Erickson, H.C., Tomlin, E.M., & Swain, M.A.P. (1983). *Modeling and role-modeling: A theory and paradigm for nursing.*
*American Journal of Nursing, 83:*155, September 1983.
*Nursing and Health Care, 4:*413, September 1983.
*Nursing Outlook, 32:*116, February 1984.

Other Sources

Bowlby, J. (1958). The nature of the child's tie to his mother. *International Journal of Psychoanalysis, 39:*89-97.

Bowlby, J. (1960). Child care and the growth of love. In M. Haimowitz, & N. Haimowitz, *Human development* (2nd ed.). New York: Thomas Y. Crowell. pp. 155-166.

Bowlby, J. (1961). Childhood mourning and its explications for psychiatry. *American Journal of Psychiatry, 118:*481-98.

Bowlby, J. (1961). Process of mourning. *International Journal of Psychoanalysis, 42:*317-40.

Bowlby, J. (1969). *Attachment.* New York: Basic Books.

Bowlby, J. (1973). *Separation.* New York: Basic Books.

Bowlby, J. (1980). *Loss.* New York: Basic Books.

Bowlby, J., Robertson, J., & Rosenbluth, D. (1952). A two-year-old goes to the hospital. *The Psychoanalytic Study of the Child, 7:*89-94.

Chinn, P.L., & Jacobs, M.K. (1983). *Theory and nursing: A systematic approach.* St. Louis: C.V. Mosby.

Engel, G.S. (1962). *Psychological development in health and disease.* Philadelphia: Saunders.

Erikson, E. (1960). The case of Peter. In M. Haimowitz, & N. Haimowitz, *Human development.* (2nd ed.). New York: Thomas Y. Crowell. pp. 355-359.

Erikson, E. (1960). Identity versus self-diffusion. In M. Haimowitz, & N. Haimowitz, *Human development.* (2nd ed.). New York: Thomas Y. Crowell. pp. 766-770.

Erikson, E. (1963). *Childhood and society.* New York: W.W. Norton.

Haley, J. (1973). *Uncommon therapy: The psychiatric techniques of Milton H. Erickson, M.D.* New York: W.W. Norton.

Klein, M. (1952). Some theoretical conclusions regarding the emotional life of the infant. In J. Riviere, *Developments in psycho-analysis.* London: Hogarth Press. pp. 198-236.

Mahler, M.S. (1967). On human symbiosis and the vicissitudes of individuation. *Journal of the American Psychoanalytic Association, 15:*740-763.

Mahler, M.S. & Furer, M. (1968). *On human symbiosis and the vicissitudes of individuation* (Vol. I). *Infantile psychosis.* New York: International Universities Press.

Maslow, A.H. (1936). The need to know and the fear of knowing. *The Journal of General Psychology, 68:*111-25.

Maslow, A.H. (1968). *Toward a psychology of being* (2nd ed.). New York: D. Von Nostrand.

Maslow, A.H. (1970). *Motivation and personality* (2nd ed.). New York: Harper & Row.

Merton, R.K. (1968). *Social theory and social structure.* New York: The Free Press.

Piaget, J. (1952). *The origins of intelligence in children.* New York: International Universities Press.

Piaget, J. (1974). The pathway between subjects' recent life changes and their near-future illness reports: Representative results and methodological issues. In B.S. Dohrenwend, & B.P. Dohrenwend, *Stressful life events: Their nature and effects.* New York: John Wiley & Sons. pp. 73-86.

Piaget, J., & Inhelder, B. (1969). *The psychology of the child.* New York: Basic Books.

Selye, H. (1974). *Stress without distress.* Philadelphia: Lippincott.

Selye, H. (1976). *The stress of life* (2nd ed.). New York: McGraw-Hill.

Selye, H. (1979). Further thoughts on stress without distress. *Resident and Staff Physician, 25:*125-34.

Winnicott, D.W. (1953). Transitional objects and transitional phenomena: A study of the first not-me possession. *International Journal of Psychoanalysis, 34:*89-97.

Winnicott, D.W. (1965). The theory of the parent-infant relationship. In D.W. Winnicott, *The maturational processes and the facilitating environment.* London, Hogarth Press.

Kathryn E. Barnard

Parent-Child Interaction Model

Jill K. Baker, Debra A. Borchers, Debra Trnka Cochran, Nancy Orcutt,
Elizabeth Godfrey Terry, Cynthia A. Wesolowski

CREDENTIALS AND BACKGROUND OF THE THEORIST

Kathryn E. Barnard was born April 16, 1938, in Omaha, Nebraska. In 1956 she enrolled in a prenursing program at the University of Nebraska and graduated with a Bachelor of Science in Nursing in June 1960. Upon graduation, she continued at the University of

Nebraska in part-time graduate studies. That summer she accepted an acting head nurse position and in the fall became an assistant instructor in pediatric nursing.[8] In 1961 Barnard moved to Boston, Massachusetts, where she enrolled in a Master's program at Boston University. She also worked as a private duty nurse. After earning her Master's of Science in Nursing in June 1962 and a certificate of Advanced Graduate Specialization in Nursing Education, she accepted a position as an instructor in maternal and child nursing at the University of Washington in Seattle. In 1965 she was named Assistant Professor. She began consulting in the

The authors wish to express appreciation to Dr. Elizabeth Choi for her assistance with data collection and to Dr. Kathryn E. Barnard for critiquing the chapter.

area of mental retardation, and coordinated training projects for nurses in child development and the care of children with mental retardation and handicaps. Barnard became the project director for a research study to develop a method for nursing child assessment in 1971. The following year she earned a Ph.D. in the Ecology of Early Childhood Development from the University of Washington.[7:1-2]

In 1972 Barnard accepted a position at the University of Washington as a professor in parent-child nursing. Since 1972 she has been the principal investigator of 14 research grants and coinvestigator of one research grant. In addition to these research efforts, Barnard has provided consultation, presented lectures internationally, and served on multiple advisory boards. She has published articles in both nursing and nonnursing journals since 1966. Her books include a four-part series on child health assessment, two editions related to teaching the mentally retarded/developmentally delayed child, and her most recent work focusing on families of vulnerable infants.[7:2-14]

Barnard[4:4] is a member of the American Nurses' Association, where she has served on the Executive Committee for the Division on Maternal and Child Health Nursing. She is a member of nine other national organizations including The Society for Research in Child Development, Sigma Theta Tau, and the American Academy of Nursing.[7:8]

In 1969 Barnard was presented with the Lucille Petry Leone Award by the National League for Nursing for her outstanding contribution to nursing education.[15:9] Since then she has been honored by several other associations, including the American Nurses' Association with the Maternal and Child Health Nurse of the Year Award, which was presented at the 1984 convention.[16:242]

THEORETICAL SOURCES FOR THEORY DEVELOPMENT

Although Barnard cites various nursing theorists, such as Florence Nightingale, Virginia Henderson, and Martha Rogers, their direct influence on her research and theory development is uncertain.[*]

Barnard refers to the Neal Nursing Construct, which has four expressions of health and illness: cognition, sensation, motion, and affiliation. Neal worked on a construct for practice and Barnard and her associate developed measures related to the period of infancy. Barnard[‡] later stated, "In reviewing both the Maryland construct and the Washington research, we were impressed with how the design and results of the Nursing Child Assessment Project (NCAP) fit into the [Neal] construct."

Barnard credits Florence Blake for the beliefs and values making up the foundation of current nursing practice. She describes Blake as:

> a great pediatric nursing clinician and educator [who] turned our minds toward an orientation on the patient rather than the procedure. Blake saw the principal function of parenthood and nursing to be the capacity to establish and maintain constructive and satisfying relationships with others. She amplified for nursing important acts such as mother-infant attachment, maternal care, and separation of child from parents. She helped nursing understand the importance of the family.[10:194]

Many of Dr. Barnard's publications were coauthored by writers such as D. King and A.W. Pattullo, indicating a variety of influences. Barnard also published a book, entitled *Teaching the Mentally Retarded Child: A Family Care Approach,* with Marcene L. Powell. Four years later they developed a second edition, *Teaching Children with Developmental Problems: A Family Care Approach.* Of greater influence were the coinvestigators and consultants of the Nursing Child Assessment Project, which includes Sandra Eyres, Charlene Snyder, and Helen Bee Douglas.[9:IV] Barnard[8] states she was influenced by child development theorists such as J. Piaget, J.S. Brunner, L. Sander, and T.B. Brazelton, in addition to nursing theorists.

---

*References 10:193-194; 4:208.
‡Reference 10:195-196.

USE OF EMPIRICAL EVIDENCE

Many researchers' findings were used as Barnard's work centering around the parent-child interaction evolved. Barnard used T. Berry Brazelton's work as well as Bettye Caldwell's. Once it was determined that the interaction/adaptation between parent and child was the area to focus on, Barnard[9:6] used the research findings of many, such as H. Als, M.F. Waldrup and J.D. Goering, and L.M.S. Dubowitz. Their findings added to the growing body of usable knowledge that could be brought to bear on the task of developing tools to adequately assess that important interactional aspect of early child development.

In addition to tapping others' research, Barnard conducted her own. She began her research in 1968 by studying mentally and physically handicapped children and adults. In the early 1970s she studied the activities of the well child and later expanded her study to include methods of evaluating growth and development of children. She also initiated a 10-year series of research projects to examine the effects of stimulation on sleep states in premature infants. The majority of these research studies were funded by grants from the U.S. Department of Health, Education, and Welfare.[7:5]

In 1976 Barnard was awarded a grant by HEW to determine "the most effective ways of disseminating research with the use of media including communication satellite."[127:5] This led to the evolution of the Nursing Child Assessment Satellite Training Project. In 1977 Barnard began researching methods for disseminating information about newborns and young children to parents. Projects have been funded by the National Foundation of the March of Dimes and Johnson & Johnson baby products. Barnard recently participated in a publication for parents entitled, "The Many Facets of Touch," which was also funded by Johnson & Johnson.

Today, Barnard continues to study the mother-infant relationship. Her most recent research projects examine the nurse's role in relation to high-risk mothers and high-risk infants.[7:6]

The Nursing Child Assessment Project (NCAP) formed the basis for Barnard's Child Health Assessment Interaction Theory. This was a longitudinal study "to identify poor [child development] outcomes before they occur and to examine the variability of the screening and assessment measures over time."[12:16] The study population included 193 infants and their parents. Using various assessment scales and interviewing tools, the child and his or her parental relationships were assessed at six stages: prenatally, postnatally, at 1 month, 4 months, 8 months, and 1 year of age. Additional funds were obtained to continue the project by reassessing the child and parent at 2 years of age, and again when the children were in the second grade.[12:16]

MAJOR CONCEPTS AND DEFINITIONS

A major focus of Barnard's work was the development of assessment tools to evaluate child health, growth, and development while viewing the parent and child as an interactive system. Barnard stated the parent-infant system was influenced by individual characteristics of each member and that the individual characteristics were also modified to meet the needs of the system. She defines modification as adaptive behavior. The interaction between parent and child is diagrammed in the Barnard Model in Figure 23-1.

Barnard[2:9-12] has defined the terms in the diagram as follows:

> *Infant's clarity to cues.* To participate in a synchronous relationship, the infant must send cues to his/her caregiver. The skill and clarity with which these cues are sent will make it either easy or difficult for the parent to "read" the cues and make the appropriate modification of his/her own behavior. Infants send cues of many kinds: sleepiness, fussiness, alertness, hunger and satiation, and changes in body activity, to name a few. Ambiguous or confusing cues sent by an infant can interrupt a caregiver's adaptive abilities.
>
> *Infant's responsiveness to the caregiver.* Just as the

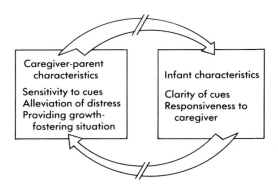

Figure 23-1. The Barnard model.
Used with permission from Barnard, K.E., et al. (1977). *The nursing child assessment training study guide: Program learning manual.* p. 8.

infant must "send" cues so that the parent can modify his/her behavior, the infant must also "read" cues so that he/she can modify his/her behavior in return. Obviously, if the infant is unresponsive to the behavioral cues of his/her caregivers, adaptation is not possible.

Parent's sensitivity to the child's cues. Parents, like infants, must be able to accurately read the cues given by the infant if they are to appropriately modify their behavior. . . . There are also other influences on the parents' sensitivity. Parents who are greatly concerned about other aspects of their lives, such as occupational or financial problems, emotional problems, or marital stress may be unable to be as sensitive as they would be otherwise. Only when these stresses are reduced are some parents able to "read" the cues of their young children.

Parents' ability to alleviate the infant's distress. Some cues sent by the infant signal that assistance from the parent is needed. . . . The effectiveness of parents in alleviating the distress of their infants depends upon several factors. First, they must recognize that distress is occurring. . . . Second, they must know (or figure out) the appropriate action which will alleviate distress. . . . Finally, they must be available to put this knowledge to work.

Parent's social and emotional growth fostering activities. . . . The ability to initiate social and emotional growth-fostering activities depends upon more global parent adaption. The parent needs to be able to play affectionately with the child, engage in social interactions such as those

associated with eating, and to provide appropriate social reinforcement of desirable behaviors. To do these things the parent must be aware of the child's level of development and be able to adjust his/her behavior accordingly. . . . This depends as much upon the parent's available energy as on his/her knowledge and skill.

Parent's cognitive growth fostering activities. . . . It has been shown in a number of studies that cognitive growth is facilitated by providing stimulation which is just above the child's level of understanding. To do this, the parent must have a good grasp of the child's present level of understanding . . . and the parent also have the energy available to use these skills.

As the NCAP continued, Barnard's model became the foundation for her Child Health Assessment Interaction Theory. Three major concepts form the basis of this theory.

CHILD. In describing the child, Barnard[12:16] used the characteristics of "newborn behavior, feeding and sleeping patterns, physical appearance, temperament and the child's ability to adapt to his/her caregiver and environment."

MOTHER. *Mother* refers to the child's mother or caregiver and his or her important characteristics. The mother's characteristics include her "psychosocial assets, her concerns about her child, her own health, the amount of life change she experienced, her expectations for her child, and most important, her parenting style and her adaptional skills."[12:17]

ENVIRONMENT. The environment represents the environment of both child and mother. Characteristics of the environment include "aspects of the physical environment of the family, the father's involvement and the degree of parent mutuality in regard to child rearing."[12:17]

MAJOR ASSUMPTIONS
Nursing

Except for nursing, Barnard does not define her major assumptions. In 1966 she defined *nursing* as "a process by which the patient is assisted in maintenance and promotion of his independence. This process may be educational, therapeutic, or restorative: it involves facilitation of change, most probably a change in the environment."[1:629] Five years later, in a 1981 keynote address to the first International Nursing Research Conference, she defined nursing as "the diagnosis and treatment of human responses to health problems."[6:2]

Person

When Barnard describes a person or human being, she speaks of the ability "to take in auditory, visual, and tactile stimuli but also to make meaningful associations from what he takes in."[11:15] This term includes infants, children, and adults.

Health

Although Barnard does not define health, she describes the family "as the basic unit of health care."[5:210] In the *Nursing Child Assessment Satellite Training Study Guide,* she states, "In health care, the ultimate goal is primary prevention."[2] Barnard emphasizes the importance of striving to reach one's maximum potential. She believes "We must promote new values in American society, which up to now has valued not health, but the absence of disease."[17:9] She wrote the definition for the scope of practice on maternal child health.

Environment

Environment is an essential aspect of Dr. Barnard's theory. In *Child Health Assessment, Part 2: The First Year of Life,* she states, "In essence, the environment includes all experiences encountered by the child: people, objects, places, sounds, visual and tactile sensations."[9:53] She makes a distinction between the animate and inanimate environments. "The inanimate environment refers to the objects available to the child for exploration and manipulation. The animate environment includes the activities of the caretaker used in arousing and directing the young child to the external world."[9:53]

THEORETICAL ASSERTIONS

Barnard's Child Health Assessment Interaction Theory is based on 10 theoretical assertions. They are:[12:6-7]

1. In child health assessment the *ultimate* goal is to identify problems at a point before they develop and when intervention would be most effective.
2. Environmental factors, as typified by the process of parent-child interaction, are important for determining child health outcomes.
3. The caregiver-infant interaction provides information that reflects the nature of the child's ongoing environment.
4. The caregiver brings a basic style and level of skills that are enduring characteristics; the caregiver's adaptive capacity is more readily influenced by responses of the infant and her environmental support.
5. In the adaptive parent-child interaction, there is a process of mutual modification in that the parent's behavior influences the infant or child and in turn the child influences the parent so that both are changed.
6. The adaptive process is more modifiable than the mother's or infant's basic characteristics; therefore, in intervention the nurse should lend support to the mother's sensitivity and response to her infant's cues rather than trying to change her characteristics or styles.
7. An important quality of promoting the child's learning is in permitting child-initiated behaviors and in reinforcing the child's attempt at a task.
8. A major issue for the nursing profession is support of the child's caregiver during the first year of life.
9. Interactive assessment is important in any comprehensive child health care model.
10. Assessment of the child's environment is important in any child health assessment model.

The Child Health Assessment Interaction Model was developed to illustrate Barnard's theory (Figure 23-2). "The smallest circle represents the child and his/her important characteristics. . . . The next largest circle represents the mother or caregiver and his/her important characteristics. . . . The largest circle repre-

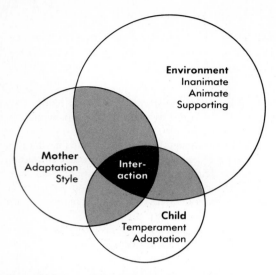

Figure 23-2. Child health assessment interaction model.

Used with permission from Barnard, K.E., et al. (1977). *The nursing child assessment training study guide: Program learning manual.* p. 19.

sents the environment of both the child and mother."[12:16-17]

Those portions of the model where two circles overlap represent interaction between the two concepts. The dark center area represents interaction among all three concepts. Barnard's theory focuses on this crucial mother-child-environment interactive process. The Nursing Child Assessment Project used this as the theoretical basis for the study of potential screening and assessment methods to be used with young children.[12:17]

LOGICAL FORM

According to Chinn and Jacobs,[13:61] "In inductive logic the reasoning method relies on observing particular instances and then combining those particulars into a larger whole." Inductive logic is the form Barnard used in developing her Child Health Assessment Interaction Theory. This theory was an outcome of the investigation and findings of the Nursing Child

Assessment Project. Barnard concluded the most important aspect of child health assessment was the interaction and adaptation that occurs between parent and child.

ACCEPTANCE BY THE NURSING COMMUNITY
Practice

The nursing satellite training project prepared about 4,000 nurses to use a series of standard assessment instruments. The exactness of the preparation in interrater reliability has increased observation skills applicable to other aspects of nursing. Now nurses use the assessment tools and their skills throughout the nation and in foreign countries.

Education

The nursing satellite training project initially used satellite communications and later videotaped classes to teach nurses how to use a series of standard assessment instruments. The concept of interrater reliability has encouraged nurses to share their knowledge and observations with co-workers. The explicitness of the observations has made the task of educating others easier.

Research

One of the outcomes of the contract to develop accurate assessment tools was the creation of a research project. The purpose of the satellite training program was to quickly disseminate current research findings. Barnard is continuing to refine the assessment scales and continues to receive funds for research. She is well recognized for her work, having been cited in the Citation Indices at least 35 times between 1976 and 1984. She has received awards recognizing her work from several organizations, including the American Nurses' Association, the American Public Health Association, and the Nurses' Association of the American College of Obstetricians and Gynecologists.

FURTHER DEVELOPMENT

The greatest deficit of Barnard's theory is lack of clarity. Barnard does not explicitly define her major assumptions about nursing, person, health, and environment. Although the identification of major concepts is implied through the Nursing Child Health Assessment Interaction Model, Barnard fails to clearly define these concepts. This is an area requiring further development.

In the Child Health Assessment Interaction theory, the mother is identified as a major concept, while the father is included in the description of the environment. Although this may accurately describe the father's role in most families, a problem exists when the father assumes the role of primary caregiver. In these instances, Barnard's theory needs modification.

Barnard says her future endeavors will focus on further investigation of the child, his or her parents, and the environment. She plans to continue work in the area of teaching parents how to improve interaction skills with their children. Although Barnard's theory is a micro theory, she does not intend to broaden her scope. Rather, she will be looking more closely at individual variables and how these affect a child's development.[8]

CRITIQUE
Clarity

Clarity in general refers to the lucidness and consistency of the theory. . . . An extremely important aspect of semantic clarity is that of definition of concepts.[13:133] Barnard does not identify or define her theoretical concepts. Rather, she describes and implies the definitions of these concepts. "In a theory with structural clarity, concepts are interconnected and organized into a coherent whole."[13:136] By using Barnard's Child Health Assessment Interaction Model, it is relatively easy for the reader to understand the interrelationships of her theoretical concepts. Barnard is consistent in the use of an inductive form of logic.

Simplicity

The Child Health Assessment Interaction Model is a simple way of communicating the main focus of Barnard's work as it relates to the parent-child interaction and the development of accurate assessment tools. However, there are several identifed characteristics for both concepts and assertions, and consequently the complexity is great. It must also be noted that the research necessary to define and support the assertions is complex.

Generality

Barnard's work with the interactive focus between parent and child is not generalizable to nursing. The original work was done on interactions between parent and child during the child's first 12 months of life. Subsequent work lengthened the time period of the child assessment to 36 months. However, one can currently only generalize to parent-child interactions in the first 3 years of life. The parent-child interaction model approaches midrange theory as defined by Chinn and Jacobs.[13] Despite the narrow scope, Barnard's theory is applicable, not only to nursing but also to other disciplines that deal with the parent-child relationship.

Empirical Precision

There is much research included in Barnard's original work. She also used alternate research concurrently to validate test results obtained by one set of raters who made home visits with test results obtained by a set of testors from another discipline. Further development of the feeding and teaching assessment tools demonstrated test-retest reliability and validity of the original scales. Original video tapes were rescored using the revised scales.

Derivable Consequences

More than 2000 nurses have been trained to use the standardized assessment scales with 85% interrater reliability. Nurses across the nation and in other countries utilize the observational skills in daily practice.[14]

Throughout her writings, Barnard emphasizes the need for strong links between nursing research, theory, and practice. In discussing research, she states "We simply must attempt to be in closer alignment with practice from the beginning."[18:169] In the Nursing Child Assessment Satellite Training Project, she identifies her goal as the dissemination of research findings and the application of these findings to practice. This is a prime example of Barnard's efforts to link research, theory, and practice.

REFERENCES

1. Barnard, K.E. (1966, Dec.). Symposium on mental retardation. *Nursing Clinics of North America, 1*:629-630.
2. Barnard, K.E. (1979, Sept. 20). Child advocates must help parents, too, *The American Nurse, 11*:4.
3. Barnard, K.E. (1980, July). Knowledge for practice: Directions for the future. *Nursing Research, 29*:208-212.
4. Barnard, K.E. (1982, Summer). The research cycle: Nursing, the profession, the discipline. *Western Journal of Nursing Research, 4*:1-12.
5. Barnard, K.E. (1984). Curriculum vitae.
6. Barnard, K.E. (1984, Nov.). Cassette tape interview.
7. Barnard, K.E. & Eyres, S.J. (Eds.). (1979). *Child health assessment, part II: The first year of life.* Hyattsville, Md.: U.S. Department of Health, Education, and Welfare.
8. Barnard, K.E. & Neal, M.V. (1977, May-June). Maternal-child nursing research: Review of the past and strategies for the future. *Nursing Research, 26*:193-200.
9. Barnard, K.E., & Powell, M.L. (1972). *Teaching the mentally retarded child: A family care approach.* St. Louis: C.V. Mosby.
10. Barnard, K.E., et al. (1977). *The nursing child assessment satellite training study guide,* Unpublished program learning manual, 1977.
11. Chinn, P., & Jacobs, M. (1983). *Theory and nursing: A systematic approach.* St. Louis: C.V. Mosby.
12. Goldman, B. (Ed.). (1984, March-April). Ross Public Health Currents 24(2).
13. Kathryn E. Barnard presented with the Lucille Petry Leone Award at NLN annual convention. *Washington State Journal of Nursing, 41*:9
14. Kathryn E. Barnard presented with the Maternal and Child Health Nurse of the Year Award, 1983, at ANA annual convention. (1984). *Nursing Outlook, 32*:242.
15. Kathryn E. Barnard presented with the 1983 Martha May Eliot Award of the American Public Health Association, Maternal and Child Health Section. (1984, March-April). *Public Health Currents, 24*:7-10.
16. King, D., Barnard, K.E., & Hoehn, R. (1981, March). Disseminating the results of nursing research. *Nursing Outlook, 29*:164-169.

BIBLIOGRAPHY
Primary Sources
Books

Barnard, K.E. (Ed.). (1983). *Structure to outcome: Making it work.* Kansas City, Mo.: American Academy of Nursing.

Barnard, K.E. (1984). *Social support and families of vulnerable infants.* White Plains, N.Y., March of Dimes Birth Defects Foundation.

Barnard, K.E. & Brazelton, T.B. (Chairpersons). (1984). *The many facets of touch.* Somerville, N.J., Johnson & Johnson.

Barnard, K.E. & Douglas, H.B. (Eds.). (1974). *Child health assessment, part I: A literature review.* Bethesda, Md.: U.S. Department of Health, Education and Welfare.

Barnard, K.E. & Erickson, M.L. (1976). *Teaching children with developmental problems: A family care approach* (2nd ed). St. Louis: C.V. Mosby.

Barnard, K.E. & Eyres, S.J. (Eds.). (1979). *Child health assessment, part II: The first year of life.* Hyattsville, Md.: U.S. Department of Health, Education, and Welfare.

Barnard, K.E. & Powell, M.L. (1972). *Teaching the mentally retarded child: A family care approach.* St. Louis: C.V. Mosby.

Book Chapters

Barnard, K.E. (1973). Nursing. In J. Wortis (Ed.), *Mental retardation and developmental disabilities: An annual review.* New York: Brunner-Mazee.

Barnard, K.E. (1975). Infant programming. In R. Koch (Ed.), *Proceedings of confidence on Down's syndrome.* New York: Brunner-Mazee.

Barnard, K.E. (1976). The state of the art: Nursing and early intervention with handicapped infants. In T. Tjossem (Ed.), *Proceedings of 1974 president's committee on mental retardation meeting on infant intervention.* Baltimore, Md.: University Park Press.

Barnard, K.E. (1978). Introduction to parent-infant interaction studies. In G.P. Sackett (Ed.), *Observing behavior* (Vol. I): *Theory and application in mental retardation.* Baltimore, Md., University Park Press.

Barnard, K.E. (1979). How focusing on the family changes the health care system. In T.B. Brazelton & V.C. Vaughan (Eds.), *The family: Setting priorities.* New York: Science & Medicine.

Barnard, K.E. (1980). How nursing care may influence prevention of development delay. In E.J. Sell (Ed.), *Follow-up of the high risk newborn: A practical approach.* Springfield, Ill.: Charles C Thomas.

Barnard, K.E. (1980). Sleep organization and motor development in prematures. In E.J. Sell (Ed.), *Follow-up of the high risk newborn: A practical approach.* Springfield, Ill., Charles C Thomas.

Barnard, K.E. (1980). How nursing care may influence prevention of development delay. In E.J. Sell (Ed.), *Follow-up of the high risk newborn: A practical approach.* Springfield, Ill., Charles C Thomas.

Barnard, K.E. (1981). An ecological approach to parent-child relations. In C.C. Brown (Ed.), *Infants at risk: Assessment and intervention.* Johnson & Johnson Pediatric Round Table.

Barnard, K.E. (1981). General issues in parent-infant interaction during the first years of life. In D.L. Yeung (Ed.), *Essays of pediatric nutrition.* Ontario, Canada: The Canadian Science Committee on Food and Nutrition, Canadian Public Health Association.

Barnard, K.E. (1981). The nursing role in the promotion of child development. In M. Tudor (Ed.), *Child development.* New York: McGraw-Hill.

Barnard, K.E. (1981). A program of temporarily patterned movement and sound stimulation for premature infants. In V.L. Smeriglio (Ed.), *Newborns and parents: Parent-infant contact and newborn sensory stimulation.* Hillsdale, N.J.: Lawrence Erlbaum Associates. pp. 31-48.

Barnard, K.E. (1984). Nursing research in relation to infants and young children. In H. Werley, & J. Fitzpatrick (Eds.), *Annual review of nursing research* (Vol. 1). New York: Springer. pp. 3-25.

Barnard, K.E., Bee, H.L., & Hammond, M.A. (1984). Home environment and cognitive development in a health, low-risk sample: The Seattle study. In A. Gottfried (Ed.), *Home environment and early cognitive development.* New York: Academic.

Barnard, K.E., et al. (1977). Premature infant refocus. In Mittler, P. (Ed.), Research to practice in mental retardation: Biomedical aspects, Vol. 3, I.A.S.S.M.D.

Barnard, K.E., et al. (In Press). An ecological paradigm for assessment and intervention. In Brazelton, T.B. & Lester, B. (Eds.), Infants at risk: Towards plasticity and intervention, Hillsdale, N.J., Erlbaum.

Mitchell, S.K., et al. (1985). Prediction of school problems and behavior problems in children followed from birth to age eight. In W.K. Frankenburg, R.N. Emde, & J. Sullivan (Eds.), *Early identification of children at risk: An international perspective.* New York: Plenum Press.

Articles

Barnard, K.E. (1966, April-May). New four-part training project is developed. *Children Limited, 15:2.*

Barnard, K.E. (1966, Dec.). Symposium on mental retardation. *Nursing Clinics of North America, 1:*629-630.

Barnard, K.E. (1968, Feb.). Teaching the mentally retarded child is a family affair. *American Journal of Nursing, 68:*305-311.

Barnard, K.E. (1969, Oct.). Are professionals educable? *Alabama Journal of Medical Sciences, 6:*388-391.

Barnard, K.E. (1973, Dec.). The effect of stimulation on the sleep behavior of the premature infant. *Communicating Nursing Research, 6:*12-33.

Barnard, K.E. (1975, Oct.). Trends in the care and prevention of developmental disabilities. *American Journal of Nursing, 75:*1700-1704.

Barnard, K.E. (1976, Oct.). Predictive nursing: The baby and parents. *Health Care Dimensions, 3:*185-202.

Barnard, K.E. (1977, Aug. 15). A challenge for nursing care. *The American Nurse, 9:*4.

Barnard, K.E. (1978, March-April). The family and

you. *American Journal of Maternal Child Nursing, 3:*82-83.

Barnard, K.E. (1979, Sept. 20). Child advocates must help parents, too. *The American Nurse, 11:*4.

Barnard, K.E. (1980, July). Knowledge for practice: Directions for the future. *Nursing Research, 29:*208-212.

Barnard, K.E. (1981, May-June). The research question. *American Journal of Maternal Child Nursing, 6:*211.

Barnard, K.E. (1981, July-August). Breast-feeding is best for U.S. babies, too. *The American Nurse, 13:*44.

Barnard, K.E. (1981, July-August). Research designs: Descriptive method. *American Journal of Maternal Child Nursing, 6:*243.

Barnard, K.E. (1981, Sept.-Oct.). Research designs: Experimental method. *American Journal of Maternal Child Nursing, 6:*321.

Barnard, K.E. (1981, Nov.-Dec.). Research designs: The historical method. *American Journal of Maternal Child Nursing, 6:*391.

Barnard, K.E. (1982, Jan.-Feb.). Research designs: Sampling. *American Journal of Maternal Child Nursing, 7:*15.

Barnard, K.E. (1982, March-April). Measurements: Reliability. *American Journal of Maternal Child Nursing, 7:*101.

Barnard, K.E. (1982, May-June). Measurement: Validity. *American Journal of Maternal Child Nursing, 7:*165.

Barnard, K.E. (1982, Summer). The research cycle: Nursing, the profession, the discipline. *Communicating Nursing Research, 15:*1-12.

Barnard, K.E. (1982, Summer). The research cycle: Nursing, the profession, the discipline. *Western Journal of Nursing Research, 4:*1-12.

Barnard, K.E. (1982, July-Aug.). Measurement descriptive statistics. *American Journal of Maternal Child Nursing, 7:*235.

Barnard, K.E. (1982, Sept.-Oct.). Determining the focus of nursing research. *American Journal of Maternal Child Nursing, 7:*299.

Barnard, K.E. (1982, Nov.-Dec.). Determining the role of nursing. *American Journal of Maternal Child Nursing, 7:*36.

Barnard, K.E. (1983, Jan.). Social policy statement can move nursing ahead. *The American Nurse, 15:*4, 14.

Barnard, K.E. (1983, Jan.-Feb.). The case study method: A research tool. *American Journal of Maternal Child Nursing, 8:*36.

Barnard, K.E. (1983, March-April). Identifying potential nursing research areas. *American Journal of Maternal Child Nursing, 8:*117.

Barnard, K.E. (1983, May-June). Nursing diagnosis: A descriptive method. *American Journal of Maternal Child Nursing, 8:*223.

Barnard, K.E. (1983, July-Aug.). Formulation of hypotheses. *American Journal of Maternal Child Nursing, 8:*263.

Barnard, K.E. (1983, Sept.-Oct.). Informed consent. *American Journal of Maternal Child Nursing, 8:*327.

Barnard, K.E. (1983, Nov.-Dec.). Control groups. *Maternal Child Nursing, 8:*431.

Barnard, K.E. (1984). Nursing research related to infants and young children. *Annual Review of Nursing Research, 1:*3-25.

Barnard, K.E. (1984, Jan.-Feb.). The family as a unit of measurement. *American Journal of Maternal Child Nursing, 9:*21.

Barnard, K.E. (1984, March-April). Commonly understood outcomes. *American Journal of Maternal Child Nursing, 9:*99.

Barnard, K.E. (1984, March-April). Children: Our greatest national resource. *Public Health Currents, 24:*8-10.

Barnard, K.E. (1984, May-June). Knowledge development. *American Journal of Maternal Child Nursing, 9:*175.

Barnard, K.E. (1984, July-Aug.). Planning experiments. *American Journal of Maternal Child Nursing, 9:*247.

Barnard, K.E. (1984, Sept.-Oct.). Determining relationships. *American Journal of Maternal Child Nursing, 9:*345.

Barnard, K.E., & Bee, H.L. (1983). The impact of temporarily patterned stimulation on the development of preterm infants. *Child Development, 54:*1156-1167.

Barnard, K.E., & Bee, H.L. (1984). Developmental changes in maternal interactions with term and preterm infants. *Infant Behavior and Development, 7:*101-113.

Barnard, K.E., Bee, J.L., & Hammond, M.A. (1984). Developmental changes in maternal interactions with term and preterm infants. *Infant Behavior and Development, 1:*101-113.

Barnard, K.E., & Neal, M.V. (1977, May-June).

Maternal-child nursing research: Review of the past and strategies for the future. *Nursing Research,* 26:193-200.

Barnard, K.E., & Collar, B.S. (1973, Feb.). Early diagnosis, interpretation and intervention: A commentary on the nurse's role. *Annals of the New York Academy of Science,* 205:373-382.

Barnard, K.E., Snyder, C., & Spietz, A. (1984). Supportive measures for high-risk infants and families. In K.E. Barnard, et al. (Eds.), *Social support and families of vulnerable infants. Birth Defects: Original Article Series* (Vol. 20, No. 5). White Plains, N.Y.: March of Dimes Birth Defects Foundation.

Barnard, K.E., et al. (1976). Predictive nursing: The baby and parents. *Health Care Dimensions, 3.* 1:185-202.

Bee, H.L., et al. (1982). Prediction of IQ and language skill from perinatal status, child performance, family characteristics, and mother-infant interaction. *Child Development,* 53:1134-1156.

Bee, H.L., et al. (1984). Predicting intellectual outcomes: Sex differences in response to early environmental stimulation. *Sex Roles, 10.*

Booth, C.L., Lyons, N.B., & Barnard, K.E. (In Press). Synchrony in mother-infant interaction: A comparison of measurement methods. *Child Study Journal.*

Hammer, S.L., & Barnard, K.E. (1966, Nov.). The mentally retarded adolescent: A review of the characteristics and problems of 44 non-institutionalized adolescent retardates. *Pediatrics,* 38:845-857.

Jacox, A., Lang, N., & Barnard, K.E. (1982, Oct.). Four nurses describe 'dramatic' changes in education. *The American Nurse, 9:8.*

Kang, R., & Barnard, K. (1979). Using the neonatal behavioral assessment scale to evaluate premature infants. *Birth Defects: Original Article Series, XV* (7):119-144. The National Foundation. New York: Alan R. Liss.

King, D., Barnard, K.E., & Hoehn, R. (1981, March), Disseminating the results of nursing research. *Nursing Outlook,* 29:164-169.

Murray, B.L., & Barnard, K.E. (1966, Dec.). The nursing specialist in mental retardation. *Nursing Clinics of North America,* 1:631-640.

Pattullo, A.W., & Barnard, K.E. (1968, Dec.). Teaching menstrual hygiene to the mentally retarded. *American Journal of Nursing,* 12:2572-2575.

Snyder, C., Eyres, S.J., & Barnard, K.E. (1979, Nov.-Dec.). New findings about mothers' antenatal expectations and their relationship to infant development. *American Journal of Maternal Child Nursing,* 4:354-357.

Whitney, L., & Barnard, K.E. (1966, June). Implications of operant learning theory for nursing care of the mentally retarded. *Mental Retardation, 4:3.*

Unpublished Papers

Barnard, K.E. (1967, April). Nursing and mental retardation: A problem solving paper. U.S. Public Health Service, Mental Retardation Division. pp. 1-70.

Barnard, K.E. (1967, April). Planning for learning experiences in university affiliated centers. Proceedings of the 4th National Workshop for Nurses in Mental Retardation, U.S. Children's Bureau.

Barnard, K.E. (1975). Predictive nursing care. In Proceedings of perinatal nursing conference, sponsored by University of Washington School of Nursing and Maternal and Child Health Services, HSMHA, Seattle, Washington.

Barnard, K.E. (1976, Feb.). A perspective on where we are in early intervention programs. Adapted from a Keynote Address at a conference on "The Nursing Role in Early Intervention Programs for Developing Disabled Children," sponsored by the University of Utah College of Nursing Division of Continuing Education and Utah State Division of Health, Denver, Colorado.

Barnard, K.E. (1977). Nursing child assessment satellite training fact sheet.

Barnard, K.E., Principal Investigator. Models of newborn nursing services. Grant #NU-00719. Division of Nursing, Bureau of Health Professions, Health Resources Administration, Public Health Service, Department of Health and Human Services. July 7, 1979-June 30, 1982.

Barnard, K.E., Principal Investigator. Clinical nursing model for infants and their families. National Institute of Mental Health, Alcohol, Drug Abuse, and Mental Health Administration, Public Health Service, Department of Health and Human Services. Grant submitted May 1981.

Barnard, K.E., Principal Investigator. Premature infant refocus. Grant #MC-R-530348. Maternal and Child Health and Crippled Children's Services, Bureau of Community Health Services, Health Services Administration, Public Health

Service, Department of Health and Human Resources. Sept. 1, 1974-April 30, 1981.

Barnard, K.E. (1981). Critical issues: Support of the caregiver Maternal Child Nursing in the 80s: Nursing Perspective. A Forum in Honor of Katherine Kendall. School of Nursing, University of Maryland.

Barnard, K.E., & Bee, H.L. The assessment of parent-infant interaction by observation of feeding and teaching.

Barnard, K.E., & Bee, H.L. (1981, Sept.). Premature infant refocus. Final report on Grant #MCR-530348. Prepared for the Maternal and Child Health and Crippled Children's Services Research Grants Program, Bureau of Community Health Services, HSA, PhS, DHHS.

Barnard, K.E., & Hoehn, R.E. (1978, Dec.). Nursing child assessment satellite training. In R.A. Duncan, (Ed.), Biomedical communications experiments, Lister Hill National Center for Biomedical Communications, Dept. of HEW, Public Health Service.

Barnard, K.E., & Kelly, J.F. (1980, May). Infant intervention: Parental consideration. State of art paper. Guidelines for Early Intervention Programs. Based on a conference Health Issues in Early Intervention Programs, Washington, D.C. Sponsored by College of Nursing, University of Utah, and School of Public Health, University of Hawaii. Office for Maternal & Child Health, Department of Health and Human Services.

Barnard, K.E., Lendzion, A., & Moser, J. (1974). Final report on the measuring interactions project, technical report #3, The first three years: Programming for atypical infants and their families. New York: United Cerebral Palsy Association.

Barnard, K.E., & Powell, M. (1967, April). Planning for learning experiences in university affiliated centers. Proceedings of the 4th National Workshop for Nurses in Mental Retardation, U.S. Children's Bureau.

Barnard, K.E., & Summer, G.A. (1981, June). The health of women with fertility-related needs. In L.V. Klerman (Ed.), Research priorities in maternal and child health: Report of a conference, Brandeis University, Waltham, Mass.

Barnard, K.E., et al. (1977). The nursing child assessment satellite training study guide. Program learning manual.

Barnard, K.E., et al. (1983, Dec.). Newborn nursing models. Final report on Grant #R01-NU-00719. Prepared for the Division of Nursing, Bureau of Manpower, Health Resources Administration, Department of Health and Human Services.

Bee, H.L., et al. (1981, April). Parent-child interaction during teaching in abusing and nonabusing families. Paper presented at the biennial meetings of the Society for Research in Child Development, Boston, Mass.

Eyres, S.J., Barnard, K.E., & Gray, C.A. Child health assessment, part III: 2-4 years.

Hammond, M.A., et al. (1983, July). Child health assessment, part IV: Follow-up at second grade. Final report of Grant #R01-NU-00816 prepared for Division of Nursing, Bureau of Health Professions, Health Resources and Services Administration, U.S. Public Health Service.

Interview

Barnard, K.E. (1984, Nov.). Cassette tape interview.

Correspondence

Barnard, K.E. Curriculum vitae. (1984, Sept.).

Videotapes

Videotape. (1984, July 27). NAACOG Invitational Research Conference, Indianapolis, Indiana.

Videotape Services, Nursing Child Assessment Satellite Training.

Secondary Sources
Book Chapters

Disbrow, M.A. (1983). Conducting interdisciplinary research: Gratifications and frustrations. In N.L. Chaska, *The nursing profession: A time to speak.* New York, McGraw-Hill.

Menke, E.M. (1983). Critical analysis of theory development in nursing. In N.L. Chaska, *The nursing profession: A time to speak.* New York: McGraw-Hill.

Book Reviews

Barnard, K.E., & Douglas, H.B. (Eds.). (1974). *Child health assessment, part I: A literature review. Journal of Continuing Education in Nursing, 6:*52, November-December 1975.
*Nursing Mirror, 141:*71, October 2, 1975.
*RN, 38:*122, September 1975.

Barnard, K.E., & Erickson, M.L. (1976). *Teaching children with developmental problems: A family care approach* (2nd ed.).
*American Journal of Nursing, 77:*499, March 1977.
*Canadian Nurse, 73:*46, July 1977.
Barnard, K.E., & Powell, M.L. (1972). *Teaching the mentally retarded child: A family care approach.*
*American Journal of Nursing, 73:*729, April 1973.
*Canadian Nurse, 69:*54, March 1973.

Research Abstracts

Barnard, K.E. (1972, Oct.). The effect of stimulation on the duration and amount of sleep and wakefulness in the premature infant. *Dissertation Abstracts International, 33:*2167-2168.

News Releases

Kathryn E. Barnard named in *National Nursing Directory* (1982). Rockville, Md.: Aspen Systems.
Kathryn E. Barnard named in *Sigma Theta Tau Directory of Nurse Researchers* (1983). Indianapolis, Indiana: Sigma Theta Tau.
Kathryn E. Barnard named in *Directory of Nurses with Doctoral Degrees* (1984). St. Louis: Missouri American Nurses Association.
Kathryn E. Barnard presented with the Lucille Petry Leone Award at NLN annual convention. (1969, May-June). *Washington State Journal of Nursing, 41:*9.
Kathryn E. Barnard presented with the Maternal and Child Health Nurse of the Year Award for 1983 at ANA annual convention. (1984). *Nursing Outlook, 32:*242.
Kathryn Elaine Barnard presented with the 1983 Martha May Eliot Award of the American Public Health Association, Maternal and Child Health Section. (1984, March-April). *Public Health Currents, 24:*7-8.

Other Sources

Als, H. (1976, May). Personal communication.
Brazelton, T.B. (1973). *The neonatal behavioral assessment scale.* London: William Heinemann, and Philadelphia: J.B. Lippincott.
Brunner, J.S. (1956). *A study of thinking.* New York: John Wiley & Sons.
Brunner, J.S. (1966). *Studies in cognitive growth.* New York: John Wiley & Sons.
Caldwell, B.M. (1965). *Daily program II: A manual for teachers.* Washington, D.C.: Office of Economic Opportunity.
Caldwell, B.M. (1967). What is the optimal learning environment for the young child? *American Journal of Orthopsychiatry, 37:*8-21.
Caldwell, B.M. (1968). On designing supplementary environments for early child development. *BAEYC Reporter 10:*1-11.
Caldwell, B.M. (1970). *Instruction manual inventory for infants* (Home Observation for Measurement of the Environment). Little Rock, Ark.
Caldwell, B.M. (1970). The rationale for early intervention. *Exceptional Children, 36:*717-726.
Caldwell, B.M. (1971, Feb. 20). A timid giant grows bolder. *Saturday Review,* pp. 47-66.
Caldwell, B.M. (1971). Impact of interest in early cognitive simulation. In H. Rie (Ed.), *Perspectives in psychopathology.* Chicago: Aldine-Atherton.
Caldwell, B.M. (1973). Do young children have a quality life in day care? *Young Children, 28:*197-208.
Caldwell, B.M. (1972). Infant day care: Fads, facts, and fancies. In R. Elardo, and B. Pagan (Eds.), *Perspective on infant day care.* Orangeburg, S.C.: Southern Association on Children under Six.
Caldwell, B.M. (1972). Kramer school: something for everybody. In S.J. Braun, and E.P. Wards (Eds.), *History and theory of early childhood education.* Worthington, Ohio, Charles A. Jones.
Caldwell, B.M., & Elardo, R. (1972). Innovative opportunities for school psychologists in early childhood education. *School Psychology Digest, 1:*8-16.
Caldwell, B.M., et al. (1963). Mother-infant interaction in monomatric and polymatric families. *American Journal of Orthopsychaitry, 33:*653-664.
Caldwell, B.M., & Richmond, J.B. (1968). The children's center in Syracuse, New York. In L.L. Dittman (Ed.) *Early child care: The new perspectives.* New York: Atherton.
Caldwell, B.M., & Smith, L.E. (1970). Day care for the very young: Prime opportunity for primary prevention. *American Journal of Public Health, 60:*690-697.
Caldwell, B.M., et al. (1970). Infant day care and attachment. *American Journal of Orthopsychiatry, 40:*397-412.
Dubowitz, L.M.S., et al. Clinical assessment of gestational age in the newborn infant. *Pediatrics, 77:*1-10.

Piaget, J. (1962). *Judgment and reasoning in the child.* New York: Humanities. (Reproduction of 1928 ed.).

Piaget, J. (1976). *The grasp of consciousness: Action and concept in young children.* Cambridge, Mass.: Harvard University Press.

Piaget, J (1983). *The child's perception of physical cau-sality.* New York: Adren Lib. (Reproduction of 1930 ed.).

Waldrop, M.F., & Goering, J.D. (1971). Hyperactivity and minor physical anomalies in elementary school children. *American Journal of Orthopsychiatry, 41(4):*602-607.

UNIT IV

Systems

Dorothy E. Johnson

Behavioral System Model

Sharon S. Conner, Judith K. Watt

CREDENTIALS AND BACKGROUND OF THE THEORIST

Dorothy E. Johnson was born Aug. 21, 1919, in Savannah, Georgia. She received her A.A. from Armstrong Junior College in Savannah, Georgia, in 1938; her B.S.N. from Vanderbilt University in Nashville, Tennessee, in 1942; and her M.P.H. from Harvard University in Boston in 1948.

The authors wish to express appreciation to Cynthia J. Allen, Sharon Evick, and Glenda Mitchell for their assistance with data collection, and to Dorothy E. Johnson for critiquing the chapter.

Most of Johnson's professional experiences involved teaching, although she was a staff nurse at the Chatham-Savannah Health Council from 1943 to 1944. She has been an instructor and an assistant professor in pediatric nursing at Vanderbilt University School of Nursing. From 1949 until her retirement in 1978 and subsequent move to Florida, Johnson was an assistant professor of pediatric nursing, an associate professor of nursing, and a professor of nursing at the University of California in Los Angeles.

In 1955 and 1956 Johnson was a pediatric nursing advisor assigned to the Christian Medical College School of Nursing in Vellore,

283

South India. In addition, from 1965 to 1967 she chaired the committee of the California Nurses' Association that developed a position statement on specifications for the clinical specialist. Johnson's publications[17] include four books, more than 30 articles in periodicals, and many reports, proceedings, and monographs.

Of the many honors she has received, the ones Johnson[16] is proudest of are the 1975 Faculty Award from graduate students, the 1977 Lulu Hassenplug Distinguished Achievement Award from the California Nurses' Association, and the 1981 Vanderbilt University School of Nursing Award for Excellence in Nursing. She is pleased that her behavioral system model has been found useful in furthering the development of a theoretical basis for nursing, but says her greatest source of satisfaction has come from following the productive careers of her students.

THEORETICAL SOURCES

Johnson's behavioral system theory springs from Nightingale's belief that nursing's goal is to help individuals prevent or recover from disease or injury.[19:117] The science and art of nursing should focus on the patient as an individual and not on the specific disease entity.

Johnson uses the work of behavioral scientists in psychology, sociology, and ethnology to develop her theory. She relies heavily on the systems theory and uses concepts and definitions from A. Rapoport, R. Chin, and W. Buckley.[15:208] The structure of the behavioral system theory is patterned after a systems model; a system is defined as consisting of interrelated parts functioning together to form a whole. In her writings, Johnson conceptualizes man as a behavioral system in which the functioning outcome is observed behavior. An analogy to the behavioral system theory is the biological system theory, which states that man is a biological system consisting of biological parts and that disease is an outcome of biological system disorder.

Developing the theory from a philosophical perspective, Johnson[15:206] writes that nursing contributes by facilitating effective behavioral functioning in the patient before, during, and following illness. She uses concepts from other disciplines, such as social learning, motivation, sensory stimulation, adaptation, and behavioral modification, to expand her theory.

Johnson notes that although the literature indicates others support the idea that man is a behavioral system, as far as she knows, the idea is original with her. Knowledge of the parts of the behavioral system is supported in the behavioral sciences, but the empirical literature supporting the notion that the behavioral system is a whole has yet to be developed. In the biological system, knowledge of the parts precedes knowledge of the whole.[15:208]

EMPIRICAL EVIDENCE

Some of the concepts Johnson has identified and defined in her theory are supported in the literature. Leitch and Escolona point out that tension produces behavioral changes and that the manifestation of tension by an individual depends on both internal and external factors.[10:66] Johnson[9:292] uses the work of Selye, Grinker, Simmons, and Wolff to support the idea that specific patterns of behavior are reactions to stressors from biological, psychological, and sociological sources, respectively.

In *Conceptual Models for Nursing Practice*, Johnson describes seven subsystems that comprise her behavioral system. To support the attachment-affiliative subsystem, she uses the work of Ainsworth and Robson.[15:210] Heathers, Gerwitz, and Rosenthal have described and explained dependency behavior, another subsystem defined by Johnson.[15:212-213] The response systems of ingestion and elimination, as described by Walike, Mead, and Sears, are also parts of Johnson's behavioral system.[15:213] The work of Kagan and Resnik is used to support the sexual subsystem.[15:213] The aggressive subsystem which functions to protect and preserve, is supported by Lorenz and Feshbach.[15:213] According to Atkinson, Feather, and Crandell, physical, creative, mechanical, and social skills are manifested by achievement behavior, another subsystem identified by Johnson.[15:214]

MAJOR CONCEPTS AND DEFINITIONS

BEHAVIOR. Johnson accepts the definition of behavior as expressed by the behavioral and biological scientists: the output of intraorganismic structures and processes as they are coordinated and articulated by and responsive to changes in sensory stimulation. She focuses on behavior affected by the actual or implied presence of other social beings that has been shown to have major adaptive significance.[15:207-208]

SYSTEM. Using Rapoport's 1968 definition of system, Johnson[15:208] states, "A system is a whole that functions as a whole by virtue of the interdependence of its parts." She accepts Chin's statement that there is "organization, interaction, interdependency, and integration of the parts and elements."[15:208] In addition, man strives to maintain a balance in these parts through adjustments and adaptations to the forces impinging on them.

BEHAVIORAL SYSTEM. A behavioral system encompasses the patterned, repetitive, and purposeful ways of behaving. These ways of behaving form an organized and integrated functional unit that determines and limits the interaction between the person and his environment and establishes the relationship of the person to the objects, events, and situations within his environment. Usually the behavior can be described and explained. Man as a behavioral system tries to achieve stability and balance by adjustments and adaptations that are successful to some degree for efficient and effective functioning. The system is usually flexible enough to accommodate the influences affecting it.[15:208-209]

Subsystems. Because the behavioral system has many tasks to perform, parts of the system evolve into subsystems with specialized tasks. A subsystem is "a minisystem with its own particular goal and function that can be maintained as long as its relationship to the other subsystems or the environment is not disturbed."[15:221] The seven subsystems identified by Johnson are open, linked, and interrelated. Motivational drives direct the activities of these subsystems, which are continually changing because of maturation, experience, and learning. The systems described appear to exist cross-culturally and are controlled by biological, psychological, and sociological factors. The seven identified are attachment-affiliative, dependency, ingestive, eliminative, sexual, achievement, and aggressive.[15:209-212]

Attachment-affiliative subsystem. The attachment-affiliative subsystem is probably the most critical, because it forms the basis for all social organization. On a general level, it provides survival and security. Its consequences are social inclusion, intimacy, and formation and maintenance of a strong social bond.[15:212]

Dependency subsystem. In the broadest sense, the dependency subsystem promotes helping behavior that calls for a nurturing response. Its consequences are approval, attention or recognition, and physical assistance. Developmentally, dependency behavior evolves from almost total dependence on other to a greater degree of dependence on self. A certain amount of interdependence is essential for survival of social groups.[15:213]

Biological subsystems. The biological subsystems of ingestion and elimination "have to do with when, how, what, how much, and under what conditions we eat, and when, how, and under what conditions we eliminate."[15:213] These responses are associated with social and psychological as well as biological considerations.[15:213]

Sexual subsystem. The sexual subsystem has the dual functions of procreation and gratification. Including, but not limited to, courting and mating, this response system begins with the development of gender role identity and includes the broad range of sex role behaviors.[15:214]

Aggressive subsystem. The aggressive subsystem's function is protection and preservation. This follows the line of thinking of ethologists such as Lorenz[4] and Feshbach[18] rather than the behavioral reinforcement school of thought. It holds that aggressive behavior is not only learned, but has a primary intent to harm others. However, society demands that limits be placed on modes of self-protection and that people and their property be respected and protected.[15:213]

Achievement subsystem. The achievement subsystem attempts to manipulate the environment. Its function is control or mastery of an aspect of self or environment to some standard of excellence. Areas of achievement behavior include intellectual, physical, creative, mechanical, and social skills.[15:214]

Johnson goes on to identify other concepts that further describe the theory of man as a behavioral system. The point that differentiates between what is inside from what is outside the system is the boundary. It is the point at which the system has little control over or impact on outcomes.[5:220] Equilibrium is defined "as a stabilized but more or less transitory, resting state in which the individual is in harmony with himself and with his environment."[10:65] Homeostasis is the process of maintaining stability in the behavioral system.[5:221] Stability is the maintenance of a certain level or range of acceptable behaviors.[5:221] Instability occurs when the system overcompensates in dealing with stress. When extra energy output is used to respond to a strain, the energy source needed to maintain stability is depleted.[19:221] Stressors are internal or external stimuli that produce tension and result in instability. Tension is a state of being stretched or strained. It results from disequilibrium and is a potential source of change.[10:65]

ASSUMPTIONS
Nursing

Nursing, as perceived by Johnson, is an external force acting to preserve the organization of the patient's behavior while the patient is under stress by means of imposing regulatory mechanisms or by providing resources.[19:118] An art and a science, it supplies external assistance both before and during system balance disturbance and therefore requires knowledge of order, disorder, and control.* Nursing activities do not depend on medical authority but are complementary to medicine.

Person

Johnson[15:209] views man as a behavioral system with patterned, repetitive, and purposeful ways of behaving that link him to the environment. Man's specific response patterns form an organized and integrated whole.[12:207] *Person* is a system of interdependent parts that requires some regularity and adjustment to maintain a balance.[15:208]

Johnson[15:208] further assumes that a behavioral system is essential to man and when strong forces or lower resistance disturb behavioral system balance, man's integrity is threatened.[19:126] Man's attempt to reestablish balance requires an extraordinary expenditure of energy, which leaves a shortage of energy to assist biological processes and recovery.[19:126]

Health

Johnson perceives health as an elusive, dynamic state influenced by biological, psychological, and social factors. Health is a desired value by health professionals and focuses on the person rather than the illness.[19:119]

Health is reflected by the organization, interaction, interdependence, and integration of the

---

*References 15:209; 13:207.

subsystems of the behavioral system.[15:208] Man attempts to achieve a balance in this system, which will lead to functional behavior. A lack of balance in the structural or functional requirements of the subsystems leads to poor health. When the system requires a minimal amount of energy for maintenance, a larger supply of energy is available to affect biological processes and recovery.[19:126]

Environment

In Johnson's theory the environment consists of all the factors that are not part of the individual's behavioral system but that influence the system and can be manipulated by the nurse to achieve the health goal for the patient.[19:126] The individual links himself to and interacts with the environment. The behavioral system at-tempts to maintain equilibrium in response to environmental factors by adjusting and adapting to the forces that impinge upon it. Excessively strong environmental forces disturb the behavioral system balance and threaten the person's stability. An unusual amount of energy is required in order for the system to reestablish equilibrium in the face of continuing forces.[19:126] When the environment is stable, the individual is able to continue with his successful behaviors.

THEORETICAL ASSERTIONS

Johnson's behavioral system theory addresses two major components: the patient and nursing (Figure 24-1). The patient is a behavioral system with seven interrelated subsystems.

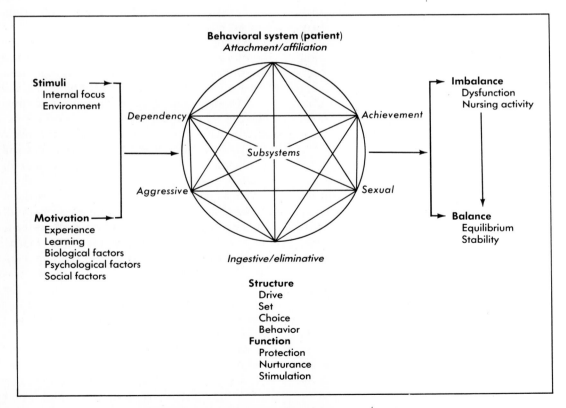

Figure 24-1. Johnson's Behavioral Systems Model.
Conceptualized by Ann Marriner.

Each subsystem can be described and analyzed in terms of structure and functional requirements. The four structural elements that have been identified include: (1) drive, or goal; (2) set, predisposition to act; (3) choice, alternatives for action; and (4) behavior.[15:210-211]

Each of the subsystems has the same functional requirements: protection, nurturance, and stimulation.[19:123] The system and subsystems tend to be self-maintaining and self-perpetuating as long as internal and external conditions remain orderly and predictable. If the conditions and resources necessary to their functional requirements are not met, or the interrelationships among the subsystems are not harmonious, dysfunctional behavior will result.[15:212]

The responses by the subsystems are developed through motivation, experience, and learning and are influenced by biological, psychological, and social factors.[15:209] The behavioral system attempts to achieve balance by adapting to internal and environmental stimuli. The resulting behavior reflects the system's successful adjustment to stressors even when the behavior is dysfunctional.[19:118] Because little information is available regarding the role of the patient, it is difficult to assess whether the relationship between the behavioral system and nursing is interactive or reactive.

A state of instability in the behavioral system results in a need for nursing intervention. Identification of the source of the problem in the system leads to appropriate nursing action that results in the maintenance or restoration of behavioral system balance.[19:129] Nursing is seen as an external regulatory force that acts to restore the balance in the behavioral system.[15:214]

LOGICAL FORM

By observing specifics in her practice, nursing literature, and research, Johnson has used the logical form of inductive reasoning to develop her theory. She states that a common core exists in nursing, which practitioners use in many settings and with varying populations.[8:200] Johnson used her observations of behavior over many years to formulate a general theory of man as a behavioral system.

ACCEPTANCE BY THE NURSING COMMUNITY
Practice

According to Johnson,[15] the behavioral system theory provides direction for practice, education, and research. Because the goal of the theory is to maintain and restore balance in the patient by helping him achieve a more optimal level of functioning, a goal also valued by nursing, the theory is acceptable to nursing. Knowledge of the behavioral system theory allows the nurse to be aware of the importance of providing a constant supply of protection, nurturing, and stimulation.

In 1974 Judy Grubbs[5:245,250] adapted the theory to the nursing process by developing an assessment tool and a nursing process sheet based on the seven subsystems. Questions and observations related to each subsystem provided powerful tools with which to collect important data. By using these tools, the nurse can discover other choices of behavior that will enable the patient to accomplish his goal of health.

That same year Bonnie Holaday[6:256] used the theory as a model to develop an assessment tool when caring for children. This tool allowed the nurse to objectively describe the child's behavior and to guide nursing action. Holaday concluded that the user of Johnson's theory was provided with a guide for planning and giving care based on scientific knowledge.

In 1980 Antionette Rawls[21:14-15] presented her attempt to use and evaluate the Johnson behavioral system theory in clinical practice. She used the theory to systematically assess a patient who was facing the loss of function in one arm and hand. Rawls concluded that Johnson's theory provided a tool that predicted the results of nursing intervention, formulated standards for care, and administered holistic care.

Education

Carol Loveland-Cherry and Sharon Wilkerson[19:133] analyzed Johnson's theory and concluded that it has utility in nursing education. A curriculum based on man as a behavioral system would have definite goals and straightforward course planning. Study would center on the patient as a behavioral system and its dysfunction, which would require use of the nursing process. In addition to an understanding of systems theory, the student would need knowledge in the biological fields and emphasis on psychology and sociology.

Research

The behavioral system theory leads the researcher in one of two directions. One researcher might investigate the functioning of the system and subsystems by focusing on the basic sciences, while another researcher might concentrate on investigating problem solving activities as they influence the behavioral system.[19:132]

Nurse researchers have demonstrated the usefulness of Johnson's theory in clinical practice. Beverly Small[23:264] used Johnson's theory as a conceptual framework to use when caring for visually impaired children. By evaluating and comparing the perceived body image and spacial awareness of normally sighted children with those of visually impaired children Small found that the sensory deprivation of visual impairment affected the normal development of the child's body image and the awareness of his body in space. She concluded that when the human system is subjected to excessive stress, the goals of the system cannot be maintained.

Karla Damus[3:276] tested the validity of Johnson's theory by comparing SGPT values in patients exposed to hepatitis B with the number of nursing diagnoses. Damus correlated the physiological disorder of elevated SGPT values

with behavioral disequilibrium and found that disorder in one area reflected disorder in another area.

Believing the model has potential in preventive care, Majesky[20] used it to construct a tool to measure patient indicators of nursing care. Holaday, Rawls, and Stamler[24] have done research using one subsystem.

FURTHER DEVELOPMENT

Although Johnson's behavioral system theory seems to focus on man as a passive being, Johnson believes people are active beings seeking constantly not only to adjust to their environments, but also to adjust environments to the end of better functioning for themselves. She also views the behavioral system as active rather than merely reactive.[16] Because the model allows for this belief, work can be done regarding it.

The theory has been associated primarily with individuals. Johnson believes groups of individuals can be considered as groups of interactive behavioral systems. Use of her theory with families and other groups needs more visibility.

As a result of the current emphasis on health promotion and maintenance and on illness and injury prevention, the theory could be developed further by recognizing behavior disorders in these areas.

> It should be noted that preventive nursing, i.e., to prevent behavioral system disorder, is not the same as preventive medicine, i.e., to prevent biological system disorders; and that disorders in both cases must be identified and explicated before approaches to prevention can be developed. At this point not even medicine has developed very many specific preventive measures (immunizations for some infectious diseases, and protection against some vitamin deficiency diseases are notable exceptions). There are a number of general approaches to better health, of course—adequate nutrition, safe water, exercise, etc.—which are applicable contributing to prevention of some

disorders. Small wonder then that preventive nursing remains to be developed, and this is true no matter what model or theory for nursing is used.[16]

Further development could identify nursing actions that would facilitate appropriate functioning of the system toward disease prevention and health maintenance. Instead of spending energy developing nursing interventions for the consequences of disequilibrium, nurses need to determine how to intervene with the precursors of disequilibrium in order to prevent a crisis in health.

How can Johnson's theory be used in community health nursing? Assuming that a community is a geographical area, a subpopulation, or any aggregate of people, and assuming that a community can benefit from nursing interventions, the behavioral system framework can be applied to community health. A community can be described as a behavioral system with interacting subsystems that have structural elements and functional requirements. Communities have goals, norms, choices, and actions in addition to needing protection, nurturance, and stimulation. The community reacts to internal and external stimuli, which results in functional or dysfunctional behavior. An example of an external stimulus is health policy and an example of dysfunctional behavior is a high infant mortality. Somewhere between is the behavioral system, consisting of yet undefined subsystems that are organized, interacting, interdependent, and integrated. Biological, psychological, and sociological factors also impact on community behavior.

CRITIQUE
Simplicity

Johnson's theory is relatively simple in relation to the number of concepts. Man is described as a behavioral system composed of seven subsystems. Nursing is an external regulatory force. However, the theory is potentially complex because of the number of possible interrelationships between and among the behavioral system and its subsystems and the forces impinging on them. However, at this point only a few of the potential relationships have been explored.

Generality

Johnson's theory is relatively unlimited when applied to sick individuals. But it has not been used as much with well individuals or groups. Johnson perceives man as a behavioral system comprised of seven subsystems, aggregates of interactive behavioral systems. The role of nursing in nonillness situations is not clearly defined in the theory, but Johnson does address it.[19:132]

Empirical Precision

Empirical precision is difficult to achieve when a theory contains highly abstract concepts and has only potential generality. Empirical precision can improve when subconcepts that are well defined and have reality indicators are introduced. The units and the relationships between the units in Johnson's theory are consistently defined and used. However, Johnson's theory has only a moderate degree of empirical precision because the highly abstract concepts need to be better defined. Throughout Johnson's writings terms such as *balance, stability and equilibrium, adjustments and adaptations, disturbances, disequilibrium,* and *behavioral disorders* are used interchangeably, which confounds their meanings. The introduction of subsystems improves the theory's empirical precision.

Derivable Consequences

The theory should guide practice, education, and research, generate new ideas, and differentiate nursing from other professions. Johnson's theory guides nursing practice, education, and research. Because of the many interacting concepts it generates new ideas for practice and research. By focusing on behavior rather than biology, the theory clearly differentiates nursing from medicine although the concepts overlap with the psychosocial professions.

Johnson's behavioral systems theory provides a conceptual framework for nursing education, practice, and research. It has generated many questions for research and continues to be used as a basis for the development of curricula. Practitioners and patients have judged the resulting nursing actions to be satisfactory.[15:215] The theory has potential for continued utility in nursing in order to achieve valued nursing goals.

REFERENCES

1. Chin, R. (1961). The utility of system models and developmental models for practitioners. In K. Benne, et al. (Eds.), *The planning for change.* New York: Holt, Rinehart & Winston.
2. Chinn, P.L., & Jacobs, M.K. (1983). *Theory and nursing: A systematic approach.* St. Louis: C.V. Mosby.
3. Damus, K. (1980). An application of the Johnson behavioral system model for nursing practice. In J.P. Riehl, & C. Roy (Eds.), *Conceptual models for nursing practice* (2nd ed.). New York: Appleton-Century-Crofts.
4. Feshback, S. (1970). Aggression. In P. Mussen (Ed.), *Carmichael's manual of child psychology* (3rd ed.). New York: John Wiley & Sons.
5. Grubbs, J. (1980). An interpretation of the Johnson behavioral system model for nursing practice. In J.P. Riehl, & C. Roy (Eds.), *Conceptual models for nursing practice* (2nd ed.). New York: Appleton-Century-Crofts.
6. Holaday, B. (1980). Implementing the Johnson model for nursing practice. In J.P. Riehl, & C. Roy (Eds.), *Conceptual models for nursing practice* (2nd ed.). New York: Appleton-Century-Crofts.
7. Johnson, D.E. (1954). Collegiate nursing education. *Coll. Publ. Rel. Quarterly, 5:*32-35.
8. Johnson, D.E. (1959, April). A philosophy of nursing. *Nursing Outlook, 7:*198-200.
9. Johnson, D.E. (1959, May). The nature of a science of nursing. *Nursing Outlook, 7:*291-294.
10. Johnson, D.E. (1961, Nov.). The significance of nursing care. *American Journal of Nursing, 61:*63-66.
11. Johnson, D.E. (1964, Dec.). Nursing and higher education. *International Journal of Nursing Studies, 1:*219-225.
12. Johnson, D.E. (1968, May-June). Theory in nursing: Borrowed and unique. Nursing Research, 17:206-209.
13. Johnson, D.E. (1974, Sept.-Oct.). Development of theory: A requisite for nursing as a primary health profession. *Nursing Research, 23:*372-377.
14. Johnson, D.E. (1978). State of the art of theory development in nursing. In *Theory development: What, why, how?* New York: National League for Nursing. NLN publication 15-1708.
15. Johnson, D.E. (1980). The behavioral system model for nursing. In J.P. Riehl, & C. Roy (Eds.), *Conceptual models for nursing practice* (2nd ed.). New York: Appleton-Century-Crofts.
16. Johnson, D.E. (1984). Personal correspondence.
17. Johnson, D.E. (1984). Curriculum vitae.
18. Lorenz, K. (1966). *On aggression.* New York: Harcourt.
19. Loveland-Cherry, C., & Wilkerson, S. (1983). Dorothy Johnson's behavioral systems model. In J. Fitzpatrick, & A. Whall (Eds.), *Conceptual models of nursing: Analysis and application.* Bowie, Md.: Robert J. Brady.
20. Majesky, S.J., Brester, M.H., & Nishio, K.T. (1978). Development of a research tool: Patient indicators of nursing care. *Nursing Research, 27*(6):365-371.
21. Rawls, A. (1980). Evaluation of the Johnson behavioral model in clinical practice: Report of a test and evaluation of the Johnson theory. *Image, 12:*13-16.
22. Rapoport, A. (1968, Feb.). *Foreward to modern systems research for the behavioral scientist.* Chicago: Aldine.
23. Small, B. (1980). Nursing visually impaired children with Johnson's model as a conceptual framework. In J.P. Riehl, and C. Roy (Eds.). *Conceptual models for nursing practice* (2nd ed). New York: Appleton-Century-Crofts.
24. Stamler, C. (1971). Dependency and repetitive visits to nurses' office in elementary school children. *Nursing Research, 20*(3):254-255.

BIBLIOGRAPHY
Primary Sources
Book Chapters

Johnson, D.E. (1964 June 19-26). Is there an identifiable body of knowledge essential to the development of a generic professional nursing program? In M. Maker (Ed.), *Proceedings of the first inter-*

university faculty work conference. Stowe, Vt.: New England Board of Higher Education.

Johnson, D.E. (1973). Medical-surgical nursing: Cardiovascular care in the first person. *In ANA Clin Sess:* New York: Appleton-Century-Crofts. 127-134.

Johnson, D.E. (1976). Foreword. In J.R. Auger, *Behavioral systems and nursing.* Englewood Cliffs, N.J.: Prentice-Hall.

Johnson, D.E. (1980). The behavioral system model for nursing. In J.P. Riehl, & C. Roy (Eds.). *Conceptual models for nursing practice* (2nd ed.). New York: Appleton-Century-Crofts.

Johnson, D.E., et al. (1978). State of the art of theory development in nursing. In *Theory development: What, why, how?* New York, National League for Nursing. NLN publication 15-1708.

Articles

Johnson, D.E. (1943, March). Learning to know people. *American Journal of Nursing, 43:*248-252.

Johnson, D.E. (1954). Collegiate nursing education. *Coll. Publ. Rel. Quarterly, 5:*32-35.

Johnson, D.E. (1959, April). A philosophy of nursing. *Nursing Outlook, 7:*198-200.

Johnson, D.E. (1959, May). The nature of a science of nursing. *Nursing Outlook, 7:*291-294.

Johnson, D.E. (1961, Oct.). Patterns in professional nursing education. *Nursing Outlook, 9:*608-611.

Johnson, D.E. (1961, Nov.). The significance of nursing care. *American Journal of Nursing, 61:*63-66.

Johnson, D.E. (1962, July-Aug.). Professional education for pediatric nursing. *Children, 9:*153-156.

Johnson, D.E. (1964, Dec.). Nursing and higher education. *International Journal of Nursing Studies, 1:*219-225.

Johnson, D.E. (1965, Sept.). Today's action will determine tomorrow's nursing. *Nursing Outlook, 13:*38-41.

Johnson, D.E. (1965, Oct.). Crying in the newborn infant. *Nursing Science, 3:*339-355.

Johnson, D.E. (1966, Jan. 16). Year round programs set the pace in health careers promotion. *Hospitals, 40:*57-60.

Johnson, D.E. (1966, Oct.). Competence in practice: Technical and professional. *Nursing Outlook, 14:*30-33.

Johnson, D.E. (1967, April). Powerlessness: A significant determinant in patient behavior? *Journal of Nursing Educators, 6:*39-44.

Johnson, D.E. (1967). Professional practice in nursing. *NLN Convention Papers, 23:*26-33.

Johnson, D.E. (1968, April). Toward a science in nursing. *So. Medical Bulletin, 56:* 13-23.

Johnson, D.E. (1968, May-June). Theory in nursing: Borrowed and unique. *Nursing Research, 17:*206-209.

Johnson, D.E. (1968). Critique: Social influences on student nurses in their choice of ideal and practiced solutions to nursing problems. *Communicating Nursing Research, 1:*150-155.

Johnson, D.E. (1974, Sept. & Oct.). Development of theory: A requisite for nursing as a primary health profession. *Nursing Research, 23:*372-377.

Johnson, D.E., Wilcox, J.A., & Moidel, H.C. (1967, Nov.). The clinical specialist as a practitioner. *American Journal of Nursing, 67:*2298-2303.

Johnson, D.E., & McCaffery, M. (1967, Fall). Effect of parent group discussion upon epistemic responses. *Nursing Research, 16:*352-358.

Audiotape

Johnson, D.E. (1978, Dec.). Paper presented at the Second Annual Nurse Educator Conference, New York. Audiotape available from Teach 'em Inc., 160 E. Illinois Street, Chicago, Ill. 60611.

Unpublished Lecture

Johnson, D.E. (1968). *One conceptual model of nursing.* Lecture given at Vanderbilt University.

Correspondence

Johnson, D.E. (1984, Feb.). Curriculum vitae.

Johnson, D.E. (1984, Feb.). Personal correspondence.

Secondary Sources
Books

Auger, J.R. (1976). *Behavioral systems and nursing.* Englewood Cliffs, N.J.: Prentice-Hall.

Chinn, P.L. (1983). *Advances in nursing theory development.* Rockville, Md.: Aspen Systems.

Chinn, P.L., & Jacobs, M.K. (1983). *Theory and nursing: A systematic approach.* St. Louis: C.V. Mosby.

Feshbach, S. (1970). Aggression. In P. Mussen (Ed.), *Carmichael's manual of child psychology* (3rd ed.). New York: John Wiley & Sons.

Fitzpatrick, J.J., & Whall, A.L. (1983). *Conceptual models of nursing: Analysis and application.* Bowie, Md.: Robert J. Brady.

Fitzpatrick, J.J., et al. (1982). *Nursing models and their psychiatric mental health applications.* Bowie, Md.: Robert J. Brady.

Infante, M.S. (1982). *Crisis theory: A framework for nursing practice.* Reston, Va.: Reston Publishing.

Kim, H.S. (1983). *The nature of theoretical thinking in nursing.* Norwalk, Conn.: Appleton-Century-Crofts.

Riehl, J.P., & Roy, C. (1980). *Conceptual models for nursing practice.* New York: Appleton-Century-Crofts.

Walker, L.O., & Avant, K.C. (1983). *Strategies for theory construction in nursing.* Norwalk, Conn.: Appleton-Century-Crofts.

Dissertation

Lovejoy, N.C. (1981). *An empirical verification of the Johnson behavioral system model for nursing.* Doctoral dissertation. University of Alabama in Birmingham.

Book Chapters

Damus, K. (1974). An application of the Johnson behavioral system model for nursing practice. In J.P. Riehl, & C. Roy (Eds.), *Conceptual models for nursing practice.* New York: Appleton-Century-Crofts. pp. 218-233.

Damus, K. (1980). An application of the Johnson behavioral system model for nursing practice. In J.P. Riehl, & C. Roy (Eds.), *Conceptual models for nursing practice* (2nd ed.). New York: Appleton-Century-Crofts. pp. 274-289.

Fawcett, J. (1984). Johnson's behavioral systems model. In J. Fawcett, *Analysis and evaluation of conceptual models of nursing.* Philadelphia: F.A. Davis. pp. 53-84.

Glennin, C.G. (1980). Formulation of standards of nursing practice using a nursing model. In J.P. Riehl, & C. Roy (Eds.), *Conceptual models for nursing practice* (2nd ed.). New York: Appleton-Century-Crofts. pp. 290-301.

Grubbs, J. (1974). An interpretation of the Johnson behavioral systems model for nursing practice. In J.P. Riehl, & C. Roy (Eds.), *Conceptual models for nursing practice.* New York: Appleton-Century-Crofts. pp. 160-194.

Grubbs, J. (1980). An interpretation of the Johnson behavioral system model for nursing practice. In J.P. Riehl, & C. Roy (Eds.), *Conceptual models for nursing practice* (2nd ed.). New York: Appleton-Century-Crofts. pp. 217-249.

Holaday, B. (1974). Implementing the Johnson model for nursing practice. In J.P. Riehl, & C. Roy (Eds.), *Conceptual models for nursing practice* (2nd ed.). New York: Appleton-Century-Crofts. pp. 197-206.

Holaday, B. (1980). Implementing the Johnson model for nursing practice. In J.P. Riehl, & C. Roy (Eds.), *Conceptual models for nursing practice* (2nd ed.). New York: Appleton-Century-Crofts. pp. 255-263.

Loveland-Cherry, C., & Wilkerson, S.A. (1983). Dorothy Johnson's behavioral systems model. In J.P. Fitzpatrick, & A.L. Whall (Eds.), *Conceptual models of nursing: Analysis and application.* Bowie, Md.: Robert J. Brady. pp. 117-135.

Meleis, A.I. (1985). Dorothy Johnson. In A.I. Meleis, *Theoretical nursing: Development and progress.* Philadelphia: J.B. Lippincott. pp. 195-205.

Riehl, J.P., & Roy, C. (1980). Appendix-Nursing assessment tool using Johnson model. In J.P. Riehl, & C. Roy (Eds.), *Conceptual models for nursing practice* (2nd ed.). New York: Appleton-Century-Crofts. pp. 250-254.

Skolny, M.S., & Riehl, J.P. (1974). Hope: Solving patient and family problems by using a theoretical framework. In J.P. Riehl, & C. Roy (Eds.), *Conceptual models for nursing practice.* New York: Appleton-Century-Crofts. pp. 206-218.

Small, B. (1980). Nursing visually impaired children with Johnson's model as a conceptual framework. In J.P. Riehl, & C. Roy (Eds.), *Conceptual models for nursing practice* (2nd ed.). New York: Appleton-Century-Crofts. pp. 264-273.

Steven, B.J. (1979). Criteria for evaluating theories. In B.J. Stevens, *Nursing theory: Analysis, application, evaluation.* Boston: Little, Brown. pp. 49-67.

Directional and Biographical Soruces

Henderson, J. (1957-1959). *Nursing studies index* (Vol. IV). Philadelphia: J.B. Lippincott.

Articles

Abdellah, F.G. (1969). Dept. HEW-Health administration center of health services research and development health services. *Nursing Research, 18*(5):390-393.

Adam, E. (1983). Frontiers of nursing in the 21st century: Development of models and theories on the concept of nursing. *Journal of Advanced Nursing, 8:*41-45.

Ainsworth, M. (1964). Patterns of attachment behavior shown by the infant in interaction with mother. *Merrill Palmer Quarterly, 10*(1):51-58.

Arndt, C. (1970). Role sharing in diversified role set director of nursing service. *Nursing Research, 19*(3):253-259.

Bates, B. (1970). Doctor and nurse, changing nurse, and relations. *New England Journal of Medicine, 283:*129-130.

Brandt, E.M. (1967). Comparison of on job performance of graduates with school of nursing objectives. *Nursing Research, 16*(1):50-60.

Brester, M.H., Majesky, S.J., & Nishio, K.T. (1978, Nov.-Dec.). Development of a research tool: Patient indicators of nursing care. *Nursing Research, 27:*365-371.

Broncatello, K.F. (1980). Anger in action: Application of the model. *Advances in Nursing Science, 2*(2):13-24.

Bullough, B. (1976). Influences on role expansion. *American Journal of Nursing, 76*(9):1476-1481.

Chance, K.S. (1982). Nursing models: A requisite for professional accountability. *Advances in Nursing Science, 4*(2):57-65.

Conway, B. (1971). Effects of hospitalization on adolescence. *Adolescence, 6*(21):77-92.

Crawford, G. (1982). The concept of pattern in nursing conceptual development and measurement. *Advances in Nursing Science, 5*(1):1-6.

Craig, S.L. (1980). Theory development and its relevance for nursing. *Journal of Advanced Nursing, 5*(4):349-355.

Darnell, R.E. (1973). Promotion of interest in role of physician association as a potential career opportunity for nurses alternative strategy. *Social Science and Medicine, 7*(7):495.

Dee, U., & Auger, J.A. (1983, May). A patient classification system based on behavioral system model of nursing. Part 2. *Journal of Nursing Administration, 13:*18-23.

Derdiarian, A.K. (1983, July-Aug.). An instrument for theory and research development using the behavioral systems model for nursing: The cancer patient. Part I. *Nursing Research, 32:*196-201.

Derdiarian, A.K., & Forsythe, A.B. (1983, Sept.-Oct.). An instrument for theory and research development using the behavioral systems model for nursing: The cancer patient. Part II. *Nursing Research, 32:*260-266.

Evans, R.T. (1969). Exploration of factors involved in maternal adaption to breastfeeding. *Nursing Research, 18*(1):28-33.

Flint, R.T. (1969). Recent issues in nursing manpower review. *Nursing Research, 18*(3):217-222.

Fritz, E. (1966). Baccalaureate nursing education: What is its job? *American Journal of Nursing, 66*(6):1312-1316.

Georgopo, B.S. (1970). Nursing kardex behavior in an experimental study of patient units with and without clinical nurse specialists. *Nursing Research, 19*(3):196-218.

Godley, S.T. (1976). Community based orientation and mobility programs. *Nursing Outlook, 70*(10):429-432.

Gortner, S.R. (1977). Overview of nursing research in United States. *Nursing Research, 26*(1):16-23.

Gray, S.E. (1977). Do graduates of technical and professional nursing programs differ in practice? *Nursing Research, 26*(5):368-373.

Greaves, F. (1980). Objectively toward curriculum improvement in nursing education in England and Wales. *Journal of Advanced Nursing, 5:*591-599.

Hadley B.J. (1969). Evolution of a conception of nursing. *Nursing Research, 18*(5):400-405.

Hall, B.P. (1981). The change paradigm in nursing: Growth versus persistence. *Advances in Nursing Science, 3*(4):1-6.

Hogstel, M.O. (1977). Associate degree and baccalaureate graduates: Do they function differently. *American Journal of Nursing, 77*(10):1598-1600.

Holaday, B. (1974). Achievement behavior in chronically ill children. *Nursing Research, 23:*25-30.

Holaday, B. (1981). Maternal response to their chronically ill infants' attachment behavior of crying. *Nursing Research, 30:*343-348.

Holaday, B. (1982). Maternal conceptual set development: Identifying patterns of maternal response to chronically ill infant crying. *Maternal-Child Nursing Journal, 11*(1):47-58.

Iveson-Iveson, J. (1982). Standards of behavior . . . theories of nursing practice . . . the Johnson model. *Nursing Mirror, 155*(20):38.

Ketefian, S. (1981). Critical thinking: Educational preparation and development of moral judgment among selected groups of practicing nurses. *Nursing Research, 30*(2):98-103.

Kohnk, M.F. (1973). Do nursing educators practice what is preached? *American Journal of Nursing, 73*(9):1571.

Lovejoy, N. (1983). The leukemic child's perceptions of family behaviors. *Oncology Nursing Forum, 10*(4):20-25.

Majesky, S.J. (1978). Development of a research

tool: Patient indicators of nursing care. *Nursing Research, 27*(6):365-371.

Mauksch, I.G. (1972). Prescription for survival. *American Journal of Nursing, 72*(12):2189-2193.

McCain, R.F. (1965, April). Systematic investigation of medical-surgical nursing content. *Journal of Nursing Education, 4*:23-31.

McFarlane, E.A. (1980). Nursing theory: Comparison of four theoretical proposals. *Journal of Advanced Nursing, 5*:3-19.

McQuaid, E.A. (1979). How do graduates of different types of programs perform on state boards? *American Journal of Nursing, 79*(2):305-308.

Rawls, A.C. (1980, Feb.). Evaluation of the Johnson behavioral model in clinical practice. *Image, 12*: 13-16.

Rickelma, B.L. (1971). Bio-psych-social linguistics conceptual approach to nurse-patient interaction. *Nursing Research, 20*(5):398-403.

Rogers, C.G. (1973). Conceptual models as guides to clinical nursing specialization. *Journal of Nursing Education, 12*(4):2-6.

Rogers, J.C. (1982, Jan.). Order and disorder in medicine and occupational therapy. *American Journal of Occupational Therapy, 36*:29-35.

Scher, M.E. (1975). Stereotyping and role conflicts between medical students and psychiatric nurses. *Hospital and Community Psychiatry, 26*(4): 219-221.

Secrest, H.P. (1968). Nurses and collaborative peritonatal research project. *Nursing Research, 17*:292.

Smith, M.C. (1974). Perceptions of head nurses, clinical nurse specialists, nursing educators and nursing office personnel re: performance of selected nursing activities. *Nursing Research, 23*(6):505-510.

Smith, M.C. (1976). Patient responses to being transferred during hospitalization. *Nursing Research, 25*(3):192-196.

Smithern, C. (1969). Vocal behavior of infants as related to nursing procedures of rocking. *Nursing Research, 18*(3):256-258.

Stamler, C. (1971). Dependency and repetitive visits to nurses' offices in elementary school children. *Nursing Research, 20*(3):254-255.

Stevens, B.J. (1971). Analysis of structural forms used in nursing curricula. *Nursing Research, 20*(5):388-397.

Taylor, S.D. (1975). Bibliography on nursing research 1950-1975. *Nursing Research, 24*(3): 207-225.

Vaillot, M.C. (1970). Hope; restoration of being. *American Journal of Nursing, 10*(2):268.

Waltz, C.F. (1978). Faculty influence on nursing students' preference in practice. *Nursing Research, 27*(2):89-97.

Waters, V.H. (1972). Nursing practice: Implemental and supplemental. *Nursing Research, 21*(2): 124-131.

White, M.B. (1972). Importance of selected nursing activities. *Nursing Research, 21*(1):4-14.

Zbilut, J.P. (1978). Epistemologic constraints to development of a theory of nursing. *Nursing Research, 27*(2):128-129.

Other Sources

Ainsworth, M. (1964). Patterns of attachment behavior shown by the infant in interaction with mother. *Merrill-Palmer Quarterly, 10*(1):51-58.

Ainsworth, M. (1972). Attachment and dependency: A comparison. In J. Gewirtz (Ed.), *Attachment and dependency.* Englewood Cliffs, N.J.: Prentice-Hall.

Atkinson, J.W. (1966). *Feather NT: A theory of achievement maturation.* New York: John Wiley & Sons.

Buckley, W. (Ed.) (1968). *Modern systems research for the behavioral scientist.* Chicago: Aldine.

Chin, R. (1961). The utility of system models and developmental models for practitioners. In K. Benne, W. Bennis, & R. Chin (Eds.), *The planning of change.* New York: Holt, Rinehart, & Winston.

Crandal, V. (1963). Achievement. In H.W. Stevenson (Ed.), *Child psychology.* Chicago: University of Chicago Press.

Feshbach, S. (1970). Aggression. In P. Mussen (Ed.), *Carmichael's manual of child psychology* (3rd ed. Vol. 2). New York: John Wiley & Sons.

Gerwitz, J. (Ed.). (1972). *Attachment and dependency,* Englewood Cliffs, N.J.: Prentice-Hall.

Grinker, R.R. (Ed.). (1956). *Toward a unified theory of human behavior.* New York: Basic Books.

Heathers, G. (1955). Acquiring dependence and independence: A theoretical orientation. *Journal of General Psychology, 87*:277-291.

Kagan, J. (1964). Acquisition and significance of sex typing and sex role identity. In Hoffman M.L., & Hoffman L.W., (Eds.), *Review of child development research.* New York: Russell Sage Foundation.

Leitch, M., & Escalona, E. (1949). The reaction of infants to stress. In *Psychoanalytic study of the child*

(Vols. 3-4). New York: International Universities Press.

Lorenz, K. (1966). *On aggression*. New York: Harcourt.

Mead, M. (1953). *Cultural patterns and technical change*. World Federation for Mental Health, UNESCO.

Rapoport, A. (1968). Foreword. In W. Buckley (Ed.), *Modern systems research for the behavioral scientist*. Chicago: Aldine.

Resnik, H.L.P. (1972). *Sexual behaviors*. Boston: Little, Brown.

Robson, K.S. (1967). *Patterns and determinants of maternal attachment. Journal of Pediatrics 77:* 976-985.

Rosenthal, M. (1967). The generalization of dependency from mother to a stranger. *Journal of Child Psychology and Psychiatry, 8:*177-183.

Sears, R., Maccoby, E., & Levin, H. (1954). *Patterns of child rearing*. White Plains, N.Y.: Row, Peterson.

Selye, H. (1956). *The stress of life*. New York: McGraw-Hill.

Simmons, L.W., & Wolff, H.G. (1954). *Social science in medicine*. New York: Russell Sage Foundation.

Walike, B., Jordan, H.A., & Stellar, E. (1969). Studies of eating behavior. *Nursing Research, 18:* 108-113.

Sister Callista Roy

25

Adaptation Model

Carolyn L. Blue, Karen M. Brubaker, Katherine R. Papazian,
Cynthia M. Riester

CREDENTIALS AND BACKGROUND OF THE THEORIST

Sister Callista Roy, a member of the Sisters of Saint Joseph of Carondelet, was born October 14, 1939, in Los Angeles, California. She received a Bachelor of Arts in Nursing in 1963 from Mount Saint Mary's College in Los Angeles and a Master of Science in Nursing from the University of California at Los Angeles in

1966. After earning her nursing degrees, Roy began her education in sociology, receiving a Ph.D. in Sociology from the University of California in 1977.

While working toward her master's degree, Roy was challenged in a seminar with Dorothy E. Johnson to develop a conceptual model for nursing. Roy had worked as a pediatric staff nurse and had noticed the great resiliency of children and their ability to adapt in response to major physical and psychological changes. The adaptation concept impressed Roy as an appropriate conceptual framework for nursing. The basic concepts of the model were devel-

The authors wish to express their appreciation to Sister Callista Roy for critiquing the chapter.

oped while Roy was a graduate student at UCLA from 1964 to 1966.

Roy began operationalizing her model in 1968 when Mount Saint Mary's College adopted the adaptation framework as the philosophical foundation of the nursing curriculum. Roy was an associate professor and chairperson of the Department of Nursing at Mount Saint Mary's College until 1982. From 1983 to 1985, she was a Robert Wood Johnson Post Doctoral Fellow at the University of California in San Franciso as a clinical nurse scholar in neuroscience.

Roy has published many books, chapters, and periodical articles and has presented numerous lectures and workshops focusing on her nursing adaptation theory. She is a member of Sigma Theta Tau, having received the National Founder's Award for Excellence in Fostering Professional Nursing Standards in 1981. Roy has been recognized in the *World Who's Who of Women, Personalities of Americas,* and as a Fellow of American Academy of Nursing. Most recently, she was awarded an Honorary Doctorate of Humane Letters by Alverno College.

THEORETICAL SOURCES

Roy's Adaptation Model for Nursing was derived in 1964 from Harry Helson's work in psychophysics. In Helson's Adaptation Theory, adaptive responses are a function of the incoming stimulus and the adaptive level. The adaptation level is made up of the pooled effect of three classes of stimuli: (1) focal stimuli, which immediately confront the individual; (2) contextual stimuli, which are all other stimuli present; and (3) residual stimuli, those factors that are relevant but that cannot be validated. Helson's work developed the concept of the adaptation level zone, which determines whether a stimuli will elicit a positive or negative response. According to Helson's theory, adaptation is a process of responding positively to environmental changes.[26]

Roy[26] combines Helson's work with Rapoport's definition of a system and views the person as an adaptive system. With Helson's Adaptation Theory as a foundation, Roy[26] developed and further refined the model using concepts and theory from B.P. Dohrenwend, M.J. Driever, R.S. Lazarus, N. Malaznik, D. Mechanic, M. Pousch and J. Van Landingham, B. Randell, and H. Selye. In the years following the development of her theory, Roy developed the model as a framework for nursing practice, research, and education.[30] According to Roy,[15] more than 1500 faculty and students have contributed to the theoretical development of the Adaptation Model.

In *Introduction to Nursing: An Adaptation Model* Roy addressed self-concept. She and her collaborators used the work of A. Coombs and D. Snygg regarding self-consistency and major influencing factors of self-concept. Social interaction theories provided a theoretical basis. Cooley indicates in Epstein's publication that self-perception is influenced by one's perceptions of other's responses. Mead expanded the idea by hypothesizing that self-appraisal uses the "generalized other." Sullivan suggests that self arises from social interaction. Gardner and Erickson provide developmental approaches.* The other modes—physiological, role functioning, and interdependence—were drawn similarly from biological and behavioral sciences for an understanding of the person.

Roy is developing the humanism value base of her model. The model uses concepts from A.H. Maslow to explore beliefs and values of persons. According to Roy, humanism in nursing is the belief in the person's own creative power or the belief that the person's own coping abilities will enhance wellness. Roy's holistic approach[23] to nursing is grounded in humanism.

USE OF EMPIRICAL EVIDENCE

The use of Roy's Adaptation Model in nursing practice led to further clarification and refine-

*References 23:263-265.

ment. A 1971 pilot research study and a survey research study from 1976 to 1977 led to some tentative confirmations of the model.[22]

From this beginning, the adaptation model has been supported through research in practice and in education.* B. Rambo[10] and B. Randell[11] have expanded Roy's model for nursing implementation. According to Roy[23] there is increasing testing through research related to the model.

Fitzpatrick and Whall[5] categorize Roy's underlying assumptions according to foundations in previous research. Available empirical data indicate Roy's general theory base has substance. However, Roy's assumption, which conceptualizes the person as having four modes of adaptation—physiological needs, self-concept, role function, and interdependence relations, is based on experience of Roy and others.[5] Roy[14,20,22] admits the assumption needs empirical data for support. In a 1983 address, she noted that these categories have been refined and established as useful and valid for nursing assessment.

MAJOR CONCEPTS AND DEFINITIONS

SYSTEM. A system is "a set of units so related or connected as to form a unity or whole and characterized by inputs, outputs, and control and feedback processes."[23:27]

ADAPTATION LEVEL. A person's adaptation level is "a constantly changing point, made up of focal, contextual, and residual stimuli, which represent the person's own standard of the range of stimuli to which one can respond with ordinary adaptive responses."[23:27-28]

ADAPTATION PROBLEMS. Adaptation problems are "the occurrences of situations of inadequate response to need deficits or excesses."[19:4] In the second edition of *Introduction to Nursing,*

Roy goes on to say "It can be noted at this point that the distinction being made between adaptation problems and nursing diagnosis is based on the developing work in both of these fields. At this point, adaptation problems are seen not as nursing diagnosis, but as areas of concern for the nurse related to adapting person or group (within each adaptive mode)."[23:89-90]

FOCAL STIMULUS. A focal stimulus is "the degree of change or stimulus most immediately confronting the person and the one to which the person must make an adaptive response, that is, the factor that precipitates the behavior."[23:43]

CONTEXTUAL STIMULI. Contextual stimuli are "all other stimuli present that contribute to the behavior caused or precipitated by the focal stimuli."[23:43]

RESIDUAL STIMULI. Residual stimuli are "factors that may be affecting behavior but whose effects are not validated."[23:43]

REGULATOR. A regulator is a "subsystem coping mechanism which responds automatically through neural-chemical-endocrine processes."[23:28]

COGNATOR. A cognator is a "subsystem coping mechanism which responds through complex processes of perception and information processing, learning, judgment, and emotion."[23:28]

ADAPTIVE (EFFECTOR) MODES. Adaptive, or effector, modes are a "classification of ways of coping that manifest regulator and cognator activity, that is, physiologic, self-concept, role function, and interdependence."[23:28]

ADAPTIVE RESPONSES. Adaptive responses are "responses that promote integrity of the person in terms of the goals of survival, growth, reproduction, and mastery."[23:28]

---

*References 1, 4, 8, 9, 25, 29.

300

INEFFECTIVE RESPONSES. Ineffective responses are "responses that do not contribute to adaptive goals, that is, survival, growth, reproduction, and mastery."[23:28]

PHYSIOLOGICAL MODE. "Physiological needs involve the body's basic needs and ways of dealing with adaptation in regard to fluid and electrolytes; exercise and rest; elimination; nutrition; circulation and oxygen; and regulation, which includes the senses, temperature, and endocrine regulation."[26:43]

SELF-CONCEPT MODE "Self-concept is the composite of beliefs and feelings that one holds about oneself at a given time. It is formed from perceptions, particularly of other's reactions, and directs one's behavior. Its components include: (1) the physical self, which involves sensation and body image; and (2) the personal self, which is made up of self-consistency, self-ideal or expectancy, and the moral, ethical self (Driever, 1976)."[26:43-44]

ROLE PERFORMANCE MODE "Role function is the performance of duties based on given positions in society. The way one performs a role is dependent on one's interaction with the other in the given situation. The major roles that one plays can be analyzed by imagining a tree formation. The trunk of the tree is one's primary role, that is, one's developmental level—for example, generative adult female. Secondary roles branch off from this—for example, wife, mother, and teacher. Finally, tertiary roles branch off from secondary roles—for example, the mother role might involve the role of P.T.A. president for a given period of time (Malaznik 1976). Each of these roles is seen as occurring in a dyadic relationship, that is, with a reciprocal role."[26:44]

INTERDEPENDENCE MODE. "The interdependence mode involves one's relations with significant others and support systems. In this mode one maintains psychic integrity by meeting needs for nurturance and affection (Poush and Van Landingham, 1977)."[26:44]

MAJOR ASSUMPTIONS

Roy has discussed her scientific and philosophical assumptions at the International Nursing Theory Conferences in Edmonton, Alberta, May 2-3, 1984, and at other conferences. She outlines scientific assumptions from systems theory and Helson's Adaptation Level Theory and philosophical assumptions from humanistic values.

Assumptions from Systems Theory:

1. A system is a set of units so related or connected as to form a unity or whole.
2. A system is a whole that functions as a whole by virtue of the interdependence of its parts.
3. Systems have inputs, outputs, and control and feedback processes.
4. Input, in the form of a standard or feedback, often is referred to as information.
5. Living systems are more complex than mechanical systems and have standards and feedback to direct their functioning as a whole.

Assumptions from Helson's Theory:

1. Human behavior represents adaptation to environmental and organismic forces.
2. Adaptive behavior is a function of the stimulus and adaptation level, that is, the pooled effect of the focal, contextual, and residual stimuli.
3. Adaptation is a process of responding positively to environmental changes. This positive response decreases the response necessary to cope with the stimuli and increases sensitivity to respond to other stimuli.
4. Responses reflect the state of the organism as well as the properties of stimuli and hence are regarded as active processes.

Assumptions from Humanism:

1. Persons have their own creative power.
2. A person's behavior is purposeful and not merely a chain of cause and effect.
3. Person is holistic.
4. A person's opinions and viewpoints are of value.
5. The interpersonal relationship is significant.

Nursing

Nursing is defined broadly as a "theoretical system of knowledge which prescribes a process of analysis and action related to the care of the ill or potentially ill person."[19:4] Roy[23:3-4] differentiates nursing as a science from nursing as a practice discipline. Nursing science is "a developing system of knowledge about persons that observes, classifies, and relates the processes by which persons positively affect their health status."[23:3-4] Nursing as a practice discipline is "nursing's scientific body of knowledge used for the purpose of providing an essential service to people, that is, promoting ability to affect health positively."[23:3-4]

Roy's goal[23] of nursing is to help man adapt to changes in his physiological needs, his self-concept, his role function, and his interdependence relations during health and illness. Nursing fills a unique role as a facilitator of adaptation by assessing behavior in each of these four adaptive modes and intervening by managing the influencing stimuli.[23]

Roy[23] uses the nursing process—assessment, making the nursing diagnosis, goal setting, intervention, and evaluation—to facilitate the adaptation of the person.

Person

According to Roy,[19:7] a person is a "biopsychosocial being in constant interaction with a changing environment." Roy[23,24] defined the person, the recipient of nursing care, as a living, complex, adaptive system with internal processes (the cognator and regulator) acting to maintain adaptation in the four adaptive modes (physiological needs, self-concept, role function, and interdependence). The person as a living system is "a whole made up of parts or subsystems that function as a unity for some purpose."[24:53]

Health

Health is "a state and a process of being and becoming integrated and whole."[23:22] Roy[23:24] derived this definition from the thought that adaptation is a process of promoting physiological, psychological, and social integrity, and that integrity implies an unimpaired condition leading to completeness or unity. In her earlier work, Roy viewed health along a continuum flowing from death and extreme poor health to high-level wellness and peak wellness. As man moves along the health-illness continuum, he will encounter problems to which he must adapt.[1] However, Roy's more recent writings have focused more on health as a process.

Health and illness are one inevitable dimension of the person's total life experience.[13] Nursing is concerned with this dimension. When mechanisms for coping are ineffective, illness results. Health ensues when man continually adapts. As people adapt to stimuli, they are free to respond to other stimuli. The freeing of energy from ineffective coping attempts can promote healing and enhance health.[23:26]

Environment

According to Roy,[23:22] environment is "all the conditions, circumstances, and influences surrounding and affecting the development and behavior of persons or groups." Environment is the input into the person as an adaptive system involving both internal and external factors. These factors may be slight or large, negative or positive. However, any environmental change demands increasing energy to adapt to the situation. Factors in the environment that affect the person are categorized as focal, contextual, and residual stimuli.

THEORETICAL ASSERTIONS

Roy's model focuses on the concept of adaptation of man. Her concept of nursing, person, health, and environment are all interrelated to this central concept. The person continually scans the environment for stimuli so he can respond and ultimately adapt. Nursing has a unique goal to assist the person in his adaptation effort by managing the environment. The result is attainment of an optimum level of wellness by the person.*

As an open, living system, the person receives inputs or stimuli from both the environment and the self. The adaptation level is determined by the combined effect of the focal, contextual, and residual stimuli. Adaptation occurs when the person responds positively to environmental changes. This adaptive response promotes the integrity of the person, which leads to health. Ineffective responses to stimuli leads to disruption of the integrity of the person.†

There are two interrelated subsystems in Roy's model (Figure 25-1). The primary, functional, or control processes subsystem consists of the regulator and the cognator. The secondary, effector subsystem consists of four adaptive

modes: physiological needs, self-concept, role-function, and interdependence.*

Roy views the regulator and cognator as methods of coping. Perception of the person links the regulator with the cognator in that "input into the regulator is transformed into perceptions. Perception is a process of the cognator. The responses following perception are feedback into both the cognator and the regulator."[6:67]

The four adaptive modes of the second subsystem in Roy's model provide form or manifestations of cognator and regulator activity. Responses to stimuli are carried out through these four modes. The mode's purpose is to achieve physiological, psychological, and social integrity. Interrelated propositions of the cognator and regulator subsystems link the systems of the adaptive modes.[4]

Man as a whole is made up of six subsystems. These subsystems—the regulator, cognator, and the four adaptive modes—are interrelated to form a complex system for the purpose of the adaptation of man. Relationships between the four adaptive modes occur when internal and external stimuli affect more than one mode; when disruptive behavior occurs in more

---

*References 11, 14, 15, 22, 23, 24, 26.
†References 11, 14, 15, 22, 23, 24.

*References 11, 14, 15, 22, 23, 24.

Figure 25-1. Person as an adaptive system.

From Sister Callista Roy (1984), *Introduction to Nursing: An Adaptation Model* (2nd ed.). p. 30. Reprinted by permission of Prentice-Hall, Inc., Englewood Cliffs, N.J.

than one mode; or when one mode becomes the focal, contextual, or residual stimulus for another mode.[1,2,8]

LOGICAL FORM

Roy's Adaptation Model for Nursing is both deductive and inductive. It is deductive in that much of Roy's theory is derived from Helson's psychophysics theory. Helson developed the concepts of focal, contextual, and residual stimuli, which Roy redefined within nursing to form a typology of factors related to adaptation levels of persons. Roy also uses other concepts and theory outside the discipline of nursing and relates these to her adaptation theory.

Roy's adaptation theory is inductive in that she developed the four adaptive modes from research and the practice experiences of herself, her colleagues, and her students. Roy[19,22,23] built on the conceptual framework of adaptation and as a result developed a step-by-step model by which nurses use the nursing process to administer nursing care to promote adaptation in situations of health and illness.

ACCEPTANCE BY THE NURSING COMMUNITY
Practice

H.T.F. Brower and B.J. Baker[1] consider Roy's model useful for nursing practice because it outlines the features of the discipline and provides direction for practice as well as for education and research. The model considers goals, values, the client, and practitioner interventions.

It is a valuable theory for nursing practice because it includes a goal that is specified as the aim for activity and prescriptions for activities to realize the goal.[3] The goal of the model is the person's adaptation in four adaptive modes in situations of health and illness. The prescriptions or interventions are the management of stimuli by removing, increasing, decreasing, or altering them. These prescriptions can be obtained by listing practice-related hypotheses generated by the model.[23]

The nursing process is well suited for use in a practice setting. The two-level assessment is unique to this model and leads to the identification of adaptation problems or nursing diagnosis. Beginning work is being done on a typology of nursing diagnoses.[23,26] Intervention is based specifically on the model, but there is a need to develop an organization of categories of nursing interventions.[26]

The model was used in practice by graduate nursing students in 1976. They found some blurring in the categories of self-concept, role function, and interdependence when deciding where a given behavior belonged. They also found the nursing process lengthy and repetitive, taking much time to complete. The model was useful in inpatient settings, except in intensive care units where there were rapid changes in the patient's condition. The students also found it easier to use the model in outpatient settings such as clinics and physician's offices.[29]

The model has also been used by nurses who cared for young, hospitalized children and in a community setting. The model provided a system that accounted for physical needs as well as psychosocial needs. It was particularly useful in the pediatric setting, because it allowed for assessment of covert psychological needs of children. The model also provides for setting needs, setting priorities, setting goals, intervening, and reevaluating the patient's needs.[6,27]

In May 1979 three nursing administrators initiated a pilot study using the model in an 18-bed unit in Arlington, Virginia. Evaluation and revision of the nursing assessment tools were conducted. By April 1980, the model was in practice. Early research suggests that it enhanced patient satisfaction and improved health outcomes. Consistent with the model, the nurses began to enhance their professionalism by writing complete care plans and phrasing patient problems in terms of nursing diagnosis. A year after initiation, the model was still supported by the staff. The group directors admitted that the model's abstractness required diligence in applying it to practice. They also contended that further validation of the theory was needed.

In September 1981 a research study was published that dealt with problems associated with nursing home applications for elderly persons. The research was done within the framework of the adaptation model. The research design was used to identify adaptation problems and hypotheses were formulated. The study concluded that, "As a broad conceptual framework, the Roy Adaptation Nursing Model served as a useful tool for systematically gathering responses regarding adaptation problems experienced by the elderly persons and their significant others."[4]

Another research study, published in August 1983, used the model to analyze the content of 20 interviews of parents whose children had been recently diagnosed as having cancer. Although operational definitions of Roy's adaptation modes were used in the study, the origins of the definitions remain unclear. The authors of the study found the framework applicable as a result of its ability to treat multiple patient variables.[28]

During the 1980s a number of health care agencies have begun implementing the Roy Adaptation Model as a basis for nursing practice. Roy has compiled a list of experienced resource persons who can assist with this work in the United States and Canada (see Appendix A).

Education

The Adaptation Model has also been useful in the educational setting and is currently in use at Mount Saint Mary's College, Department of Nursing.[23] Mount Saint Mary's program demonstrates the relationship of nursing theory to nursing education. Three vertical strands run throughout the curriculum. These include two theory strands (the adapting person and health-illness) and one practice strand (nursing man-

agement). There are two horizontal strands in the curriculum—nursing process and student adaptation/leadership. The horizontal strands enhance the theory and practice of the vertical strands. All strands within the curriculum build in complexity from one level to the next.[21] In addition, the model allows for increasing knowledge in both the areas of theory and practice.[16]

Roy[16,21] states that the model defines for students the distinct purpose of nursing, which is to promote man's adaptation in each of the adaptive modes in situations of health and illness. The model also distinguishes nursing science and medical science by having the content of these areas taught in separate courses. Roy[21] believes that curriculum based on this model helps in theory development by the students, who also learn how to test theories and develop new theoretical insights.

In 1976 the model was used for curriculum development of a practitioner program at the University of Miami in Florida. Organization of curriculum content and selections of student learning experiences were derived from the model. Course objectives included identifying adaptive problems and distinguishing between effective and noneffective coping mechanisms. Application of the model resulted in decreased anxiety in the students and provided a framework to give direction to the education of practitioners.[1]

Throughout the 1970s and into the 1980s the Roy model has been implemented as a basis for curriculum development in associate degree, diploma, baccalaureate, and higher degree programs in many countries. Roy and her colleagues have provided consultation for this work in more than 30 schools in the United States, Canada, and abroad.

Research

If research is to affect practitioners' behavior, it must be directed at testing and retesting conceptual models for nursing practice. Roy[23] has stated that theory development and the testing of developed theories are nursing's highest priority. The model must be able to generate testable hypotheses for it to be researchable.

As previously stated, Roy's theory has generated a number of general propositions. From these general propositions, specific hypotheses can be developed and tested. B.J. Hill and C.S. Roberts[7] have demonstrated the development of testable hypotheses from the model, as has Roy. Data to validate or support the model would be created by the testing of such hypotheses. But to date there has been little research in this area.[5]

Roy[14] has identified a set of concepts forming a model from which the process of observation and classification of facts would lead to postulates. The postulates concern the occurrence of adaptation problems, coping mechanisms, and interventions based on laws derived from factors making up the response potential of the focal, contextual, and residual stimuli. Roy[16,17,18] is in the early stages of outlining a typology of adaptation problems or nursing diagnoses. Research and testing are needed in the areas of typology and categories of interventions that fit into the model. General propositions have been developed that need to be tested.[24]

A group of graduate students at DePaul University tested the model in a number of practice situations. The students adapted an assessment tool and tested the model in episodic settings in a variety of units in different hospitals. They also used distributive settings in physicians' offices, industrial health settings, and outpatient clinics. The students concluded that the model provided a good framework for ordering a variety of observations and was flexible enough to be used in both episodic and distributive settings.[28] The study provided empirical support for the model in the area of the process of assessment within the four adaptive modes.

During presentations, Roy outlines the research to be done as focusing on the basic nursing science of adaptive systems of persons as individuals and as groups and on nursing practice that affects adaptation of the client and changes the profession of nursing and the delivery of health care (see Appendix B).

Some research has been done on the model, but more is needed for further validation. The model does generate many testable hypotheses related to practice and theory.[5]

FURTHER DEVELOPMENT

The Roy Adaptation Model is an approach to nursing that has made and can continue to make a significant contribution to nursing's body of knowledge, but a few needs remain in the development of the theory. Some assumptions about the model should be validated, such as the assumption that the person has four modes of adaptation. A more thoroughly defined typology of nursing diagnosis and an organization of categories of interventions are needed. There is some overlapping of the categories of self-concept, role function, and interdependence. A clearer definition of health would also be useful. Adaptive mechanisms of the comatose patient in response to tactile and verbal stimuli need to be incorporated in the model. There appear to be problems involved in using the model in an intensive care unit where situations change rapidly. Roy notes that it is helpful to use a system for setting priorities with the model. When a priority setting system is used in conjunction with the model, it might be better suited for use in a critical care setting.[20:690] A chapter regarding life closure was added to the 1984 edition of *Introduction To Nursing: An Adaptation Model*. Support and encouragement of adaptation to the dying process is an integral component of nursing. Roy's model is useful and contributes to the science and practice of nursing.

EVALUATION OF THE THEORY
Simplicity

The Roy model includes the concepts of nursing, person, health-illness, environment, adaptation and nursing activities. It also includes the subconcepts of regulator, cognator, and the four effector modes of physiological, self-concept, role function, and interdependence. Because this theory has several major concepts and subconcepts, it is complex.

Generality

Roy[23] defines her model as drawn from multiple middle range theories and advocates multiple middle range theories for use in nursing. Middle range theories are testable, but have sufficient generality to be scientifically interesting.[30] Roy's model is generalizable to all settings in nursing practice, but is limited in scope because it primarily addresses the concept of person-environment adaptation.

Empirical Precision

Increasing complexity within theories often helps increase empirical precision. When subcomponents are designated within the theory, the empirical precision increases, assuming the broad concepts are based in reality.[2]

Because Roy's broad concepts stem from theory in physiological psychology, psychology, sociology, and nursing, empirical data to indicate that this general theory base has substance. Roy[14,22] studied and analyzed 500 samples of patient behaviors collected by nursing students. From this analysis, Roy proposed her four adaptive modes in man. This is the least supported of Roy's concepts.[5]

Roy's assumptions can also be analyzed to determine what type of statements they are. The eight assumptions of the Adaptation Model of Nursing follow:

1. The person is a biopsychosocial being.
2. The person is in constant interaction with a changing environment.
3. To cope with a changing world, the person uses both innate and acquired mechanisms, which are biological, psychological, and sociological in origin.
4. Health and illness are one inevitable di-

mension of the person's life.
5. To respond positively to environmental changes, the person must adapt.
6. The person's adaptation is a function of the stimulus he is exposed to and his adaptation level.
7. The persons' adaptation level is such that it comprises a zone indicating the range of stimulation that will lead to a positive response.
8. The person is conceptualized as having four modes of adaptation: physiological needs, self-concept, role function, and interdependence relations.[22:180-182]

Of the eight basic assumptions presented in the model, assumptions 1 through 5 are existence statements. Assumptions 6 and 7 are associational statements. As defined by Reynolds,[12] relational statements can be either associational or causal. The relational statements are the relations that may be tested.

Roy[24,26] identifies many propositions in relation to the regulator and cognator mechanisms and the self-concept, role function, and interdependence modes. These propositions have varying degrees of support from general theory and empirical data. The majority of the propositions are relational statements and can also be tested.[5] Testable hypotheses have been derived from the model.[7]

Derivable Consequences

Derivable consequences refer to how practically useful, important, and generally sufficient the theory is in relation to achieving valued nursing outcomes. The theory needs to guide research and practice, generate ideas, and differentiate the focus of nursing from other service professions.[2]

The Roy adaptation model has a clearly defined nursing process and can be useful in guiding clinical practice. The model is also capable of generating new information through the testing of the hypotheses that have been derived from it.[5]

REFERENCES

1. Brower, H.T.F., & Baker, B.J. (1976, Nov.). The Roy adaptation model: Using the adaptation model in a practitioner curriculum. *Nursing Outlook, 24:*686-689.
2. Chinn, P.L., & Jacobs, M.K. (1983). *Theory and nursing: A systematic approach.* St. Louis: C.V. Mosby.
3. Dickoff, J., James, P., & Widenbach, E. (1968, May). Theory in practice discipline, part I, practice oriented theory. *Nursing Research, 17:*413-415.
4. Farkas, L. (1981, March). Adaptation problems with nursing home application for elderly persons: An application of the Roy adaptation nursing model. *Journal of Advanced Nursing, 6:*363-368.
5. Fitzpatrick, J.J., & Whall, A.L. (Eds.). (1983). *Conceptual models of nursing: Analysis and application.* Bowie, Md.: Robert J. Brady.
6. Galligan, A.C. (1979, Jan.). Using Roy's concept of adaptation to care for young children. *The American Journal of Maternal Child Nursing, 4:*24-28.
7. Hill, B.J., & Roberts, C.S. (1981). Formal theory construction: An example of the process. In C. Roberts, & S.L. Roberts (Eds.), *Theory construction in nursing: An adaptation model.* Englewood Cliffs, N.J.: Prentice-Hall.
8. Mastal, M., & Hammond, H. (1980, July). Analysis and expansion of the Roy model: A contribution to holistic nursing. *Advances in Nursing Science, 3:*7-78.
9. Mastal, M., Hammond, H., & Roberts, M. (1982, June). Theory into hospital practice: A pilot implementation. *The Journal of Nursing Administration, 12:*9-15.
10. Rambo, B. (1983). *Adaptation nursing: Assessment and intervention.* Philadelphia: W.B. Sanders.
11. Randell, B., Tedrow, M.P., & Van Landingham, J. (1982). *Adaptation nursing: The Roy conceptual model applied.* St. Louis: C.V. Mosby.
12. Reynolds, P.D. (1971). *A primer in theory construction.* Indianapolis: Ind.: Bobbs-Merrill.
13. Riehl, J.P., & Roy, C. (Eds.). (1980). *Conceptual models for nursing practice* (2nd ed.). New York: Appleton-Century-Crofts.
14. Roy, C. (1970, March). Adaptation: A conceptual framework in nursing. *Nursing Outlook, 18:*42-45.
15. Roy, C. (1971, April). Adaptation: A basis for nursing practice. *Nursing Outlook, 19:*254-257.
16. Roy, C. (1973, March). Adaptation: Implications for curriculum change. *Nursing Outlook, 21:*163-168.
17. Roy, C. (1975, Feb.). A diagnostic classification system for nursing. *Nursing Outlook, 23:*90-94.
18. Roy, C. (1976, Summer). The impact of nursing diagnosis. *Nursing Digest, 4:*67-69.
19. Roy, C. (1976). *Introduction to nursing: An adaptation model.* Englewood Cliffs, N.J.: Prentice-Hall.
20. Roy, C. (1976, Nov.). The Roy adaptation model: Comment. *Nursing Outlook, 24:*690-691.
21. Roy, C. (1979, Feb.). Relating nursing theory to nursing education: A new era. *Nurse Educator, 4:*16-21.
22. Roy, C. (1980). The Roy adaptation model. In J.P. Riehl, & C. Roy (Eds.), *Conceptual models for nursing practice* (2nd ed.). New York: Appleton-Century-Crofts. pp. 179-188.
23. Roy, C. (1984). *An introduction to nursing: An adaptation model* (2nd ed.). Englewood Cliffs, N.J.: Prentice-Hall.
24. Roy, C., & McLeod, D. (1981). Theory of the person as an adaptive system. In C. Roy, & S.L. Roberts (Eds.), *Theory construction in nursing: An adaptation model.* Englewood Cliffs, N.J.: Prentice-Hall.
25. Roy, C., & Obloy, M. (1978, Oct.). The practitioner movement. *American Journal of Nursing, 78:*1698-1702.
26. Roy, C., & Roberts, S. (1981). *Theory construction in nursing: An adaptation model.* Englewood Cliffs, N.J.: Prentice-Hall.
27. Schmitz, M. (1980). The Roy adaptation model: Application in a community setting. In J.P. Riehl, & C. Roy (Eds.), *Conceptual models for nursing practice* (2nd ed.). New York: Appleton-Century-Crofts.
28. Smith, C.E., et al. (1983, Aug.). Content analyses of interviews using a nursing model: A look at parents adapting to the impact of childhood cancer. *Cancer Nursing, 6:*269-275.
29. Wagner, P. (1976, Nov.). The Roy adaptation model: Testing the adaptation model in practice. *Nursing Outlook, 24:*682-685.

30. Walker, L.O., & Avant, K.C. (1983). *Strategies for theory construction in nursing.* Norwalk, Conn.: Appleton-Century-Crofts.

BIBLIOGRAPHY
Primary Sources
Books

Andrews, H., & Roy, C. (1985). *Essentials of the Roy adaptation model.* Englewood Cliffs, N.J.: Prentice-Hall.

Riehl, J.P., & Roy, C. (Eds.). (1974). *Conceptual models for nursing practice.* Englewood Cliffs, N.J.: Prentice-Hall.

Riehl, J.P., & Roy, C. (Eds.). (1980). *Conceptual models for nursing practice* (2nd. ed.). New York: Appleton-Century-Crofts.

Roy, C. (1976). *Introduction to nursing: An adaptation model:* Englewood Cliffs, N.J.: Prentice-Hall.

Roy, C. ((1982). *Introduction to nursing: An adaptation model.* Japanese translation by Yuriko Kanematsu. Japan: UNI Agency.

Roy, C. (1984). *Introduction to nursing: An adaptation model* (2nd ed.). Englewood Cliffs, N.J.: Prentice-Hall.

Roy, C., & Roberts, S. (1981). Theory construction in nursing: An adaptation model, Englewood Cliffs, N.J.: Prentice-Hall, Inc.

Book Chapters

Roy, C. (1974). The Roy adaptation model. In J.P. Riehl, & C. Roy (Eds.), *Conceptual models for nursing practice.* New York: Appleton-Century-Crofts.

Roy, C. (1975, June). Adaptation framework. In *Curriculum innovation through framework application.* Loma Linda, Calif.: Loma Linda University.

Roy, C. (1978). The stress of hospital events: Measuring changes in level of stress. In M.V. Batey (Ed.), *Symposium on stress.* In Conference on Communicating Nursing Research. Boulder, Colo: Western Interstate Commission on Higher Education (WICHE), Vol. 11.

Roy, C. (1978, Jan. 12-13). Conceptual framework for primary care in baccalaureate programs. In *Primary Care Conference,* U.S. Department of Health, Education, and Welfare. Denver, Col.

Roy, C. (1979). Health-illness (powerlessness) questionnaire and hospitalized patient decision-making. In M.J. Ward, & C.A. Lindeman (Eds.), *Instruments for measuring nursing practice and other health care variables* (Vol. 1). Hyattsville, Md.: U.S. Department of Health, Education, and Welfare.

Roy, C. (1980). Expose de Callista Roy sur theorie. Expose de Callista Roy sur l'utilisation de sa theorie dans l'enseignement. In Acta Nursological 3, Ecole Genevoise D. Infirmieres Le Bon Secours, Geneve.

Roy, C. (1980). Expose de Callista Roy sur theorie. Expose de Callista Roy sur l'utilisation de sa theorie au neveau de la recherche. In Acta Nursological 3, Ecole Genevoise D. Infirmieres Le Bon Secours, Geneve.

Roy, C. (1980). The Roy adaptation model. In J.P. Riehl, & C. Roy (Eds.), *Conceptual models for nursing practice.* (2nd ed.). New York: Appleton-Century-Crofts.

Roy, C. (1981). A systems model of nursing care and its effect on the quality of human life. *Proceedings of the International Congress on Applied Systems Research and Cybernetics.* London: Pergamon Press.

Roy, C., & McLeod, D. (1981). Theory of the person as an adaptive system. In C. Roy, & S.L. Roberts (Eds.). *Theory construction in nursing: An adaptation model.* Englewood Cliffs, N.J.: Prentice-Hall.

Roy, S.C. (1983). Theory development in nursing: A proposal for direction. In N. Chaska (Ed.), *The nursing profession: A time to speak.* New York: McGraw-Hill.

Roy, S.C. (1983). A conceptual framework for clinical specialist practice. In A. Harris, & J. Sproos (Eds.), *The clinical nurse specialist in theory and practice.* New York: Grune & Stratton.

Roy, S.C. 1983). Roy's adaptation model and application to family case studies. In I. Clements, & F. Roberts (Eds.), *Theoretical approaches to family health.* New York: John Wiley & Sons.

Roy, C. (1983). Roy adaptation model, the expectant family—analysis and application of the Roy adaptation model, and the family in primary care—analysis and application of the Roy adaptation model. In I. Clements, & F. Roberts (Eds.), *Family health: A theoretical approach to nursing care.* New York: John Wiley & Sons.

Roy, C. (1984, May 20-23). The Roy adaptation model: Applications in community health nursing. In *Proceedings of the Annual Community Health Nursing Conference.* The University of North Carolina, Chapel Hill, N.C.

Roy, C. (In press). Concepts of nursing practice: Roy's adaptation model. In L.M. Malarkey, & M.E. McMorrow (Eds.), *Medical-Surgical Nursing: A nursing process approach.* Englewood Cliffs, N.J.: Prentice-Hall.

Articles

Roy, C. (1967, Feb.). Role cues and mothers of hospitalized children. *Nursing Research, 16:*178-182.

Roy, C. (1970, March). Adaptation: A conceptual framework in nursing. *Nursing Outlook, 18:*42-45.

Roy, C. (1971, April). Adaptation: A basis for nursing practice. *Nursing Outlook, 19:*254-257.

Roy, C. (1973). Adaptation: Implications for curriculum change. *Nursing Outlook, 21:*163-168.

Roy, C. (1975, Feb.). Adaptation: Implications for curriculum change. *Nursing Outlook, 23:*90-94.

Roy, C. (1975, Feb.). A diagnostic classification system for nursing. *Nursing Outlook, 23:90-94.*

*Roy, S.C. (1975, May). The impact of nursing diagnosis. AORN Journal, 21:*1023-1030.

Roy, C. (1976). Comment. *Nursing Outlook, 24:*690-691.

Roy, C. (1976, Summer). The impact of nursing diagnosis. *Nursing Digest, 4:*67-69.

Roy, C. (1976, Nov.). The Roy adaptation model: Comment. *Nursing Outlook, 24:*690-691.

Roy, C., & Obloy, M. (1978, Oct.). The practitioner movement. *American Journal of Nursing, 78:* 1698-1702.

Roy, C. (1979, Feb.). Relating nursing theory to nursing education: A new era. *Nurse Educator, 4:*16-21.

Roy, C. (1979, Dec.). Nursing diagnosis from the perspective of a nursing model. *Nursing Diagnosis Newsletter,* Vol. 6. St. Louis School of Nursing.

Roy, C. (1983). To the Editor. *Nursing Research, 23:*320.

Dissertation

Roy, C. (1977). *Decision-making by the physically ill and adaptation during illness.* Doctoral dissertation. University of California, Los Angeles.

Booklet

Roy, S.C., et al. (1979). *Getting our act together.* New York, National League of Nursing. Publication No. 52-1805.

Audiotape

Roy, C. (1978, Dec.). Paper presented at the second Annual Nurse Educator Conference. Audiotape available from Teach 'em Inc., 160 E. Illinois Street, Chicago, Ill. 60611.

Roy, C. (1984, May). Nurses' Theorist Conference at Edmonton, Alberta. Audiotape available from Kennedy Recordings, R.R. 5, Edmonton, Alberta TSP 4B7.

Correspondence

Roy, S.C. (1984, March 26). Curriculum vitae.

Interview

Roy, S.C. (1984, March 25). Telephone interview.

Secondary Sources
Book Reviews

Riehl, J.P., & Roy, S.C. (1974). *Conceptual models for nursing practice.*
*Nursing Outlook, 23:*457, July 1975.
*Nursing Research, 24:*306-307, July-August 1975.

Roy, S.C. (1976). *Introduction to nursing: An adaptation model.*
*American Journal of Nursing, 77:*1359, August 1977.
*Nursing Outlook, 25:*658, October 1977.

Roy, S.C., & Roberts, S. (1981). *Theory construction in nursing.*
*Nursing Outlook, 30:*141, February 1982.

Books

Chinn, P.L., & Jacobs, M.K. (1983). *Theory and nursing: A systematic approach.* St. Louis: C.V. Mosby.

Fitzpatrick, J.J., & Whall, A.L., (1983). *Conceptual models of nursing: Analysis and application.* Bowie, Md.: Robert J. Brady.

Fitzpatrick, J.J., et al. (1982). *Nursing models: Applications to psychiatric mental health nursing.* Bowie, Md.: Robert J. Brady.

Kim, H.S. (1983). *The nature of theoretical thinking in nursing.* Norwalk, Conn.: Appleton-Century-Crofts.

Potter, D.O. (Ed.). (1984). *Practices nurses' reference library.* Springhouse, Penn.: Nursing 84 Books Springhouse Corporation.

Rambo, B. (1983). *Adaptation nursing: Assessment and intervention.* Philadelphia: W.B. Saunders.

Randell, B., Tedrow, M.P., & Van Landingham, J. (1982). *Adaptation nursing: The Roy conceptual model applied.* St. Louis: C.V. Mosby.

Reynolds, P.D. (1971). *A primer in theory construction.* Indianapolis, Ind.: Bobbs-Merrill.

Walker, L.O., & Avant, K.C. (1983). *Strategies for theory construction in nursing.* Norwalk, Conn.: Appleton-Century-Crofts.

Book Chapters

Downey, C. (1974). Adaptation nursing applied to an obstetric patient. In J.P. Riehl & C. Roy (Eds.), *Conceptual models for nursing practice,* New York: Appleton-Century-Crofts.

Fawcett, J. (1984). Roy's adaptation model. In Fawcett, J., *Analysis and evaluation of conceptual models of nursing.* Philadelphia: F.A. Davis.

Fawcett, J. (1981). Assessing and understanding the cesarean father. In C.F. Kehoe (Ed.), *The cesarean experience: Theoretical and clinical perspectives for nurses.* New York: Appleton-Century-Crofts.

Fitzpatrick, J.J., et al. (1982). *Nursing models: Applications to psychiatric mental health nursing.* Bowie, Md.: Robert J. Brady.

Galbreath, J.G. (1980). Sister Callista Roy. In Nursing Theories Conference Group, J.B. George, Chairperson, *Nursing theories: The base for professional nursing practice.* Englewood Cliffs, N.J.: Prentice-Hall.

Gordon, J. (1974). Nursing assessment and care plan for a cardiac patient. In J.P. Riehl, & C. Roy (Eds.), *Conceptual models for nursing practice.* New York: Appleton-Century-Crofts.

Hill, B.J., & Roberts, C.S. (1981). Formal theory construction: An example of the process. In C. Roberts, & S.L. Roberts (Eds.), *Theory construction in nursing: An adaptation model.* Englewood Cliffs, N.J.: Prentice-Hall.

Idle, B.A. (1978). SPAL: A tool for measuring self-perceived adaptation level appropriate for an elderly population. In Sigma Theta Tau, *Clinical nursing research: Its strategies and findings. Proceedings from the Fifth Annual Nursing Research Conference, Tuscon, Arizona, Sept. 15-16, 1977.* Indianapolis: Sigma Theta Tau. Monograph, Series 79-Two. University of Arizona.

Kehoe, C.F. (1981). Identifying the nursing needs of the postpartum cesarean mother. In C.F. Kehoe (Ed.), *The cesarean experience: Theoretical and clinical perspective for nurses.* New York: Appleton-Century-Crofts.

Kehoe, C.F., & Fawcett, J. (1981). An overview of the Roy adaptation model. In C.F. Kehoe (Ed.), *The cesarean experience: Theoretical and clinical perspectives for nurses.* New York: Appleton-Century-Crofts.

Levesque, L. (1980, Oct. 22-24). Rehabilitation of the chronically-ill elderly: A method of operationalizing a conceptual model for nursing. In R.C. MacKay, & E.G. Zilm (Eds.), *Research for practice: Proceedings of the National Nursing Research Conference,* Halifax, Nova-Scotia.

Lewis, F., et al. (1978). Measuring adaptation of chemotherapy patients. In J.C. Krueger, A.H. Nelson, & M. Opal, *Nursing Research: Development, collaboration, utilization.* Rockville, Md.: Aspen Systems.

Meleis, A.I. (1985). Sister Callista Roy. In A.I. Meleis, *Theoretical nursing: Development and progress.* Philadelphia: J.B. Lippincott.

Schmitz, M: (1980). The Roy adaptation model: Application in a community setting. In J.P. Riehl, & C. Roy (Eds.), *Conceptual models for nursing practice* (2nd ed.). New York: Appleton-Century-Crofts.

Starr, S.L. (1980). Adaptation applied to the dying patient. In J.P. Riehl, & C. Roy (Eds.), *Conceptual models for nursing practice* (2nd ed.). New York: Appleton-Century-Crofts.

Tiedeman, M.E. (1983). The Roy adaptation model. In J. Fitzpatrick, & A. Whall, (Eds.), *Conceptual models of nursing: Analysis and application.* Bowie, Md.: Robert J. Brady.

Articles

Andreoli, K.G., & Thompson, C.E. (1977, June). The nature of science in nursing. *Image, 9*(2):33-37.

Beckstrand, J. (1980). A critique of several conceptions of practice theory in nursing. *Research in Nursing and Health, 3:*69-79.

Brower, H.T.F., & Baker, B.J. (1976, Nov.). The Roy adaptation model: Using the adaptation model in a practitioner curriculum. *Nursing Outlook, 24:*686-689.

Camooso, C., Green, M., & Reilly, P. (1981). Students' adaptation according to Roy. *Nursing Outlook, 29:*108-109.

Chance, K.S. (1982). Nursing models: A requisite for professional accountability. *Advances in Nursing Science, 4*(2):57-65.

Dickoff, J., James, P., & Widenbach, E. (1968, May). Theory in a practice discipline. Part I. Practice oriented theory. *Nursing Research, 17:*413-435.

Farkas, L. (1981, March). Adaptation problems with nursing home application for elderly persons: An application of the Roy adaptation nursing model. *Journal of Advanced Nursing, 6:*363-368.

Fawcett, J. (1981). Needs of cesarean birth parents. *Journal of Obstetrics, Gynecologic, and Neonatal Nursing, 10*:371-376.

Gartner, S.R., & Nahm, H. (1977, Jan.-Feb.). An overview of nursing research in the United States. *Nursing Research, 26*:10-29.

Galligan, A.C. (1979, Jan.). Using Roy's concept of adaptation to care for young children. *The American Journal of Maternal Child Nursing, 4*:24-28.

Goodwin, J.O. (1980). A cross-cultural approach to integrating nursing theory and practice. *Nurse Educator, 5*(6):15-20.

Janelli, L.M. (1980). Utilizing Roy's adaptation model from a gerontological perspective. *Journal of Gerontological Nursing, 6*(3):140-150.

Johnson, D.E. (1974), Sept.-Oct.). Development of theory: A requisite for nursing as a primary health profession. *Nursing Research, 23*:372-377.

Kasemwatana, S. (1982). An application of Roy's adaptation model. *Thai Journal of Nursing, 31*(1):25-46.

Laros, J. (1977). Deriving outcome criteria from a conceptual model. *Nursing Outlook, 25*:333-336.

Lewis, F.M., Firsich, S.C., & Parsell, S. (1979). Clinical tool development for adult chemotherapy patients: Process and content. *Cancer Nursing, 2*:99-108.

Mastal, M., & Hammond, H. (1980, July). Analysis and expansion of the Roy adaptation model: A contribution to holistic nursing. *Advances in Nursing Science, 2*:71-81.

Mastal, M., Hammond, H., & Roberts, M. (1982, June). Theory into hospital practice: A pilot implementation. *The Journal of Nursing Administration, 12*:9-15.

Norris, S., Campbell, L., & Brenkert, S. (1982). Nursing procedures and alternations in transcutaneous oxygen tension in premature infants. *Nursing Research, 31*:330-336.

Park, K.O. (1982). Study of Roy's adaptation model. *Trehan Kanho, 21*(3):49-58 (Japan).

Porth, C.M. (1977). Physiological coping: A model for teaching pathophysiology. *Nursing Outlook, 25*:781-784.

Richard, L. (1982). Roy's adaptation model, *Infirmiere Candienne (Montreal), 24*(9):12-13.

Robitaille-Tremblay, M. (1983). Les soins infirmiers en psychiatrie a l'ere d'un modele conceptuel. *L'infirmiere Canadienne, 6*:37-40.

Silva, M.C. (1977, Oct.). Philosophy science theory: Interrelationships and implications for nursing research. *Image, 9*(3):59-63.

Smith, C.E., Garvis, M.S., & Martinson, I.M (1983, Aug.). Content analysis of interviews using a nursing model: A look at parents adapting to the impact of childhood cancer. *Cancer Nursing, 6*:269-275.

Wagner, P. (1976, Nov.). The Roy adaptation model: Testing the adaptation model in practice. *Nursing Outlook, 24*(11):682-685.

Other Sources

Coombs, A., & Snygg, D. (1959). *Individual behavior: A perceptual approach to behavior.* New York: Harper Brothers.

Dohrenwend, B.P. (1961). The social psychological nature of stress. A framework for causal inquiry. *Journal of Abnormal and Social Psychology, 62*(2):294-302.

Driever, M.J. (1976). Theory of self-concept. In C. Roy (Ed.), *Introduction to nursing: An adaptation model.* Englewood Cliffs, N.J.: Prentice-Hall.

Ellis, R. (1968, May-June). Characteristics of significant theories. *Nursing Research, 17*:217-223.

Epstein, S. (1973, May). The self-concept revisited or a theory of a theory. *American Psychologist, 28*:(5):404-416.

Erickson, E.H. (1963). *Childhood and society* (2nd ed.). New York: W.W. Norton.

Gardner, B.D. (1964). *Development in early childhood.* New York: Harper & Row.

Helson, H. (1964). *Adaptation-level theory: An experimental and systematic approach to behavior.* New York: Harper & Row.

Lazarus, R.S. (1966). *Psychological stress and the coping process.* New York: McGraw-Hill.

Lazarus, R.S., Averill, J.R., & Opton, E.M., Jr. (1974). The psychology of coping: Issues of research and assessment. In G.V. Coelho, D.A. Hamburg, & J.E. Adams (Eds.), *Coping and adaptation.* New York: Basic Books.

Malaznik, N. (1976). Theory of role function. In C. Roy (Ed.), *Introduction to nursing: An adaptation model.* Englewood Cliffs, N.J.: Prentice-Hall.

Maslow, A.H. (1968). *Toward a psychology of being* (2nd ed.). New York: Van Nostrand Reinhold.

Mead, G.H. (1934). *Mind, self, and society.* Chicago: University of Chicago.

Mechanic, D. (1974). Social structure and personal adaptation: Some neglected dimensions. In G.V.

Coelho, D.A. Hamburg, & J.E. Adams (Eds.), *Coping and adaptation*. New York: Basic Books.

Mechanic, D. (1970). Some problems in developing a social psychology of adaptation to stress. In J. McGrath (Ed.), *Social and psychological factors in stress*. New York: Holt, Rinehart, & Winston.

Miller, J.G. (1965, July). Living systems: Basic concepts. *Behavioral Science, 10:*193-237.

Pousch, M., & Van Landingham, J. (1977). *Interdependence mode module*. Class handout, Mount St. Mary's College, Los Angeles.

Randell, B. (1976). Development of role function. In C. Roy (Ed.), *Introduction to nursing: An adaptation model*. Englewood Cliffs, N.J.: Prentice-Hall.

Reynolds, P.D. (1971). *A primer in theory construction*. Indianapolis, Ind.: Bobbs-Merrill.

Selye, H. (1978). *The stress of life*. New York: McGraw-Hill.

Sullivan, H.S. (1953). *The interpersonal theory of psychiatry*. New York: W.W. Norton.

Appendix A

RESOURCES FOR IMPLEMENTING ROY ADAPTATION MODEL IN CLINICAL PRACTICE

Joanne Gray, R.N., M.S.
Director of Education
South Coast Medical Center
31872 Coast Highway
South Laguana, California

Helen Hammond, R.N., M.S.N., C.C.R.N.
Executive Director
Educational Networks Associates, Inc.
Gaithersburg, Maryland

Maureen T. Jakocko, R.N., M.N.
Director of Inservice Education
Children's Hospital of Orange County
P.O. Box 5700
Orange, California

Lois McMillan, R.N., M.A., C.N.A.A.
Nursing Consultant, Adventist Health System
Eastern Middle America, Inc.
Shawnee Mission Medical Center
Shawnee Mission, Kansas

Linda Sowden, R.N., M.N.
Clinical Nurse Specialist
Children's Hospital of Orange County
P.O. Box 5700
Orange, California

Marthe R. Tremblay, R.N., M.A.
Nurse Clinician Specialist
Centre-Hospitalier Pierre Janet
20, rue Pharand
Hull, Quebec, Canada

Appendix B

RESEARCH BASED ON THE ROY ADAPTATION MODEL

I. Nursing as a basic science
   A. Persons or groups as adaptive systems
   B. Adaptive processes that affect health status
II. Nursing as a practice discipline
   A. Function of nursing—promoting adaptation
      1. Nursing diagnosis
      2. Nursing intervention
      3. Outcomes for persons or groups
   B. Role of nursing—model based practice
      1. Teaching the use of the model
      2. Implementing the model in nursing care systems
      3. Outcomes
         A. For nurses
         B. For relation to other disciplines

Betty Neuman

Systems Model

Mary E. Hermiz, Mary Meininger

26

CREDENTIALS AND BACKGROUND OF THE THEORIST

Betty Neuman was born in 1924 on a farm near Lowell, Ohio. Her father was a farmer and her mother a homemaker. She developed a sense of love for the land while growing up in rural Ohio, and it was because of this rural background that her compassion for people in need evolved. Neuman's first nursing education

The authors wish to express appreciation to Judy K. Cowling for her assistance with data collection and to Betty Neuman for critiquing the chapter.

was completed at Peoples Hospital School of Nursing (now General Hospital) in Akron, Ohio, in 1947. She then moved to Los Angeles to live with relatives. In California she held various positions, including head and hospital staff nurse and a school and industrial nurse. She was also involved in clinical teaching in the medical-surgical, communicable disease, and critical care areas. Because she had always had an interest in people's behavior and reaction to struggles, she attended the University of California at Los Angeles with a focus on public health and psychology. She completed her baccalaureate degree in nursing in 1957 and then helped establish and manage her husband's ob-

313

stetrical and gynecological practice. In 1966 she received her master's degree in mental health, public health consultation from UCLA. She is currently pursuing doctoral studies in educational administration in the higher degree programs at Ohio University.*

Neuman was a pioneer in nursing involvement in mental health. She developed her first explicit teaching and practice model for mental health consultation in the late 1960s, before the creation of her systems model. Neuman designed a conceptual model for nursing in 1970 in response to requests from UCLA graduate students, who wanted a course that emphasized breadth rather than depth in evaluating nursing problems. The model extended beyond the medical model and included the new behavioral science concepts such as problem-finding and prevention. Neuman[21:265] first published her model in 1972. She spent the following decade refining and defining various aspects of the model in preparation for her first book, *The Neuman Systems Model.*[17]

Since developing her model, Neuman has been involved in various professional activities, including professional paper presentations, consultations, and conferences, and has served as a group facilitator, lecturer, and instructor. Many universities and schools of nursing are using her model in their programs. Neuman‡ maintains her role as consultant across the country for schools or institutions adopting her model.

THEORETICAL SOURCES

The model has some similarity to Gestalt theory.[17:14] Gestalt theory maintains that the homeostatic process is the process by which an organism maintains its equilibrium, and consequently its health, under varying conditions. Homeostasis is thus the process by which the organism satisfies its needs. Because there are many needs and each upsets the equilibrium,

the homeostatic process is continuous. All life is characterized by this ongoing play of balance and imbalance in the organism. When the homeostatic process fails to some degree, or when the organism remains in state of disequilibrium for too long and is consequently unable to satisfy its needs, sickness develops. When the homeostatic process fails completely, the organism dies.[22:4] The Gestalt approach then, considers the individual as a function of the organism-environmental field and considers his behavior a reflection of his relatedness within that field.[22:25]

The model is also derived from philosophical views of deChardin and Bernard Marx.[17:14] Marxist philosophy suggests that the properties of parts are determined partly by the larger wholes within dynamically organized systems. Along with this, Neuman[17:14] confirmed that the patterns of the whole influence awareness of the part, which is drawn from deChardin's philosophy of the wholeness of life. She used H. Selye's definition of stress, which is the nonspecific response of the body to any demand made on it.[24:14] Stress increases the demand for readjustment. This demand is nonspecific; it requires adaptation to a problem, irrespective of what the problem is. The essence of stress is therefore the nonspecific demand for activity.[24:15] Stressors are tension-producing stimuli with the potential for causing disequilibrium and situational or maturational crises.[16:14]

Neuman's model also gained ideas from the general systems theory of the nature of living open systems. This theory states that all the elements are in interaction in a complex organization.[17:3] From G. Caplan's conceptual model for levels of prevention Neuman identifies the levels and views them as encompassing one another on a continuing basis. Caplan defines the three levels of prevention to include primary, secondary, and tertiary prevention. Primary prevention involves counteracting harmful circumstances before production of illness.[4:26] Secondary prevention attempts to reduce the prevalence of disease in two ways: (1) by alter-

---

*References 18:239-240; 20; 21.
‡References 17:239-240; 20.

ing the factors which led to the disorder, or (2) by early diagnosis and effective treatment.[4:89] Tertiary prevention attempts to reduce the rate of the residual effects of the disorder.[4:113] Neuman's model not only stems from a synthesis of knowledge from several other disciplines, but it also incorporates observations made during her clinical experiences in mental health nursing.[8:36]

USE OF EMPIRICAL EVIDENCE

Neuman does not cite any research that she draws from for her conceptual framework. However, the theories she uses have been tested and are a sound theoretical basis for her model. She wrote the conceptual framework and then evaluated it by use of an evaluation tool given to her students in the program for which the model was designed. The raw interval and nominal data were recorded in the 1972 issue of *Nursing Research,* but no statistical figures were presented to support her conclusions.

The evaluation tool combined a Likert-type scale, and a yes or no response, with written response. Reorganizing the evaluation tool could have helped support the concept with statistical evidence. But because the tool was only for evaluation and not for statistical evidence, this was not done. Because statistical evidence can provide indirect support for abstract statements, statistical test of significance could have been used to support this model's validity.[23:137] Empirical evidence is not a strong point of this conceptual model.

MAJOR CONCEPTS AND DEFINITIONS

Neuman uses a total person approach incorporating the holistic concept and an open-systems approach. The major concepts she identifies in the model (Figure 26-1) are stressors, basic structure, lines of resistance, lines of defense, degree of reaction, intervention, levels of prevention, and reconstitution.

TOTAL PERSON APPROACH. The Neuman health care system's model is a total person approach to client care aimed at providing a unifying focus for approaching varied nursing problems and for understanding man and his environment. The model is also appropriate for other health care providers.

HOLISTIC CONCEPT. The holistic concept is evident in the Neuman model because it "depicts the parts and subparts and their interrelationships for the whole of man, as a complete system."[17:11] Because it considers all variables affecting an individual, such as physiological, psychological, sociocultural, and developmental influences at any point in time, it is described as multidimensional.

OPEN-SYSTEM APPROACH. Neuman uses the open-system approach, which implies that the system is never at rest. She maintains that in any system a tendency to maintain balance (homeostasis) among the disrupting forces exists. She labels these forces *stressors,* which can be either noxious or beneficial "depending on their nature, timing, degree, and potential for ultimate positive change."[17:9] Neuman[17:9] believes "The identification of stressors and the nature of reaction or possible reaction to them is critical to systems analysis." It is the goal of nursing to identify and reduce these stressors affecting the client to provide optimal functioning.

STRESSORS. Neuman[17:14] uses Selye's definition of "stressors as tension-producing stimuli with the potential of causing disequilibrium, situational or maturational crises, or the experience of stress within an individual's life." Neuman[17:14-15] views stressors as:

1. Intrapersonal—forces occurring within the individual, e.g., conditioned responses.
2. Interpersonal—forces occurring between one or more individuals, e.g., role expectations.
3. Extrapersonal—forces occurring outside the individual, e.g., financial circumstances.

Figure 26-1. The Betty Neuman model: A total person approach to viewing patient problems.

From Neuman, B.M., & Young, R.J. (1972, May-June). A model for teaching total person approach to patient problems. *Nursing Research*, 21:265. Used with permission of B.M. Neuman.

The model represents an individual's relationship to stressors, although it could be used to study the response of a group or community to stressors. In this chapter the model will be discussed in terms of the individual.

BASIC STRUCTURE ENERGY RESOURCES. The Neuman model represents the individual by a series of circles surrounding a central core. The person is viewed as an open system in interaction with his environment. Graphically, the inner circle of the model, "basic structure energy resources," represents the basic survival factors or energy resources that are unique to the individual but within a common range of response (see Figure 26-1). These factors include mechanisms for maintenance of a normal temperature range, a genetic response pattern, and the strengths and weaknesses of the various body parts or organs.[17]

FLEXIBLE LINES OF RESISTANCE. The series of broken rings surrounding the core vary in size and distance from the center and are called the "flexible lines of resistance." These represent the internal factors that help the person to defend against a stressor. An example of this is the body's immune response system.

NORMAL LINE OF DEFENSE. The "normal line of defense" is the outer solid circle. It represents a state of wellness of the individual, or the state of adaptation the individual has maintained over time that is considered normal for him.

> This is a result or composite of several variables and behaviors such as the individual's usual coping patterns, lifestyle, developmental stage, and so forth; it is basically the way in which an individual deals with stressors while functioning within the cultural pattern in which he was born and to which he attempts to conform.[17:15]

FLEXIBLE LINES OF DEFENSE. The outer broken ring is called the "flexible line of defense." It is dynamic and can be rapidly altered over a short period of time. It is perceived as a protective buffer for preventing stressors from breaking through the solid line of defense. The relationship of the variables (physiological, psychological, sociocultural, and developmental) can affect the degree to which an individual is able to use his flexible line of defense against possible reaction to a stressor or stressors, such as loss of sleep. It is important to strengthen this flexible line of defense to prevent a possible reaction.[17]

DEGREE OF REACTION. "The model is based upon an individual's relationship to stress—his reaction to stress and factors of reconstitution—and is thought of as dynamic in nature."[17:14] Reaction variables are basic structure idiosyncrasies, natural and learned resistance, and the time of encounter with stressor.[17:13]

INTERVENTIONS. Neuman supports beginning intervention when a stressor is either suspected or identified. Interventions can occur before or after resistance lines are penetrated in both reaction and reconstitution phases. Interventions are based on degree of reaction, resources, goals, and the anticipated outcome.[17:13]

LEVELS OF PREVENTION. Neuman defines three levels of prevention: primary, secondary, and tertiary.

Primary prevention. Primary prevention (Figure 26-2) is carried out when a stressor is suspected or identified. A reaction has not yet occurred, but the degree of risk is known. Neuman[17:15] states, "The actor or intervener would perhaps attempt to reduce the possibility of the individual's encounter with the stressor or in some way attempt to strengthen the individual's flexible line of defense to decrease the possibility of a reaction."

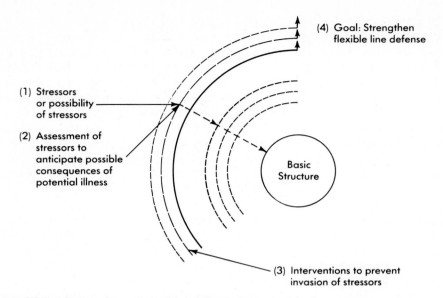

(4) Goal: Strengthen
flexible line defense

(1) Stressors
or possibility
of stressors

(2) Assessment of
stressors to
anticipate possible
consequences of
potential illness

Basic
Structure

(3) Interventions to prevent
invasion of stressors

Figure 26-2. Format for primary prevention/intervention mode.
From Neuman, B. (1982). *The Neuman systems model*. Norwalk, Conn.: Appleton-Century-Crofts. p. 24. Copyright ©
1980 by Betty Neuman. Used with permission of B.M. Neuman.

Secondary prevention. Secondary prevention (Figure 26-3) involves interventions or treatment initiated after symptoms have occurred. The individual's external and internal resources would be used in an attempt to stabilize him, or to help strengthen his internal lines of resistance to reduce the reaction.

Tertiary prevention. Tertiary prevention (Figure 26-4) is intervention following the active treatment or secondary prevention stage. It focuses on readaptation. A primary goal is to strengthen resistance to stressors by reeducation to help prevent recurrence of reaction or regression. This leads back in a circular fashion toward primary prevention. An example would be avoidance of stressors known to be hazardous to the person.

RECONSTITUTION. Reconstitution is the state of adaptation to stressors in the internal and external environment.[17:16] Reconstitution

can begin at any degree or level of reaction and may progress beyond, or stabilize somewhat below the person's previous normal line of defense. Included in reconstitution are interpersonal, intrapersonal, and extrapersonal factors that are considered within the context of physiological, psychological, sociocultural, and developmental variables.[17:13]

MAJOR ASSUMPTIONS
Nursing

Neuman believes nursing is concerned with the total person. She views nursing as a "unique profession in that it is concerned with all of the variables affecting an individual's response to stress."[17:14] Because the nurse's perception influences the care given, Neuman states that the care giver's perceptual field must be assessed as well as the client's. She has developed an assessment and intervention tool to help with this task.

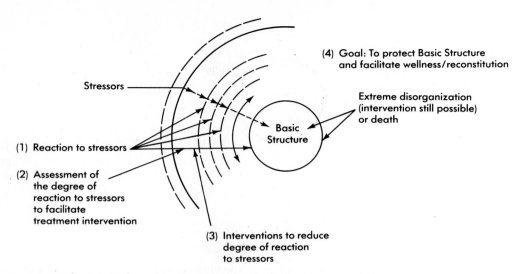

Figure 26-3. Format for secondary prevention/intervention mode.

From Neuman, B. (1982). *The Neuman systems model.* Norwalk, Conn.: Appleton-Century-Crofts. p. 24. Copyright © by Betty Neuman. Used with permission of B. Neuman.

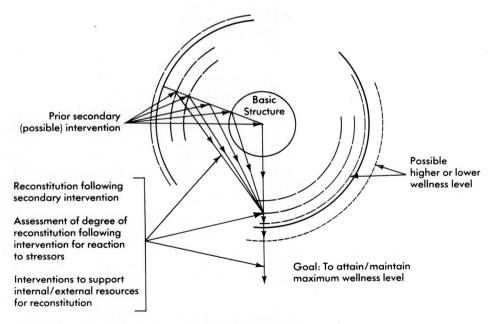

Figure 26-4. Format for tertiary prevention/intervention mode.

From Neuman, B. (1982). *The Neuman systems model.* Norwalk, Conn.: Appleton-Century-Crofts. p. 24. Copyright © 1980 by Betty Neuman. Used with permission of B. Neuman.

Person

Neuman's model presents the client as a total person. Man is a dynamic composite of inter-relationships between physiological, psychological, sociocultural, and developmental factors. Man is viewed as being in constant change or motion, "in reciprocal action with the environment."[17:9]

Health

Neuman[16:9] defines health or wellness as "the condition in which all parts and subparts (variables) are in harmony with the whole of man. Disharmony reduces the wellness state." Man is an interacting open system with his environment and is either in a dynamic state of wellness or is experiencing some degree of ill health. Health is reflected in the level of wellness. "If man's total needs are met, he is in a state of optimal wellness. Conversely, a reduced state of wellness is the result of needs not met."[17:9]

Environment

Environment is critical to Neuman's model. She states that there are both internal and external environments. The person maintains varying degrees of harmony and balance between the internal and external environment. "Environment has been conceptualized as all factors affecting and affected by the system."[17:9] It thus seems safe to assume that stressors, which are an important part of the model, make up the environment. The emphasis is on all the stressors (intrapersonal, interpersonal, extrapersonal) that might disturb the normal line of defense.

THEORETICAL ASSERTIONS

Theoretical assertions are the relationships among the essential concepts of the model. The Neuman model depicts the nurse as an active participant with the client and as "concerned with all the variables affecting an individual's response to stressors."[17:14] The client is in a re-ciprocal relationship with the environment in that "he interacts with this environment by adjusting himself to it or adjusting it to himself."[17:14]

Neuman links the four essential concepts of person, environment, health, and nursing in her statements regarding primary, secondary, and tertiary prevention.

L.O. Walker and K.C. Avant have presented additional relational statements that are specified in the model but not stated in the theory (see box on p. 321).

LOGICAL FORM

Neuman used both deductive and inductive logic in developing her model. As previously discussed, Neuman derived her model from other theories and disciplines. The model is also a product of Neuman's observations during her clinical experience in mental health nursing.[8:36]

ACCEPTANCE BY THE NURSING COMMUNITY

Neuman's model has been described as a grand nursing theory by Walker and Avant. A grand theory consists of a comprehensive conceptual framework that defines broad perspectives for practice, and includes ways of viewing nursing phenomena based on these perspectives.[25:4] Grand theories can provide a comprehensive perspective for nursing practice, education, and research and Neuman's model does.[19:7]

Practice

The Neuman systems model has been applied and adapted to various specialties and subspecialties of nursing practice. The specialties include family therapy, public health, rehabilitation, and hospital nursing. The subspecialties include pulmonary, renal, critical care, and hospital medical units. This model is an example of a conceptual framework that provides structure for development and analysis of an individual or a group of patients in the commu-

LOGICAL ADEQUACY

	RC	BER	DR	RS	TECS	PP	S	NLD	A	DEV
RC	(+)	+	(-)	(+)	(-)	?	(-)	(+)	?	?
BER		(+)	-	(+)	?	(+)	(-)	(+)	?	?
DR			(+)	-	+	(+)	(-)	(+)	?	?
RS				(+)	(-)	?	(-)	(+)	?	?
TECS					(+)	(-)	?	(-)	(-)	(-)
PP						(+)	-	(+)	?	(+)
S							(+)	(-)	?	?
NLD								(+)	?	?
A									(+)	(+)
DEV										(+)

Figure 26-5. Matrix of variables.

1. The schematic model gives some indication of relationships which are not specified verbally. Some additional relational statements which are specified in the model but not in the verbal theory are listed and diagrammed below.

    a. Reconstitution *(RC)* is positively related to basic energy resource *(BER)*

$$RC \overset{+}{\rightarrow} BER$$

    b. Degree of reaction *(DR)* is related to basic energy resources *(BER)*, resistance *(RS)*, and time of encounter with stressor *(TECS)*

$$DR \Rightarrow BER$$
$$DR \Rightarrow RS$$
$$DR \overset{+}{\rightarrow} TECS$$

Used with permission from Walker, L.O., & Avant, K.C. (1983). *Strategies for theory construction in nursing.* Norwalk, Conn.; Appleton-Century-Crofts. *Continued.*

LOGICAL ADEQUACY—cont'd

---

c. Primary prevention *(PP)* is related to a decreased encounter with stressors *(S)*

$$PP \Rightarrow S$$

d. Normal line of defense *(NLD)* varies with age *(A)* and development *(DEV)*

$$NLD \xrightarrow{?} A \qquad NLD \xrightarrow{?} DEV$$

2. The schematic is confusing.
3. There are no predictions made by the theorist herself.
4. Predictions which *could* be drawn would be highly abstract since no operational measures are specified.
5. We doubt if agreement about predictions could be reached with theory at this level of development.
6. Since this theory is derived, there is some support from Gestalt research but no testing has been done on this new derivation. In addition, it is difficult to tell if the theory is intended to be deductive.

---

nity or in an organization. One of the model's strengths is that it can be used in a variety of settings.

Using this conceptual model permits comparison of a nurse's interpretation of a problem with that of the patient, so the patient and nurse do not work on two separate problems. The role of the nurse in the model is to work with the patient to move him as far as possible along a continuum toward wellness.[15:88] Because this model requires individual interaction with the total health care system, it is indicative of the futuristic direction the nursing profession is taking. The patient is being relabeled as a consumer with individual needs and wants.[2:166]

Neuman has designed a nursing process format for use with her model. The format is systematized into three steps: nursing diagnosis, nursing goals, and nursing outcomes. Nursing diagnosis consists of obtaining a data base to determine variances from wellness. Nursing goals are then established by negotiation with the client for desired prescriptive changes to correct variances from wellness. Nursing outcomes are determined by nursing intervention through one of the three prevention modes. Evaluation then takes place either to confirm the desired outcome goals or to reformulate subsequent nursing goals.

Specifically, the Neuman model has been used in the Hospice of Windsor in Ontario, Canada, where it provided an excellent approach for organizing effective multidisciplinary assessments and interventions for individuals and families faced with life-threatening and terminal illness.[7:257] In Arlington, Pennsylvania, Diane Breckenridge adapted the model for clients with renal disorders because it provided a framework that emphasized prevention and focused on the client's perception of an optimal level of wellness. The framework was put into operation in a renal transplant unit.[3:274] The model also has been a highly successful and adaptable framework for use with clinical practice of family psychiatry. Its usefulness was demonstrated in the treatment of disordered families.[9:217,221]

Professor Patricia Babcock, chairperson for Purdue University School of Nursing in West-ville, Indiana, modified and used this model while pursuing her doctorate in education ad-ministration from Ball State in Muncie, Indiana. She applied the model in a cardiac step-down and oncology unit and found it to be an excellent structure for development in ap-proaching patient problems. She found that the guidelines from the assessment tool created an open rapport with the patient, thereby enhanc-ing overall communication. Babcock com-mented that patients are smart consumers. They no longer listen to just what the nurse or doc-tor has to say, and they desire an approach of partnership, which leads to better cooperation.[1] Because Neuman systems model can provide what patients and families desire and require, it has been accepted and adopted by the nursing community for practice. These examples are evidence of the universal appeal of this model.

Education

The model has also been widely accepted in ac-ademic circles. It has often been selected as a curriculum guide for a conceptual framework oriented more toward wellness than toward a medical model and has been used at various lev-els of nursing education.[2:170] In the associate degree program at Indiana University/Purdue University at Ft. Wayne, Indiana, one of the objectives for nursing graduates is to demon-strate ability to use the Neuman health care sys-tem in nursing practice.[11] This helps prepare the students for developing a frame of reference centered on holistic care.

Neuman's model has been selected for bac-calaureate programs on the basis of its theoret-ical and comprehensive foundation for a holistic curriculum.[13:128] In 1977 freshmen students at the University of Pittsburgh were admitted to a curriculum based on this model. The faculty had developed an integrated curriculum built around four key components of the Neuman model that helped unify their concepts: (1)

man as an open system with physiological, psy-chological, sociocultural, and developmental variables; (2) levels of prevention; (3) lines of defense; and (4) stress.*

At Northwestern State University in Shreve-port, Louisiana, the faculty determined that a systems model approach was preferred for their master's program because of the universality of its application. They chose to adapt the Neu-man model in their program for the master's clinician, the role being one of mediator be-tween stressors and the various lines of defense and resistance of the client or client system.† Many universities have adopted this model and use its conceptual framework. Acceptance by the nursing community for education therefore is evident.

Research

In 1980 a study was published by Riehl and Roy to test the usefulness of the Neuman model in nursing practice. There were two ma-jor objectives of the study:

> (1) to test the model/assessment tool for its use-fulness as a unifying method of collecting and an-alyzing data for identifying client problems; (2) to test the assessment tool for its usefulness in the identification of congruence between the client's perception of stressors and the care giver's percep-tion of client stressors.[6:163]

The study took place in a home-health agency. Results indicated that the model can help cat-egorize data for assessing and planning care and for guiding decision making and can supply a mechanism for using other health professionals' input in the assessment of the client situation.

Neuman's model can easily generate nursing research. It does this by providing a framework to develop goals for desired outcomes. An ex-ample, which Neuman suggested, of using the model is to evaluate the effects of primary pre-vention in school children. Neuman wonders

---

*Reference 12:117, 118.
†Reference 14:168-169.

how effectively the health education needs of school children are being met by the present system. If the needs are not being met, then what creative ways can nurses use to meet these needs? Another suggestion by Neuman was directed toward health alternatives available for people. She suggested that researchers devise a way to gather information about health alternatives and make it available to the client on an ongoing basis. This suggestion reflects her sensitivity to the client's needs in a dynamic state, to maintain equilibrium. Neuman's final suggestion was to institute primary prevention and aim it at the people in the 40 to 60 age range. She feels there is a gap of concern for this age group when talking in terms of offsetting disease, and sees potential for nursing research in this area. Her suggestions reflect the whole person approach with an emphasis on primary prevention.[20] Unpublished research projects are currently underway. Acceptance by the nursing community for research applying this model is in the beginning stages and positive.

FURTHER DEVELOPMENT

Three suggestions for further development are: (1) to simplify the schematic model, if appropriate based on proven research; (2) to support Neuman's conceptual framework with empirical research; and (3) to elaborate on man's response to various stressors using Gestalt's theory.

Models are simplified representations of a theory.[10:104] Because Neuman's complete schematic model is somewhat complex and occasionally arduous to follow, it is not a simplified representation of her conceptual framework. As her framework develops into a theory, perhaps her model will simplify to the point of enhanced understanding.

Because research evidence to support validity is a fundamental prerequisite to deciding whether a theory can be applied to practice, development of sound statistical research is suggested.[5:177] A suggestion would be to develop

an evaluation tool using a Likert-type scale and have faculty and students in various schools of nursing answer specific questions concerning various aspects of the model. The questionnaire would have to be broken down into concepts, and the questions reflect evaluation of how well the model was serving their needs. This study could potentially enhance the empirical precision of the framework if the inferences were favorable. A tool has been designed and implemented at Cesil Community College in North East, Maryland.

Another area of development could be expanding the model regarding identification of what a patient does when stressors come into existence simultaneously. Researchers could use Gestalt theory and define how an organism operates within a hierarchy of values or priorities. With Gestalt theory, the dominant need of the organism, at any time, becomes the foreground figure. The other needs recede, at least temporarily, into the background.[22:7]

CRITIQUE

Neuman developed this model as a frame of reference for nursing. The theme of stress and man's adaptation to stress permeates her framework. Her model is abstract and general. Therefore it is classified as a grand theory.

Clarity

Neuman[21:267] states that the simple terminology of the framework enabled students to adapt it to a wide variety of settings. The terminology is simple, but a few of the concepts were not well defined. For example, her definition of environment included internal and external forces. Because these forces are not clearly defined, it is unclear what *internal* and *external* mean. The concept of reconstitution is confusing as a result of its various innerlocking parts. Neuman borrowed concepts from other disciplines and defined them clearly, using their definitions and concepts. The diagram representing the various concepts is complex, but it becomes clear when broken down and examined. Based on the diagram, the model can be followed from Primary to Tertiary prevention, then back to Primary prevention. Neuman sets out to provide a frame of reference for nursing related to universal stressors, reaction to stressors, and reconstitution factors following a reaction. The theme of stressors and reaction to them remain consistent in the framework. Because of the lack of explanation of some definitions, this model is considered semiclear.

Simplicity

Many relationships comprise this model; they are organized in a complex fashion and tend to overlap one another. The concepts are coalesced, but a loss of theoretical meaning would occur if they were completely separated. The model can be used to describe the systems concept of nursing and can describe various other systems as well. It can be used to explain man's dynamic state of equilibrium and the reaction of stressors as a result of environmental conflict, but this explanation renders itself complex. Using primary prevention within the framework, one can predict the origin of stressors. The model can be used to describe, explain, or predict, but not in a simplified manner. Because of the complex nature of this model, it cannot be described as a simple framework.

Generality

This framework has been used in various nursing situations and is general enough to be useful in most health care settings. The nursing care settings it is applicable to include anything from critical care to community nursing in any time frame. Other related fields can use this framework because of its encompassing emphasis on man as a whole. The goal of the model is to set forth a structure that depicts the part and subparts and their relationships for the whole of man as a complete system. This is a justifiable nursing goal because it views man as a whole and can easily be incorporated into the nursing process. Some concepts are broad and represent the phenomenon of man, but others are more definitive and identify specific modes of action, such as primary prevention. The subgoals can be identified as broad nursing actions. Because of the broad scope of this framework, it can be considered general.

Empirical Precision

To date, the framework has not been thoroughly tested. It contains highly abstract concepts. Some concepts are identifiable and could be tested to determine empirical validation. The testing that has occurred using this model has found it to be favorable. The conclusions from the research, however, are based only on observation, and no recorded statistical inferences. As a result of minimal research reports, Neuman's framework lacks empirical evidence.

Derivable Consequences

To achieve valued nursing outcomes, this conceptual framework provides a complete evaluation of the whole person. It provides the nurse with a framework for a dynamic patient relationship that is in constant change, thereby making the consequences important to nursing. It provides growth in nursing by using the systems theory, whereby everything is in progressive development. It is a useful guide for research because the nurse can evaluate care based on what stressors were affected by intervention. If nursing practice were based on this framework, better nurse-patient communication would evolve. The development of ideas is evident with the concept of energy as input and output, providing a basis for new ideas. The model can provide a framework for nursing as a separate entity or for other related health care fields. Because of the framework's generality, it is questionable whether it contributes to nursing as a unique body of knowledge.

The nursing issue in Neuman's work is traditionalism versus progressive development. Her framework easily provides a basis for progressive development by enabling man to create and shape reality in his desired direction.

REFERENCES

1. Babcock, P., (1984, June 10). Telephone interview.
2. Beitler, B., Tkachuck, B., & Aamodt, D. (1980). The Neuman model applied to mental health, community health, and medical-surgical nursing. In J.P. Reihl, & C. Roy (Eds.), *Conceptual models for nursing practice* (2nd ed.). New York: Appleton-Century-Crofts.
3. Breckenridge, D.M. (1982). Adaptation of the Neuman systems model for the renal client. In B. Neuman, *The Neuman systems model: Application to nursing education and practice*. Norwalk, Conn.: Appleton-Century-Crofts.
4. Caplan, G. (1964). *Principles of preventive psychiatry*. New York: Basic Books.
5. Chinn, P.L., & Jacobs, M.K. (1983). *Theory and nursing: A systematic approach*. St. Louis: C.V. Mosby.
6. Craddock, R.B., & Stanhope, M.K. (1980). The Neuman health care systems model: Recommended adaptation. In J.P. Reihl, & C. Roy, *Conceptual models for nursing practice,* New York, Appleton-Century-Crofts, pp. 159-169.
7. Echlin, J.D. (1982). Pallative care and the Neuman model. In B. Neuman, *The Neuman systems model: Application to nursing education and practice*. Norwalk, Conn.: Appleton-Century-Crofts.
8. Fawcett, J., et al. (1982). A framework for analysis and evaluation of conceptual models of nursing with an analysis and evaluation of the Neuman systems model. In B. Neuman, *The Neuman systems model: Application to nursing education and practice*. Norwalk, Conn.: Appleton-Century-Crofts.
9. Graff, G.D., & Graff, H. (1982). The Neuman model adapted to family therapy. In B. Neuman, *The Neuman systems model: Application to nursing education and practice*. Norwalk, Conn.: Appleton-Century-Crofts.
10. Hardy, M. (1974, March-April). Theories: Components, development, evaluation. *Nursing Research,* 23(2):100-107.
11. Indiana University, Purdue University at Ft. Wayne. (1983). *Behavioral objectives for the associate degree program.*
12. Knox, J.E., Kilchenstein, L., & Yakulis, I.M. (1982). Utilization of the Neuman model in an integreated baccalaureate program: University of Pittsburgh. In B. Neuman, *The Neuman systems model: Application to nursing education and practice*. Norwalk, Conn.: Appleton-Century-Crofts.
13. Lebold, M.M., & Davis, L.H. (1982). A baccalaureate nursing curriculum based on the Neuman systems model: Saint Xavier College. In B. Neuman, *The Neuman systems model: Application to nursing education and practice*. Norwalk, Conn.: Appleton-Century-Crofts.
14. Moxley, P.A., & Allen, M.H. (1982). The Neuman systems model approach in a master's degree program: Northwestern State University. In B. Neuman, *The Neuman systems model: Application to nursing education and practice*. Norwalk, Conn.: Appleton-Century-Crofts.
15. Neal, M.C. (1982). Nursing care plans and the Neuman systems model II. In B. Neuman, *The Neuman systems model: Application to nursing education and practice*. Norwalk, Conn.: Appleton-Century-Crofts.
16. Neuman, B.M. (1977, Jan. 17). An explanation of the Betty Neuman Nursing Model. Paper presented to Indiana University-Purdue University at Fort Wayne, Indiana.
17. Neuman, B. (1982). *The Neuman systems model: Application to nursing education and practice*. Norwalk, Conn.: Appleton-Century-Crofts.
18. Neuman, B. (1983). Family interaction using the Betty Neuman health care systems model. In I.W. Clements, & F.B. Roberts, *Family health: A theoretical approach to nursing care*. New York: John Wiley & Sons.
19. Neuman, B. (1983). Curriculum vitae.
20. Neuman B. (1984, June 3). Telephone interview.
21. Neuman, B.M., & Young, R.J. (1972, May-June). A model for teaching total person approach to patient problems. *Nursing Research,* 21:264-269.
22. Perls, F. (1973). *The Gestalt approach: Eye witness to therapy*. Palo Alto, Calif.: Science and Behavior Books.
23. Reynolds, P.D. (1971). *A primer in theory construction*. Indianapolis, Ind.: Bobbs-Merrill.
24. Selye, H. (1974). *Stress without distress*. Philadelphia: J.B. Lippincott.
25. Walker, L.O., & Avant, K. (1983). *Strategies for theory construction in nursing*. Norwalk, Conn.: Appleton-Century-Crofts.

BIBLIOGRAPHY
Primary Sources
Books

Neuman, B. (1982). *The Neuman systems model: Application to nursing education and practice.* Norwalk, Conn.: Appleton-Century-Crofts.

Neuman, B., Deloughery, G.W., & Gebbie, M. (1971). *Consultation and community organization in community mental health nursing.* Baltimore: Williams & Williams.

Book Chapters

Neuman, B. (1983). Analysis and application of Neuman's health care model. In I.W. Clements, & F.B. Roberts, *Family health: A theoretical approach to nursing care.* New York: John Wiley & Sons. pp. 353-367.

Neuman, B. (1983). Family interaction using the Betty Neuman health care systems model. In I.W. Clements, & F.B. Roberts, *Family health: A theoretical approach to nursing care.* New York: John Wiley & Sons. pp. 239-254.

Neuman, B. (1980). The Betty Neuman health care systems model: A total person approach to patient problems. In J.P. Riehl, & C. Roy (eds.), *Conceptual models for nursing practice* (2nd ed.). New York: Appleton-Century-Crofts. pp. 119-134.

Neuman, B. (1974). The Betty Neuman health care systems model: A total person approach to patient problems. In J.P. Riehl, & C. Roy, (eds.), *Conceptual models for nursing practice.* New York: Appleton-Century-Crofts. pp. 94-104.

Neuman, B., & Wyatt, M. (1980). The Neuman stress/adaptation systems approach to education for nurse administrators. In J.P. Riehl, & C. Roy (Eds.), *Conceptual models for nursing practice* (2nd ed.). New York: Appleton-Century-Crofts. pp. 142-150.

Articles

Neuman, B. (1974, Jan.). Teaching organizational concepts to nurses in community mental health. *Journal of Nursing Education, 13:*1.

Neuman, B.M., Deloughery, G.W., & Gebbie, K.M. (1970, Jan.-Feb.). Levels of utilization: Nursing specialists in community mental health. *Journal of Psychiatric Nursing and Mental Health Services, 8*(1):37-39.

Neuman, B.M., Deloughery, G.W., & Gebbie, K.M. (1970). Changes in problem solving ability among nurses receiving mental health consultation: A pilot study. *Communicating Nursing Research, 3:*41-52.

Neuman, B.M., Deloughery, G.W., & Gebbie, K.M. (1971, Oct). Nurses in community mental health: An informative interpretation for employees of professional nurses. *Public Personnel Review, 32*(4).

Neuman, B.M., Deloughery, G.W., & Gebbie, K.M. (1972, Feb.). Mental health consultation as a means of improving problem solving ability in work groups: A pilot study. *Comparative Group Studies, 3*(1):81-97.

Neuman, B., & Wyatt, M.A. (1981, Jan.). Prospects for change: Some evaluative reflections by faculty members from one articulated baccalaureate program. *Journal of Nursing Education, 20:*40-46.

Neuman, B.M., & Young, R.J. (1972, May-June). A model for teaching total person approach to patient problems. *Nursing Research, 21:*264-269.

Professional Papers

Emerging leadership in mental health: Preparation of community mental health sapecialists. Presented at World Mental Health Assembly, Washington, D.C., November 19, 1969.

Improved utilization of nurses in community mental health. Position paper presented to the task force for Development of the California State Plan for Health, Sacramento, November 13, 1970.

A pilot study to measure change in problem solving ability among nurses receiving mental health consultation. Presented at the Western Interstate Commission for Higher Education Conference on Communicating Research in Nursing, Salt Lake City, Utah, April 30, 1970, and at the State Department of Mental Health Center for Training in Community Psychiatry, Los Angeles, California, May 11, 1970.

Toward healthy, productive group interaction. Presented to the Psychiatric Mental Health Conference Group, California Nurses' Association Convention, Anaheim, California, March 4, 1971.

A systems approach to the integrity of the client/client system based on the Neuman model. Presented at the International Congress on Applied Systems Research and Cybernetics, Acapulco, Mexico, December 12-15, 1980.

Correspondence

Neuman, B. (1984, June 4). Personal correspondence.

Interview

Neuman, B. (1984, June 3). Telephone interview.

Secondary Sources
Book Reviews

Hawkins, J. (1982). *The Neuman systems model: Application to nursing education and practice.* *Western Journal of Nursing Research, 5:*182-183, Spring 1983.

Varricchio, C.G. (1982). The Neuman systems model: Application to nursing education and practice. *American Journal of Nursing, 83:*963-964, June 1983.

Book Chapters

Arndt, C. (1982). Systems theory and educational programs for nursing service administration. In B. Neuman, *The Neuman systems model: Application to nursing education and practice,* Norwalk, Conn.: Appleton-Century-Crofts. pp. 182-187.

Arndt, C. (1982). Systems concepts for management of stress in complex health-care organizations. In B. Neuman, *The Neuman systems model: Application to nursing education and practice,* Norwalk, Conn.: Appleton-Century-Crofts. pp. 107-116.

Baker, N.A. (1982). The Neuman systems model as a conceptual framework for continuing education in the work place. In B. Neuman, *The Neuman systems model: Application to nursing education and practice,* Norwalk, Conn.: Appleton-Century-Crofts. pp. 241-256.

Baker, N.A. (1982). Use of the Neuman model in planning for the psychological needs of the respiratory disease patient. In B. Neuman, *The Neuman systems model: Application to nursing education and practice.* Norwalk, Conn.: Appleton-Century-Crofts. pp. 260-266.

Balch, C. (1974). Breaking the lines of resistance. In J.P. Riehl, & C. Roy, *Conceptual models for nursing practice.* New York: Appleton-Century-Crofts. pp. 130-134.

Beitler, B., Tkachuck, B., & Aamodt, D. (1980). The Neuman model applied to mental health, community health, and medical-surgical nursing. In J.P. Riehl, and C. Roy (Eds.), *Conceptual models for nursing practice* (2nd ed.). New York: Appleton-Century-Crofts. pp. 170-178.

Benedict, M.B., & Sproles, J.B. (1982). Application of the Neuman model to public health nursing practice. In B. Neuman, *The Neuman systems model: Application to nursing education and practice.* Norwalk, Conn.: Appleton-Century-Crofts. pp. 223-240.

Bower, F.L. (1982). Curriculum development and the Neuman Model. In B. Neuman, *The Neuman systems model: Application to nursing education and practice.* Norwalk, Conn.: Appleton-Century-Crofts. pp. 94-99.

Bowman, G.E. (1982). The Neuman assessment tool adapted for child day-care centers. In Neuman, B., *The Neuman systems model: Application to nursing education and practice,* Norwalk, Conn.: Appleton-Century-Crofts. pp. 324-334.

Breckenridge, D.M. (1982). Adaptation of the Neuman systems model for the renal client. In B. Neuman, *The Neuman systems model: Application to nursing education and practice,* Norwalk, Conn.: Appleton-Century-Crofts. pp. 267-277.

Cardona, V.D. (1983). Client rehabilitation and the Neuman model. In B. Neuman, *The Neuman systems model: Application to nursing education and practice.* Norwalk, Conn.: Appleton-Century-Crofts. pp. 278-290.

Clark, F. (1982). The Neuman systems model: A clinical application for psychiatric nurse practitioners. In B. Neuman, *The Neuman systems model: Application to nursing education and practice,* Norwalk, Conn.: Appleton-Century-Crofts. pp. 335-354.

Conners, V.L. (1982). Teaching the Neuman systems model: An aproach to student and faculty development. In B. Neuman, *The Neuman systems model: Application to nursing educaiton and practice.* Norwalk, Conn.: Appleton-Century-Crofts. pp. 176-181.

Conners, V., Harmon, V.M., & Langford, R.W. (1982). Course development and implementaiton using the Neuman systems model as a framework: Texas Woman's University (Houston Campus). In B. Neuman, *The Neuman systems model: Application to nursing education and practice.* Norwalk, Conn.: Appleton-Century-Crofts. pp. 153-158.

Craddock, R.B., & Stanhope, M.K. (1980). The Neuman health care systems model: Recommended adaptation. In J.P. Riehl, & C. Roy, (Eds.), *Conceptual models for nursing practice* (2nd ed.). New York: Appleton-Century-Crofts. pp. 159-169.

Cunningham, S.G. (1982). The Neuman model applied to an acute care setting: Pain. In B. Neuman,

The Neuman systems model: Application to nursing education and practice. Norwalk, Conn.: Appleton-Century-Crofts. pp. 291-296.

Davis, L.H. (1982). Aging: A social and preventive perspective. In B. Neuman, *The Neuman systems model: Application to nursing education and practice.* Norwalk, Conn.: Appleton-Century-Crofts. pp. 211-216.

Dunbar, S.B. (1982). Critical care and the Neuman ··model. In B. Neuman, *The Neuman systems model: Application to nursing education and practice.* Norwalk, Conn.: Appleton-Century-Crofts. pp. 297-307.

Echlin, D.J. (1982). Palliative care and the Neuman model. In B. Neuman, *The Neuman systems model: Application to nursing education and practice.* Norwalk, Conn.: Appleton-Century-Crofts. pp. 257-259.

Fawcett, J. (1984). Neuman systems model. In Fawcett, J., *Analysis and evaluation of conceptual models of nursing.* Philadelphia: F.A. Davis. pp. 154-174.

Fawcett, J. et al. (1982). A framework for analysis and evaluation of conceptual models of nursing with an analysis and evaluation of the Neuman Systems Model. In B. Neuman, *The Neuman systems model: Application to nursing education and practice.* Norwalk, Conn.: Appleton-Century-Crofts. pp. 30-43.

Goldblum-Graff, D., & Graff, H. (1982). The Neuman model adapted to family therapy. In B. Neuman, *The Neuman systems model: Application to nursing education and practice,* Norwalk, Conn.: Appleton-Century-Crofts. pp. 217-222.

Gunter, L.M. (1982). Application of the Neuman systems model to gerontic nursing. In B. Neuman, *The Neuman systems model: Application to nursing education and practice,* Norwalk, Conn.: Appleton-Century-Crofts. pp. 196-210.

Harty, M.B. (1982). Continuing education in nursing and the Neuman model. In B. Neuman, *The Neuman systems model: Application to nursing education and practice.* Norwalk, Conn.: Appleton-Century-Crofts. pp. 100-106.

Hoffman, M.K. (1982). From model to theory construction: An analysis of the Neuman health-care systems model. In B. Neuman, *The Neuman systems model: Application to nursing education and practice.* Norwalk, Conn.: Appleton-Century-Crofts. pp. 44-54.

Johnson, M.N., et al. (1982). Use of the Neuman health-care systems model in the master's curriculum: Texas Woman's University. In B. Neuman, *The Neuman systems model: Application to nursing education and practice.* Norwalk, Conn.: Appleton-Century-Crofts. pp. 130-152.

Knox, J.E., Kilchenstein, L., & Yakulis, I.M. (1982). Utilization of the Neuman model in an integrated baccalaureate program: University of Pittsburgh. In B. Neuman, *The Neuman systems model: Application to nursing education and practice.* Norwalk, Conn.: Appleton-Century-Crofts. pp. 117-123.

Lebold, M., & Davis, L. (1980). A baccalaureate nursing curriculum based on the Neuman health systems model. In J.P. Riehl, & C. Roy (Eds.), *Conceptual models for nursing practice* (2nd ed.). New York: Appleton-Century-Crofts. pp. 151-158.

Lebold, M.M., & Davis, L.H. (1982). A baccalaureate nursing curriculum based on the Neuman systems model: Saint Xavier College. In B. Neuman, *The Neuman systems model: Application to nursing education and practice.* Norwalk, Conn.: Appleton-Century-Crofts. pp. 124-129.

McInerey, K.A. (1982). The Neuman systems model applied to critical care nursing of cardiac surgery clients. In B. Neuman, *The Neuman systems model: Application to nursing education and practice.* Norwalk, Conn.: Appleton-Century-Crofts. pp. 308-315.

Mayers, M.A., & Watson, A.B. (1982). Nursing care plans and the Neuman systems model. In B. Neuman, *The Neuman systems model: Application to nursing education and practice.* Norwalk, Conn.: Appleton-Century-Crofts. pp. 69-84.

Moxley, P.A., & Allen, L.M.H. (1982). The Neuman systems model approach in a master's degree program: Northwestern State University. In B. Neuman, *The Neuman systems model. Application to nursing education and practice.* Norwalk, Conn.: Appleton-Century-Crofts. pp. 168-175.

Neal, M.C. (1982). Nursing care plans and the Neuman systems model: II. In B. Neuman, *The Neuman systems model: Application to nursing education and practice.* Norwalk, Conn.: Appleton-Century-Crofts. pp. 85-93.

Pinkerton, A. (1974). Use of the Neuman model in a home health-care agency. In J.P. Riehl, & C. Roy (Eds.), *Conceptual models for nursing practice.* New York: Appleton-Century-Crofts. pp. 122-129.

Reed, K. (1982). The Neuman systems model: A basis for family psychosocial assessment and intervention. In B. Neuman, *The Neuman systems model: Application to nursing education and practice*. Norwalk, Conn.: Appleton-Century-Crofts. pp. 188-195.

Rice, M.J. (1982). The Neuman systems model applied in a hospital medical unit. In B. Neuman, *The Neuman systems model: Application to nursing education and practice*. Norwalk, Conn.: Appleton-Century-Crofts. pp. 310-323.

Thibodeau, J.A. (1983). A systems model: The Neuman model. In J.A. Thibodeau, *Nursing models: Analysis and evaluation*. Monterey, Calif.: Wadsworth. pp. 105-123.

Tollett, S.M. (1982). Teaching geriatrics and gerontology: Use of the Neuman systems model. In B. Neuman, *The Neuman systems model: Application to nursing education and practice*. Norwalk, Conn.: Appleton-Century-Crofts. pp. 157-164.

Venable, J. (1974). The Neuman health-care systems model: An analysis. In J.P. Riehl, & C. Roy (Eds.), *Conceptual models for nursing practice* New York: Appleton-Century-Crofts. pp. 115-121.

Venable, J.F. (1980). The Neuman health-care systems model: An analysis. In J.P. Riehl, & C. Roy (Eds.), *Conceptual models for nursing practice* (2nd ed.), New York: Appleton-Century-Crofts. pp. 135-141.

Vokaty, D.A. (1982). The Neuman systems model applied to the clinical nurse specialist role. In B. Neuman, *The Neuman systems model: Application to nursing education and practice*. Norwalk, Conn.: Appleton-Century-Crofts. pp. 165-167.

Whall, A. (1983). The Betty Neuman health care systems model. In J. Fitzpatrick, & A.L. Whall (Eds.), *Conceptual models of nursing analysis and application*. Bowie, Md.: Robert J. Brady. pp. 204-219.

Walker, L.O., & Avant, K.C. (1983). Theory analysis: The Betty Neuman health care systems model: A total person approach to patient problems. In L.A. Walker, & K.C. Avant, *Strategies for theory construction in nursing*. Norwalk, Conn.: Appleton-Century-Crofts. pp. 133-143.

Ziegler, S.M. (1982). Taxonomy for nursing diagnosis derived from the Neuman systems model. In B. Neuman, *The Neuman systems model: Application to nursing education and practice*. Norwalk, Conn.: Appleton-Century-Crofts. pp. 55-68.

Articles

Johnson, P.T. (1983). Black hypertension: A transcultural case study using the Betty Neuman model of nursing care. *Issues in Health Care, 4*:191-210.

Tlaskund, J.H. (1980). Areas in theory development. *Advances in Nursing Science, 3*:1-7.

Utz, S.W. (1980). Applying the Neuman Model to nursing practice with hypertensive clients. *Cardiovascular Nursing, 16*:29-34.

Dissertation

Zimmer, M.M. (1982). *Providing patients with information prior to surgery and the reported frequency of coping behaviors and development of symptoms following surgery*. Doctoral dissertation. University of Pennsylvania.

Interview

Babcock, P. (1984, June 10). Telephone interview.

Unpublished papers

Babcock, B. *Euthanasia and the Neuman model.*

Beaman, C. *The leukemia client and the Neuman model.*

Burton, C. *The Neuman systems model: Application with black clients and their families.*

Crow, S. *Client advocacy using the Neuman total person approach: A nursing art.*

Edwards, B. *The Neuman model applied in a community mental health partial hospitalization program.*

Green, P. *A modified assessment-intervention tool for the Neuman systems model used with colostomy patients.*

Lassan, R. *Use of the Neuman systems model in the care of the high-risk newborn.*

Lowry, L. *Application of the Neuman systems model to a clinical study: Ego functions in normal pregnant women.*

Vanore, N. *Application of the Neuman systems model to an acute drug psychosis in a psychiatric clinical situation.*

Wardian, J. *Child abuse and the Neuman model.*

Educational Programs Using the Neuman Model

Aarhus University, School of Nursing, Aarhus, Denmark, Master's level.

Delta State College, Cleveland, Mississippi, Baccalaureate program.

Indiana University-Purdue University at Fort Wayne, Indiana, School of Nursing. Associate degree program.

Medical University of South Carolina, Charleston.

Methodist Central Hospitals of Memphis, Nursing Diploma School, Memphis, Tennessee.

Neuman College, Aston, Pennsylvania. Baccalaureate program.

Northwestern State University of Louisiana, Shreveport. Graduate program.

Saint Xavier College, School of Nursing, Chicago, Illinois. Baccalaureate program.

Texas Women's University at Dallas and Houston. Graduate program.

University of Missouri, School of Nursing, Kansas City, Missouri. Master's program.

University of Ottawa, Public Health and Perinatal Nursing, Ottawa, Canada. Master's level.

University of Pittsburgh, School of Nursing, Pittsburgh, Pennsylvania. Baccalaureate program.

University of Puerto Rico, School of Nursing, San Juan, Puerto Rico. Baccalaureate and master's programs.

Clinical Agencies Using the Neuman Model

Boston City Health Department, Community health nursing health and hospitals Boston, Mass.

Copenhagen Public Health, Department of Nursing, Copenhagen, Denmark.

Mercy Catholic Medical Center, Fitzgerald Mercy Division, Nursing Service Department, Darby, Pennsylvania.

Regional Perinatal Education Program of Eastern Ontario, Nursing Department, Ottawa, Ontario, Canada.

Rehabilitation Institute of the South, Nursing Department, Shreveport, Louisiana.

UNIT V

Energy Fields

Myra Estrin Levine

Four Conservation Principles

Karen J. Foli, Tamara Johnson, Ann Marriner, Mary Carolyn Poat,
LaDema Poppa, Susan T. Zoretich

CREDENTIALS AND BACKGROUND OF THE THEORIST

Myra Estrin Levine obtained a diploma from Cook County School of Nursing in 1944, an S.B. from the University of Chicago in 1949, an M.S.N. from Wayne State University in 1962, and has taken postgraduate courses at the University of Chicago.[27] Hutchins' curriculum was being taught to undergraduate students at

The authors wish to express appreciation to Myra Levine for critiquing the chapter.

that time. All students took a year-long survey in the biological, physical, and social sciences and the humanities. The students read and analyzed primary work under the guidance of distinguished professors. Irene Beland became Levine's mentor while she was a graduate student at Wayne State and directed her attention to many of the authors who greatly influenced her thinking.[28,29]

Levine has enjoyed a varied career. She has been a private duty nurse (1944), a civilian nurse in the U.S. Army (1945), a preclinical instructor in the physical sciences at Cook County (1947-1950), the director of Nursing at Drexel Home in Chicago (1950-1951), and a surgical supervisor at the University of Chicago Clinics (1951-1952) and at Henry Ford Hospital in Detroit (1956-1962). She worked her way up the academic ranks at Bryan Memorial Hospital in Lincoln, Nebraska (1951), Cook County School of Nursing (1963-1967), Loyola University (1967-1973), Rush University (1974-1977), and the University of Illinois (1962-1963, 1977 to present). She chaired the Department of Clinical Nursing at Cook County School of Nursing (1963-1967) and coordinated the graduate nursing program in oncology at Rush University (1974-1977). Levine was the director of the Department of Continuing Education at Evanston Hospital (March-June 1974) and a consultant to the department (July 1974-1976). She became an adjunct associate professor of Humanistic Studies at the University of Illinois in 1981. In 1974 Levine went to Tel-Aviv University, Israel, as visiting associate professor and returned as a visiting professor in 1982. She was also a visiting professor at Recanati School of Nursing, Ben Gurion University of the Negev, Beer Sheva, Israel (March-April, 1982).

Levine has received numerous honors, including being a charter fellow of the American Academy of Nursing (1973), honorary membership in the American Mental Health Aid to Israel (1976), and honorary recognition from the Illinois Nurses' Association. She was the first recipient of the Elizabeth Russell Belford Award for excellence in teaching from Sigma Theta Tau (1977). Both the first and second editions in her book, *Introduction to Clinical Nursing*, received AJN Book of the Year awards and her 1971 book, *Renewal for Nursing*, was translated into Hebrew.[27]

Levine is an active leader in the American Nurses' Association and the Illinois Nurses' Association. A dynamic speaker, she is a frequent presentor on programs, workshops, seminars, and panels, and a prolific writer regarding nursing and education. Although she never in-

tended to develop theory, she provided an organizational structure for teaching medical-surgical nursing and a stimulus for theory development. "The Four Conservation Principles of Nursing"[20] was the first statement of the conservation principles. Other preliminary work included "Adaptation and Assessment: A Rationale for Nursing Intervention,"[19] "For Lack of Love Alone,"[21] and "The Pursuit of Wholeness."[22] The first edition of her book using the conservation principles, *Introduction to Clinical Nursing*, was published in 1969. She addressed the consequences of the four conservation principles in "Holistic Nursing."[23] The second edition of the book was published in 1973. Since then, Levine[25,26] has presented about the conservation principles at nurse theory conferences, some of which have been audiotaped,[25] and at the Allentown College of St. Francis de Sales Conferences[26] in April 1984.

THEORETICAL SOURCES

Levine learned historical viewpoints of diseases and that the way people think about disease changes over time from Beland's presentation of the theory of specific causation and multiple factors. Beland directed Levine's attention to numerous authors who became influential in her thinking, including Kurt Goldstein,[12] Sir Arthur Sherrington,[35] and Rene Dubos.[5,6] Levine uses James E. Gibson's definition[11] of perceptual systems, Erik Erikson's differentiation[8,9] between total and whole, Hans Selye's stress theory,[34] and M. Bates' models[1] of external environment. Levine is proud that Martha Rogers was her first editor.[28,29]

USE OF EMPIRICAL EVIDENCE

Levine believes that specific nursing activities can be deduced from scientific principles. The scientific theoretical sources have been well researched. She based much of her work on accepted science principles and a natural law, conservation of energy.[30,31]

MAJOR CONCEPTS AND DEFINITIONS

HOLISTIC. "Whole, health, hale are all derivations of the Anglo-Saxon word, Hal."[26] Levine* quotes Erikson, who says, "Wholeness emphasizes a sound, organic, progressive, mutuality between diversified functions and parts within an entirety, the boundaries of which are open and fluent."

HOLISM. Holism means that "human beings are more than and different from the sum of their parts."† "Perceiving the 'wholes' depends upon recognizing the organization and interdependence of observable phenomena."[4:255]

INTEGRITY. Integrity is from the Latin *integer,* meaning *one.*[25]

CONSERVATION. Conservation is from the Latin word *conservatio,* meaning *to keep together.*[15,24,25]

Levine's model[24,29] stresses nursing interactions and interventions that are intended "to keep together the unique and individual resources that each individual brings to his predicament." Those interactions are based on the scientific background of the conservation principles. Nursing care is based on scientific knowledge and nursing skills. There are four conservation principles.

CONSERVATION PRINCIPLES

Conservation of energy. The individual requires a balance of energy and a constant renewal of energy in order to maintain life activities. That energy is challenged by processes such as healing and aging. This second law of thermodynamics applies to everything in the universe, including people.

Conservation of structural integrity. Healing is a process of restoring structural integrity. Nurses should limit the amount of tissue involved in disease by early recognition of functional changes and by nursing interventions.

Conservation of personal integrity. Self-worth and a sense of identity are important. Nurses can show patients respect by calling them by name, respecting their wishes, valuing personal possessions, providing privacy during procedures, supporting their defenses, and teaching them.

Conservation of social integrity. Life gains meaning through social communities, and health is socially determined. Nurses fulfill professional roles, provide for family members, assist with religious needs, and use interpersonal relationships to conserve social integrity.*

ADAPTATION. "Adaptation is a process of change whereby the individual retains his integrity within the realities of his environment."† Some adaptations are successful. Some are not. Adaptation is a matter of degree, not an all-or-nothing process.† Change is selective, not random. The outcomes of the change can sometimes be predicted; when it is, it can be observed and measured.

ENVIRONMENT. Environment is "where we are constantly and actively involved."[29] The person and his relationship to the environment is what counts.[29]

Levine also views each individual as having his own environment, both internally and externally. The internal environment can be related

---

*References 8:92; 22:94; 26.
†References 23:253; 33:146.

*References 21; 22:13-18; 29.
†References 24:11; 29.

by nurses as the physiological and pathophysiological aspects of the patient. Levine uses a definition of the external environment from Bates, who suggests there are three levels: perceptual, operational, and conceptual. The perceptual level includes the aspects of the world about us that we are able to intercept and interpret with our sense organs. The operational level contains things that affect us physically even though we cannot directly perceive them, such as microorganisms. At the conceptual level, the environment is constructed from cultural patterns, characterized by a spiritual existence, and mediated by the symbols of language, thought, and history.[24:12] There are four levels of integration that safeguard the end and help a person maintain his integrity or wholeness.[24:9]

ORGANISMIC RESPONSE. The capacity of the individual to adapt to his environmental condition has been called the organismic response. It can be divided into four levels of integration: fight or flight, inflammatory response, response to stress, and perceptual response.

Fight or flight. The most primitive response is the flight or fight syndrome. The individual perceives that he is threatened, whether or not a threat does actually exist. Hospitalization, illness, and new experiences elicit a response. The individual responds by being on the alert to find more information and to assure his safety and well-being.

Inflammatory response. This is a defense mechanism to protect the self from insult in a hostile environment. It is a way of healing. This response uses available energy to remove or keep out unwanted irritants or pathogens. But it is limited in time because it drains the individual's energy reserves. Environmental control is important.

Response to stress. Selye described the stress response syndrome as predictable nospecifically induced organismic changes. The wear and tear of life is recorded on the tissues and reflects long-term hormonal responses to life experiences that cause structural changes. It is characterized by irreversibility and influences the way patients respond to nursing care.

Sensory response. This response is based on the individual's perceptual awareness. It occurs only as the individual experiences the world around him. This response is used by the individual to seek and maintain safety for himself. It is information seeking.*

TROPHICOGNOSIS. Levine recommended trophicognosis as an alternative to nursing diagnosis. It is a scientific method to reach a nursing care judgment.[18]

MAJOR ASSUMPTIONS

Introduction to Clinical Nursing is a text for beginning nursing students that uses the conservation principles as an organizing framework. Therefore Levine does not specifically identify her assumptions.

Nursing

"Nursing is a human interaction."[24:1] "Professional nursing should be reserved for those few who can complete a graduate program as demanding as that expected of professionals in any other discipline. . . . There will be very few professional nurses."[17:214] "Nursing practice—and this includes the teaching of nurses—has always mirrored prevailing theories of health and disease."[19:2450] "It is the nurse's task to bring a body of scientific principles on which decisions depend into the precise situation which she shares with the patient. Sensitive observation and the selection of relevant data from the basis for her assessment of his nursing requirements."[19:2452] "The nurse participates actively in every patient's environment, and much

---

*References 20:95-96; 21; 29.

of what she does supports his adjustments as he struggles in the predicament of illness."[19:2452] The essence of Levine's theory is that "When nursing intervention influences adaptation favorably, or toward renewed social well-being, then the nurse is acting in a therapeutic sense; when the response is unfavorable, the nurse adds supportive care."* The goal of nursing is to promote wholeness.[23:258]

Person

Person is "who we know ourself to be: a sense of identity."

Health

Health is socially determined. It is predetermined by social groups and is not just an absence of pathological conditions.[28] "Change is characteristic of life, and adaptation is the method of change. The organism retains its integrity in both the internal and external environment through its adaptive capability."[24:10]

Environment

Environment is the "context in which we live our lives."[28] It is not a passive backdrop. We are active participants in it.[28]

THEORETICAL ASSERTIONS

Because Levine's work was intended to provide an organizational structure for teaching medical-surgical nursing rather than to develop theory, she did not explicitly identify theoretical assertions. Although many theoretical assertions can be generated from her work, the four major ones are:

1. "Nursing intervention is based on the conservation of the individual patient's energy."†[1]
2. "Nursing intervention is based on the conservation of the individual patient's structural integrity."‡

3. "Nursing intervention is based on the conservation of the individual patient's personal integrity."*
4. "Nursing intervention is based on the conservation of the individual patient's social integrity."†

LOGICAL FORM

Levine primarily uses deductive logic. In developing her model, Levine integrates theories and concepts from the humanities and the sciences of nursing, physiology, psychology, and sociology. She uses the information to analyze nursing practice situations and describe nursing skills and activities.

ACCEPTANCE BY THE NURSING COMMUNITY
Practice

Levine helps define what nursing is by identifying the activities it encompasses while giving the scientific principles behind them. Conservation principles, levels of integration, and other concepts can be used in numerous contexts. Hirschfield[15] has used the principles of conservation in care of the older adult. Taylor[36,37] used them to measure outcomes of nursing care and then again in her textbook.

Education

Levine wrote a textbook for beginning students that introduced material into curricula that had not been taught before. She presented an early discussion of death and dying and believed that women should be awakened after a breast biopsy and consulted about the next step.‡

Introduction to Clinical Nursing provides an organizational structure for teaching medical-surgical nursing. In both the 1969 and 1973 editions Levine presents a model at the end of

---

*References 24:13; 19:2452; 29.
†References 24:13; 20:47.
‡References 24:13; 20:53.

*References 24:13; 20:53.
†References 24:14; 20:56.
‡References 24:356-359; 28; 29.

each of the first nine chapters. Each model contains objectives, essential science concepts, and nursing process to give nurses a foundation for nursing activities. The nine models are:

1. "Vital signs," including temperature, pulse, and respirations.[24:34-42]
2. "Body movement and positioning," including body posture, body mechanics, bed rest, and ambulation.[24:86-92]
3. "Ministration of personal hygiene needs," including personal and environmental hygiene.*
4. "Pressure gradient systems in nursing intervention," specifically fluids.†
5. "Nursing determinants in provision for nutritional needs," including psychological, cultural, and religious, socioeconomic, and therapeutic needs for fluids and nourishment.‡
6. "Pressure gradient systems in nursing," specifically gases and pulmonary ventilation.§
7. "Local application of heat and cold," stressing patient's safety and comfort.‖
8. "The administration of medications."¶
9. "Establishing an aseptic environment," including teaching patients principles of asepsis.**

Critics argue that although the text is labeled introductory, a beginning student would need a fairly extensive background in physical and social science to use it.[3] Another critic suggests a definite strength is the emphasis of scientific principles, but a weakness of the text is it does not present adequate examples of pathological profiles when disturbances are discussed. For this reason, one reviewer recommends the text as supplementary or complementary, rather than as a primary text.[4] Levine wrote a teacher's manual to assist in the use of her book.[28]

Hall[14] indicates Levine's model is one used as a curriculum model. Several graduate students are using Levine's model for thesis and dissertations.[28]

Research

Fitzpatrick and Whall[10:115] state, "All in all, Levine's model served as an excellent beginning. Its contribution has added a great deal to the overall development of nursing knowledge." Many research questions can be generated from Levine's model. Several graduate students are using the conservation principles as a framework for their research.[28,29]

FURTHER DEVELOPMENT

Levine and others are working to use the conservation principles as the basis of a taxonomy of nursing diagnosis. Levine is also working on a theory of redundancy that still requires much discussion and critique because it is not definitive yet. Much related research is still needed.[28,29]

CRITIQUE
Clarity

Levine's model possesses clarity. Fitzpatrick and Whall[10] believe Levine's work to be both internally and externally consistent. Esposito and Leonard[7:160] state that Levine's ideas are, "organized in such a way as to be sequential and logical." They add that there are no apparent contradictions in the model.

Simplicity

Although the four conservation principles initially appear simple, they contain subconcepts and multiple variables. However, this remains one of the simpler models.

Generality

The four conservation principles can be used in all nursing contexts.

---

*Reference 24:131-139.
†Reference 24:198-208.
‡Reference 24:245-253.
§Reference 24:292-303.
‖Reference 24:332-339.
¶Reference 24:381-393.
**Reference 24:435-440.

Empirical Precision

Levine used deductive logic to develop her model, which can be used to generate research questions.

Derivable Consequences

Various authors disagree as to the level of contributions provided by Levine's model. The four conservation principles was one of the earliest models and seems to be receiving increasing recognition.

REFERENCES

1. Bates, M. (1967). A naturalist at large. *Natural History, 76*(6):8-16.
2. Beland, I. (1971). *Clinical nursing: Pathophysiological and psychosocial implications* (2nd ed.). New York: Macmillan.
3. Book Review. (1970, Jan.) *Canadian Nurse, 66:*42.
4. Book Review. (1974, May) *Canadian Nurse, 70:*39.
5. Dubos, R. (1961). *Mirage of health.* Garden City, N.Y.: Doubleday.
6. Dubos, R. (1965). *Man adapting.* New Haven, Conn.: Yale University Press.
7. Esposito, C.H., & Leonard, M.K. (1980). Myra Estrin Levine. In Nursing Theories Conference Group, J.B. George, Chairperson, *Nursing theories: The base for professional nursing practice.* Englewood Cliffs, N.J.: Prentice-Hall.
8. Erikson, E.H. (1964). *Insight and responsibility.* New York: W.W. Norton.
9. Erikson, E.H. (1968). *Identity: Youth and crisis.* New York: W.W. Norton.
10. Fitzpatrick, J.J., & Whall, A.L. (1983). *Conceptual models of nursing: Analysis and application.* Bowie, Md.: Robert J. Brady.
11. Gibson, J.E. (1966). *The senses considered as perceptual systems.* Boston: Houghton Mifflin.
12. Goldstein, K. (1963). *The organism.* Boston: Beacon Press.
13. Hall, E.T. (1966). *The hidden dimension.* Garden City, N.Y.: Doubleday.
14. Hall, K.V. (1979). Current trends in the use of conceptual frameworks in nursing education. *Journal of Nursing Education, 18*(4):26-29.
15. Hirschfeld, M.J. (1976). The cognitively impaired older adult. *American Journal of Nursing, 76:*1981-1984.
16. Levine, M.E. (1963). Florence Nightingale: The legend that lives. *Nursing Forum, 2*(4):24-35.
17. Levine, M.E. (1965, June). The professional nurse and graduate education. *Nursing Science, 3:*206.
18. Levine, M.E. (1966). Trophicognosis: An alternative to nursing diagnosis. In *Exploring progress in medical-surgical nursing practice.* New York: American Nurses' Association.
19. Levine, M.E. (1966, Nov.). Adaptation and assessment: A rationale for nursing intervention. *American Journal of Nursing, 66:*2450.
20. Levine, M.E. (1967). The four conservation principles of nursing. *Nursing Forum, 6:*45.
21. Levine, M.E. (1967, Dec.). For lack of love alone. *Minnesota Nursing Accent, 39:*179.
22. Levine, M.E. (1969, Jan.). The pursuit of wholeness. *American Journal of Nursing, 69:*93.
23. Levine, M.E. (1971, June). Holistic nursing. *Nursing Clinics of North America, 6:*253.
24. Levine, M.E. (1973). *Introduction to clinical nursing* (2nd ed.). Philadelphia: F.A. Davis.
25. Levine, M.E. (1978). Paper presented at the Second Annual Nurse Educators' Conference, New York. (Audiotape).
26. Levine, M.E. (1984, April). *A conceptual model for nursing: The four conservative principles.* In the proceedings from Allentown College of St. Francis Conference.
27. Levine, M.E. (1984). Curriculum vitae.
28. Levine, M.E. (1984). Telephone interviews.
29. Levine, M.E. (1985). Telephone interviews.
30. Levine, M.E. (1984). Personal correspondence.
31. Levine, M.E. (1985). Personal correspondence.
32. Levine, M.E., & Levine, E.B. (1965, Dec.). Hippocrates: Father of nursing too. *American Journal of Nursing, 65:*86.
33. Rogers, M.E. (1970). *An introduction to the theoretical basis of nursing.* Philadelphia: F.A. Davis.
34. Selye, H. (1956). *The stress of life.* New York: McGraw-Hill.
35. Sherrington, A. (1906). *Integrative function of the nervous system.* New York: Charles Scribner's Sons.
36. Taylor, J.W. (1974). Measuring the outcomes of nursing care. *Nursing Clinics of North America, 9:*337-348.
37. Taylor, J., & Ballenger, S. (1980). *Neurological dysfunction and nursing interventions.* New York: McGraw-Hill.

38. Tillich, P. (1961). The meaning of health. *Perspectives in Biology and Medicine, 5*:92-100.

BIBLIOGRAPHY
Primary Sources
Books

Levine, M.E. (1969). *Introduction to clinical nursing.* Philadelphia: F.A. Davis.

Levine, M.E. (1969). *Renewal for nursing.* Philadelphia: F.A. Davis.

Levine, M.E. (1973). *Introduction to clinical nursing* (2nd ed.). Philadelphia: F.A. Davis.

Book Chapters

Levine, M.E. (1964). Nursing Service. In M. Leeds, & H. Shore, *Geriatric Institutional Management.* New York: J.P. Putnam & Sons.

Levine, M.E. (1966). Trophicognosis: An alternative to nursing diagnosis. In *ANA regional conference papers* (Vol. 2: Medical-Surgical Nursing).

Levine, M.E. (1972). Benoni. In *Comprehensive Clinical Papers* (Vol. 6: The nurse and the dying patient). American Journal of Nursing Company.

Levine, M.E. (1973). Adaptation and assessment: A rationale for nursing intervention. In M.E. Hardy (Ed.), *Theoretical foundations for nursing.* New York: Irvington.

Articles

Levine, M.E. (1963). Florence Nightingale: The legend that lives. *Nursing Forum, 2*(4):24-35.

Levine, M.E. (1964, Feb.). Not to startle, though the way were steep. *Nursing Science, 2*:58-67.

Levine, M.E. (1964, Dec.). There need be no anonymity. *First, 18*(9):4.

Levine, M.E. (1965, June). The professional nurse and graduate education. *Nursing Science, 3:* 206-214.

Levine, M.E. (1965). Trophicognosis: An alternative to nursing diagnosis. *ANA Reg. Clinical Conferences, 2*:55-70.

Levine, M.E. (1966, Nov.). Adaptation and assessment: A rationale for nursing intervention. *American Journal of Nursing, 66*(11):2450-2453.

Levine, M.E. (1967). The four conservation principles of nursing. *Nursing Forum, 6*:45-59.

Levine, M.E. (1967, May). Medicine-nursing dialogue belongs at patient's bedside. *Chart, 64*(5):136-137.

Levine, M.E. (1967, July). This I believe: About patient-centered care. *Nursing Outlook, 15*:53-55.

Levine, M.E. (1967, Dec.). For lack of love alone. *Accent, 39*(7):179-202.

Levine, M.E. (1968, Feb.). Knock before entering personal space bubbles (Part 1). *Chart, 65*(2): 58-62.

Levine, M.E. (1968, March). Knock before entering personal space bubbles (Part 2). *Chart, 65*(3): 82-84.

Levine, M.E. (1968, April). The pharmacist in the clinical setting: A nurse's viewpoint. *American Journal of Hospital Pharmacy, 25*(4):168-171. (Also translated into Japanese and published in *Kyushu National Hospital Magazine for Western Japan*).

Levine, M.E. (1969, Jan.). The pursuit of wholeness. *American Journal of Nursing, 69*:93-98.

Levine, M.E. (1969, Feb.). Constructive student power. *Chart, 66*(2):42FF.

Levine, M.E. (1969, Oct.). Small hospital—big nursing. *Chart, 66*:265-269.

Levine, M.E. (1969, Nov.). Small hospital—big nursing. *Chart, 66*:310-315.

Levine, M.E. (1970). Dilemma. *ANA Clinical Conferences*, pp. 338-342.

Levine. M.E. (1970, April). Breaking through the medications mystique. Published simultaneously in *American Journal of Nursing, 70*(4):799-803, and *American Journal of Hospital Pharmacy, 27*(4): 294-299.

Levine, M.E. (1970, Oct.) The intransient patient. *American Journal of Nursing, 70*:2106-2111.

Levine, M.E. (1971, May). Considers implications for nursing in the use of physician's assistants. *Hospital Topics, 49*:60-63.

Levine, M.E. (1971, June). Holistic nursing. *Nursing Clinics of North America, 6*:253-264.

Levine, M.E. (1970, July-Dec.). Symposium on a drug compendium: View of a nursing educator. *Drug Information Bulletin*. pp. 133-135.

Levine, M.E. (1971, June). The time has come to speak of health care. *AORN Journal, 13*:37-43.

Levine, M.E. (1972, February). Nursing educators—An alientating elite? *Chart, 69*(2):56-61.

Levine, M.E. (1972, March.). Benoni. *American Journal of Nursing, 72*(3):466-468.

Levine, M.E. (1972, March.). Nursing grand rounds: Complicated case of CVA. *Nursing '72, 2*(3):3-34. (With P. Moschel, J. Taylor, & G. Ferguson).

Levine, M.E. (1972, May). Nursing grand rounds: Insulin reactions in a brittle diabetic, *Nursing '72, 2*(5):6-11. (With L. Line, A. Boyle, E. Kopacewski).

Levine, M.E. (1973). On creativity in nursing. *Image, 3*(3):15-19.

Levine, M.E. (1973, November). A letter from Myra, *Chart, 70(9).* (Also in *Israel Nurses' Journal,* December 1973, in English and Hebrew).

Levine, M.E. (1974, Oct.). The pharmacist's clinical role in interdisciplinary care: A nurse's viewpoint. *Hospital Formulary Management, 9:*47.

Levine, M.E. (1975, Jan.-Feb.). On creativity in nursing. *Nursing Digest, 3:*38-40.

Levine, M.E. (1977, May). Nursing ethics and the ethical nurse. *American Journal of Nursing, 77:*845-849.

Levine, M.E. (1978, June). Cancer chemotherapy: A nursing model. *Nursing Clinics of North America, 13*(2):271-280.

Levine, M.E. (1978, July). Kapklvoo and nursing, too. *Research in Nursing and Health, 1*(2):51). (Editorial).

Levine, M.E. (1978, Nov.). Does continuing education improve nursing practice? *Hospitals, 52*(21):138-140.

Levine, M.E. (1979). Knowledge base required by generalized and specialized nursing practice. *ANA Publications, (G-127):*57-69.

Levine, M.E. (1980). The ethics of computer technology in health care. *Nursing Forum, 19*(2):193-198.

Levine, M.E. (1982, March-April). Bioethics of cancer nursing. *Rehabilitation Nursing, 7:*27-31, 41.

Levine, M.E. (1982, March-April). The bioethics of cancer nursing. *Journal of Enterostomal Therapy, 9:*11-13.

Levine, M.E. (1984, April). A conceptual model for nursing: The four conservative principles. In the proceedings from Allentown College of St. Francis Conference.

Levine, M.E. & Levine, E.B. (1965, Dec.). Hippocrates: Father of nursing, too. *American Journal of Nursing, 65*(12):86-88.

Levine, M.E., Porter, A.L., & McDonald, A. (1973, September). Giving diabetics control of their own lives. *Nursing '73, 3:*44-49.

Levine, M.E., & Rayder, M. (1979, Nov.). Problem: A new nurse asks why preoperative teaching isn't done . . . three answers from experience. *American Journal of Nursing, 79:*1992-1995.

Audiotapes

Levine, M.E. (1978; Dec.). Paper presented at the Second Annual Nurse Educator Conference, New York: Audiotape available from Teach 'em Inc., 160 E. Illinois Street, Chicago, Ill. 60611.

Levine, M.E. (1979). Paper presented at nursing theory conference. Audiotapes (2 reels) available from Teach 'em Inc., 160 E. Illinois Street, Chicago, Ill. 60611.

Levine, M.E. (1984, May). Paper presented at Nursing Theory Conference, Boyle, Letoueneau Conference, Edmonton, Canada. Audiotapes available from Ed Kennedy, Kennedy Recording, R.R.5, Edmonton, Alberta, Canada TSP4B7 (403-470-0013).

Proceedings

Levine, M.E. (1976, Jan.). On the nursing ethnic and the negative command. *Proceedings of the Intensive Conference* (Faculty of the University of Illinois Medical Center.) Philadelphia: Society for Health and Human Values.

Levine, M.E. (1977). History of nursing in Illinois. *Proceedings of the Bicentennial Workshop of the University of Illinois College of Nursing.* University of Illinois Press.

Levine, M.E. (1977). Primary nursing: Generalist and specialist education. *Proceedings of the American Academy of Nursing.* Kansas City, Mo.

Interviews

Levine, M. (1984). Telephone interviews.
Levine, M. (1985). Telephone interviews.

Correspondence

Levine, M. (1984). Curriculum vitae.
Levine, M. (1984). Personal correspondence.
Levine, M. (1985). Personal correspondence.

Secondary Sources
Book Reviews

Levine, M.E. (1969). *Introduction to clinical nursing.*
*Bedside Nurse, 2:*4, September-October 1969
*Canadian Nurse, 66:*42, January 1970
*American Journal of Nursing, 70:*99 + January 1970
*Nursing Outlook, 18:*20, February 1970
*American Journal of Nursing, 70:*2220 + October 1970
*Nursing Mirror, 132:*43, April 2, 1971

*Bedside Nurse, 4:*2 November 1971
*Canadian Nurse, 76:*47 December 1971
*Nursing Mirror, 133:*16, December 17, 1971
*American Journal of Nursing, 74:*347 February 1974
*Canadian Nurse, 70:*39 May 1974
*Nursing Outlook, 22:*301 May 1974
Levine, M.E. (1969). *Renewal for nursing.*
*Supervisor Nurse, 2:*68, August 1971
*Bedside Nurse, 4:*2, November 1971
*AANA Journal, 49:*495, December 1971
*Canadian Nurse, 67:*47, December 1971
*Nursing Mirror, 133:*16, December 1971

Book Chapters

Chinn, P.L., & Jacobs, M.K. (1983). *Theory in nursing: A systematic approach.* St. Louis: C.V. Mosby. p. 188.

Esposito, C.H., & Leonard, M.K. (1980) Myra Estrin Levine. In Nursing Theories Conference Group. J.B. George, Chairperson, *Nursing theories: The base for professional nursing practice.* Englewood Cliffs, N.J.: Prentice-Hall. pp. 150-163.

Fawcett, J. (1984). Levine's conservation model. In J. Fawcett, *Analysis and evaluation of conceptual models of nursing.* Philadelphia: F.A. Davis. pp. 115-144.

Meleis, A.I. (1985). Myra Levine. In A.I. Meleis, *Theoretical nursing: Development and progress.* Philadelphia: J.B. Lippincott. pp. 275-283.

Pieper, B.A. (1983). Levine's nursing model. In J.J. Fitzpatrick, & A.L. Whall, *Conceptual models of nursing: Analysis and application.* Bowie, Md.: Robert J. Brady. pp. 101-115.

Profiles

Profile. (1974, May). *Nursing '74, 4:*70.

New Releases

Myra Levine elected to new National Academy of Nursing. (1973, March). *Chart, 70:*5.

Other Sources
Books

Beland, I. (1971). *Clinical nursing: Pathophysiological and psychosocial implications* (2nd ed.). New York: Macmillan.

Dubos, R. (1961). *Mirage of health.* Garden City, N.Y.: Doubleday.

Dubos, R. (1965). *Man adapting.* New Haven, Conn.: Yale University Press.

Erikson, E.H. (1964). *Insight and responsibility.* New York: W.W. Norton.

Erikson, E.H. (1968). *Identity: Youth and crisis.* New York: W.W. Norton.

Gibson, J.E. (1966). *The senses considered as perceptual systems.* Boston: Houghton Mifflin.

Goldstein, K. (1963). *The organism.* Boston: Beacon Press.

Rogers, M.E. (1970). *An introduction to the theoretical basis of nursing.* Philadelphia: F.A. Davis.

Selye, H. (1956). *The stress of life.* New York: McGraw-Hill.

Sherrington, A. (1906). *Integrative function of the nervous system.* New York: Charles Scribner & Sons.

Taylor, J., & Ballenger, S. (1980). *Neurological dysfunction and nursing interventions.* New York: McGraw-Hill.

Articles

Bates, M. (1967). A naturalist at large. *Natural History, 76*(6):8-16.

Hall, K.V. (1979). Current trends in the use of conceptual frameworks in nursing education. *Journal of Nursing Education, 18*(4):26-29.

Flaskerud, J.H., & Halloran, E.J. (1980). Areas of agreement in nursing theory development. *Advances in Nursing Science, 3*(1):1-7.

Hirschfeld, M.J. (1976). The cognitively impaired older adult. *American Journal of Nursing, 76:*1981-1984.

Taylor, J.W. (1974). Measuring the outcomes of nursing care. *Nursing Clinics of North America, 9:*337-348.

Tillich, P. (1961). The meaning of health. *Perspectives in Biology and Medicine, 5:*92-100.

Tompkins, E.S. (1980). Effect of restricted mobility and dominance on perceived duration. *Nursing Research, 29*(6):333-338.

Martha E. Rogers

28

Unitary Human Beings

Joann Sebastian Daily, Judy Sporleder Maupin, Martha Carole Satterly

CREDENTIALS AND BACKGROUND OF THE THEORIST

Martha E. Rogers was born May 12, 1914, in Dallas, Texas, the eldest of four children. She began her collegiate education at the University of Tennessee in Knoxville, where she studied science from 1931 to 1933. She received her nursing diploma from Knoxville General Hospital School of Nursing in 1936. In 1937 she received a B.S. from George Peabody College

in Nashville, Tennessee. Her other degrees include an M.A. in public health nursing supervision from Teacher's College, Columbia University, New York, in 1945; an M.P.H. in 1952 and a Sc.D. in 1954, both from Johns Hopkins University in Baltimore.

For 21 years, from 1954 to 1975, she was Professor and Head of the Division of Nursing at New York University. Since 1975, she has been Professor, and in 1979 she became Professor Emerita.

Rogers' early nursing practice was in rural public health nursing in Michigan and in visiting nurse supervision, education, and practice in Connecticut. Her publications include three

The authors wish to express appreciation to Dr. Lois Meier for her assistance, and to Dr. Martha Rogers for critiquing the chapter.

books and numerous articles; she continues to write and publish extensively. She has lectured throughout the United States and the world.

A verbal portrait of Rogers might include such descriptive terms as stimulating, challenging, controversial, idealistic, visionary, prophetic, philosophic, academic, outspoken, humorous, blunt, and ethical. She has been widely recognized and honored for her contributions and leadership in nursing. Her colleagues consider her one of the most original thinkers in nursing.[5:245]

THEORETICAL SOURCES

Rogers' early grounding in the liberal arts and sciences is apparent in the origin of her conceptual system and its ongoing development. The model was first published in 1970 as *An Introduction to the Theoretical Basis of Nursing*. Rogers has continued to clarify and define her concepts in later publications and presentations such as "The Science of Unitary Human Beings: A Paradigm for Nursing."[13]

Rogers draws on a knowledge base gained from anthropology, psychology, sociology, astronomy, religion, philosophy, history, biology, physics, mathematics, literature, and other sources to create her model of unitary human beings and the environment as energy fields integral to the life process.[4:166] A statement frequently repeated in her writings is, "Man is a unified whole possessing his own integrity and manifesting characteristics that are more than and different from the sum of his parts."[11:47] In the prologue of *An Introduction to the Theoretical Basis of Nursing* she states, "Man's biological, physical, social, psychological, and spiritual heritages become an indivisible whole as scientific facts are merged with human warmth."[11:xii]

Several sources influenced Rogers' theorizations. During the midnineteenth century, Florence Nightingale's proposals and statistical data placed man within the framework of the natural world, and "the foundation for the scope of modern nursing was laid."[11:30]

As the nineteenth century moved into the twentieth, classical physics gave way to field physics and events of the physical world had a new unity. In 1905 Einstein's theory of relativity introduced the four coordinates of space-time.[11:31]

In 1935 Burr and Northrop's "The Electro-Dynamic Theory of Life" stated the concepts of the pattern and organization of the electrodynamic field, the outcome of whose activity is wholeness, organization and continuity. Rogers[11:32] says, "An electrical field was replacing the cell as the fundamental unit of biological systems."

In the 1950s von Bertalanffy introduced general systems theory, which presented a general science of wholeness. The term *negentropy* was brought into use to signify increasing order, complexity, and heterogeneity.[11:51]

A theme of Rogers' writings and discussions may be paraphrased, "You cannot understand the *whole* by studying the parts, and the *whole* is more than and different from the sum of its parts."

USE OF EMPIRICAL EVIDENCE

As supporting evidence for her theory Rogers cites nurse researchers such as M. Neal, L. Porter, and A. Earle. Their studies support a significant relationship between imposed motion and infant growth and development.[11:105-106] More recent research based on the paradigm, "Nursing Science of Unitary Human Beings," is listed in Appendix C.

MAJOR CONCEPTS AND DEFINITIONS

In 1970 Rogers' conceptual model of nursing rested upon a set of basic assumptions that described the life process in man. The life process was characterized by wholeness, openness, unidirectionality, pattern and organization, sentience, and thought.[11:90]

In her 1983 paradigm, she postulated four building blocks for her model. These are energy field, a universe of open systems, pattern, and four dimensionality.[13]

ENERGY FIELD. An energy field constitutes the fundamental unit of both the living and the nonliving. Field is a unifying concept, and energy signifies the dynamic nature of the field. "Energy fields are infinite. Two fields are identified: the human field and the environmental field."[13] They are irreducible.

UNIVERSE OF OPEN SYSTEMS. The concept of the universe of open systems holds that energy fields are infinite and open, and integral with one another.[13]

PATTERN

Pattern identifies energy fields. It is the distinguishing characteristic of a field and is perceived as a single wave. The nature of the pattern

changes continuously and innovatively. Each human field pattern is unique and is integral with its own environmental field.[13]

FOUR-DIMENSIONALITY. Four dimensionality is defined as a nonlinear domain without spatial or temporal attributes. "All reality is postulated to be four dimensional."[13]

From this conceptual system, Rogers derives the Principles of Homeodynamics, which postulate a way of perceiving unitary man. Table 28-1 depicts the evolution of these principles from 1970 to 1983. Rogers says, "The life process is homeodynamic. . . . These principles postulate the way the life process is and predict the nature of its evolving."[11:96]

Rogers repeatedly states that change is probabilistic. According to *Webster's Ninth New Collegiate Dictionary,* "probabilism" is a theory that certainty is impossible, especially in the sci-

Table 28-1. Evolution of principles of homeodynamics—1970, 1980, 1983

An Introduction to the Theoretical Basis of Nursing 1970	*Nursing: A Science of Unitary Man* 1980	*Science of Unitary Human Beings: A Paradigm for Nursing* 1983
Resonancy—continuously propagating series of waves between man and environment	*Resonancy*—the continuous change from lower to higher frequency wave patterns in the human and environmental fields	*Resonancy*—the continuous change from lower to higher frequency wave patterns in human and environmental fields
Helicy—continuous, innovative change growing out of mutual interaction of man and environment along a spiralling longitudinal axis bound in space-time	*Helicy*—nature of change between human and environmental fields is continuously innovative, probabilistic, and increasingly diverse manifesting nonrepeating rhythmicities.	*Helicy*—the continuous, innovative, probabilistic, increasing diversity of human and environmental field patterns characterized by nonrepeating rhythmicities
Reciprocy—continuous mutual interaction between the human field and environmental field		
Synchrony—change in the human field depends on the state of human field and simultaneous state of environmental field at any given point in space-time.	*Complementarity*—the continuous, mutual simultaneous interaction between human and environmental fields	*Integrality*—the continuous mutual human field and environmental field process

Conceptualized by Joann Daily from the following sources: Rogers, M.E. (1970). *An introduction to the theoretical basis of nursing.* Philadelphia: F.A. Davis; Riehl, J.P., & Roy, C. (ed.). (1980). *Conceptual models for nursing practice.* (2nd ed.). New York: Appleton-Century-Crofts; Rogers, M.E. (1983). Science of unitary human beings: A paradigm for nursing. In I.W. Clements, & F.B. Roberts, *Family health: A theoretical approach to nursing care.* New York: John Wiley & Sons.

ences, and that probability suffices to govern action and belief.[14] Rogers[11:57] goes on to say, "Probability statistics provide a basis for practical operations. Prediction is a fundamental necessity for knowledgeable intervention that has as its goal the betterment of man."

MAJOR ASSUMPTIONS
Nursing

"Historically the term *nursing* most often has been used as a verb signifying 'to do.' When nursing is perceived as a science, the term nursing becomes a noun signifying 'a body of abstract knowledge.' "[13:1] Rogers describes nursing as a learned profession that is both a science and an art. "Nursing is a humanistic science dedicated to compassionate concern for maintaining and promoting health, preventing illness, and caring for and rehabilitating the sick and disabled."[11:vii] Nursing seeks to promote symphonic interaction between the environment and man, to strengthen the coherence and integrity of the human beings, and to direct and redirect patterns of interaction between man and his environment for the realization of maximum health potential.[11:122]

The professional practice of nursing is creative and imaginative and exists to serve people. It is rooted in intellectual judgment, abstract knowledge, and human compassion. Professional nursing practice has no dependent functions, but collaborative ones.[11:122] Professional practitioners participate "in the coordination of their knowledges and skills with those of professional personnel in other health disciplines."[11:128]

Nursing intervention is predicated upon the wholeness of man and derives its safety and effectiveness from a unified concept of human functioning. Nursing is concerned with evaluating the simultaneous state of the individual (or group) and the environment, and the preceding configurations leading up to the present. Intervention is dependent on evaluation and adds a conscious dimension to enhancing probabilistic outcomes toward a predetermined goal.[11:124]

The safe practice of nursing intervention depends on the nature and amount of scientific knowledge the individual brings to practice and the imaginative, intellectual judgment that puts such knowledge to use in the service to mankind. Nursing is a "science of unitary human being" and is therefore unique because it is the only science that deals with the whole person.[13:1]

Person

Rogers' unitary man (who represents all human beings) is as a unified being integral with the environment. Man is in continuous mutal process with his environment in his totality and "the whole cannot be understood when it is reduced to particulars."[11:44] Human beings "are not disembodied entities, nor are they mechanical aggregates. . . . They behave as a totality. . . . Man is a unified whole possessing his own integrity and manifesting characteristics that are more than and different from the sum of his parts."[11:46-47] A science of unitary human beings is basic to nursing and requires a new view and a conceptual system specific to nursing's concern. People and their environment are perceived as irreducible energy fields integral with one another and continuous and creative in their evolution.

Rogers defines *person* as an open system in continuous process with the open system that is environment. She defines *unitary man* as "an irreducible four dimensional energy field identified by pattern and manifesting characteristics that are specific to the whole and which cannot be predicted from knowledge of the parts" (Appendix B).

Rogers' primary concern is that nursing view the person as an irreducible whole. This is not to be confused with *holistic,* which is often used to mean the sum of all the parts. An irreducible whole is different from the sum of the parts. She also conceptualizes the person as a sentient being able to participate creatively in change.

Environment

Rogers[13:2] defines environment as "an irreducible, four dimensional energy field identified by pattern and manifesting characteristics different from those of the parts. Each environmental field is specific to its given human field. Both change continuously and creatively."

Environment encompasses everything outside any given human field. Environmental change is continuously innovative, probabilistic, and characterized by increasing diversity. Environmental and human fields are identified by wave pattern and organization manifesting continuous change. Interaction between environmental and human fields is continuous, mutual, and simultaneous.

Health

Rogers uses *health* in many of her earlier writings, but never really defines the term. She uses the term *positive health* to symbolize wellness and the absence of disease and major illness.[11] Her promotion of positive health connotes direction in helping people with opportunities for rhythmic consistency and for man and the environment an interchange that stimulates the flow of repatterning commensurate with the openness of nature. Enhancement of health requires an intervention that strengthens the man-environment symmetry. Positive health measures are directed at helping people develop patterns of living compatible with environmental changes rather than in conflict with them. Promotion and maintenance of health include correction of problems stemming from social inequities, technological advances, and other events.[11:123]

Health is used by Rogers as a value term defined by the culture or individual. Health and illness are manifestations of pattern and are considered "to denote behaviors that are of high value and low value."[5:248] Events taking place in the life process indicate the extent to which man achieves maximum health. Maximum health potential varies from the greatest of health potential to conditions incompatible with maintaining life. Health may not be ideal but is the maximum health state that is potential for an individual.

THEORETICAL ASSERTIONS

In 1970 Rogers identified five assumptions that are also theoretical assertions supporting her model derived from literature on man, physics, mathematics, and behavioral science:

1. Man is a unified whole possessing his own integrity and manifesting characteristics that are more than and different from the sum of his parts (energy field).[11:47]
2. Man and environment are continuously exchanging matter and energy with one another (openness).[11:54]
3. The life process evolves irreversibly and unidirectionally along the space-time continuum (helicy).[11:59]
4. Pattern and organization identify man and reflect his innovative wholeness (pattern and organization).[11:65]
5. Man is characterized by the capacity for abstraction and imagery, language and thought, sensation, and emotion (sentient, thinking being).[11:73]

Ten years later Rogers developed "Nursing: A Science of Unitary Man." The science of nursing seeks to study the nature and direction of unitary human development integral with the environment. Rogers[11:57] believes "man lives in a probabilistic universe" and therefore is subject to the laws of probability. Probability statistics provide a basis for prediction that is a fundamental necessity for knowledgeable intervention with the goal of the betterment of man.[11:57] Professional practice of nursing flows from the application of knowledge.

Rogers sees the need for predictive principles that guide nursing practice. These principles emerge from nursing's conceptual system. Nursing science seeks to make intelligible knowledge about man and his world that has significance for nursing practice. The phenomena central to nursing's conceptual system is man's life process. "The life process in man is a phenomena of wholeness, of continuity, of dynamic and creative change."[11:84] Nursing is an empirical science that seeks to describe, explain, and predict the life process in man. If the life process in man is to be studied and understood, the normal and the pathological must be treated equally. The life process has its own unity, inseparable from environment, and is characterized as the whole.[11:85]

Rogers' prerequisite to the process of nursing is the development of the science of nursing with the goal of providing a body of knowledge that stems from scientific research and logical analysis and is capable of being translated into nursing practice. Rogers' conceptual model of unitary man is a clear, direct statement about the unique focus of nursing: a flexible and creative, individualized, and socially oriented compassionate and skillful practice.

LOGICAL FORM

Rogers' model of unitary man is clearly deductive and logical. The Theory of Relativity, General Systems Theory, and Electro-Dynamic Theory of Life contributed ideas for Rogers' model. The central components of the model, unitary man and environment, are integral with one another. The basic building blocks of her model are energy field, openness, pattern, and four dimensionality and when synthesized provide for a new conceptual system—a new world view. These concepts form the basis of nursing's abstract conceptual system, which relates to nursing and health. From the abstract conceptual system Rogers derives the principles of helicy, resonancy, and integrality. These broad generalizations postulate the nature and direction of unitary man's development. Other theories have been derived from the abstract conceptual system, such as the theory of accelerating evolution, paranormal events, and rhythmical correlates of change. The derived

theories are intended to explain, predict, and prescribe phenomena related to the life process of man.

ACCEPTANCE BY NURSING COMMUNITY
Practice

Rogers believes the theories derived from her conceptual model are translatable to practice, but the examples are not specific. She envisions changes in nursing practice based on theories evolving from her model. Although the abstract conceptual model is not directly useful to practice, it does provide a base for research and theory development, which provide the knowledge base for practice. Falco and Lobo[4] attempted to develop a care plan using the principles of homeodynamics (see Appendix A), and Whelton[15] made an effort to operationalize Rogers' theory throughout the nursing process. But the results of these applications remain general rather than specific. The model has served as a basis for explication of other nursing conceptualizations by Newman, Parse, and Fitzpatrick. "Rogers' model does not require that one discard previous knowledge, but it does require that such knowledge be viewed differently."[7:21]

Education

Rogers repeatedly discusses rebuilding the nursing education programs to reflect nursing as a learned profession. The education of nurses is based on theory and committed to human service.

In the early 1960s Rogers proposed that the basic entry position of professional nursing should be at the baccalaureate level. At that time her goal seemed idealistic, but today her assertions are becoming the standard rather than the exception.

She said, "The only people competent to teach nursing or to teach what nurses are supposed to do are qualified nurses."[12:65] Her advocacies are evidenced in nursing education today as more nurses have been prepared to teach nurses at all levels of nursing education.

Research

Rogers' theories are directly related to research and theory development in nursing science. The conceptual model provides a stimulus and direction for scientific activity. Principles of homeodynamics are being studied. Investigation into the nature of field patterning and the search for indices of patterning have begun. The integral nature of the man-environment relationship and the growing complexity of life have been used in recent studies using Rogers' model. Although hypotheses are difficult to develop, the theory is being tested with research.[5:6]

FURTHER DEVELOPMENT

Several areas may be identified as needing further development.

TYPOLOGY. A typology is "a method of organizing and categorizing."[8:4] Whatever method of categorizing is used should include the criteria of exhaustiveness, mutual exclusiveness, and consistency with the concepts used in the theory.[8:5] Rogers has developed many new constructs that need to be organized and categorized.

OPERATIONAL DEFINITIONS AND HYPOTHESES. Operational definitions are missing. There is a real need to be able to concretize both concepts and relational statements in order to empirically test this theory. For example, Rogers[11:113] identifies a need for "an operational definition of the human field." Further development in these areas should be given a high priority.

COMPLEXITY. The complexity of Rogers' work has made the concepts and relationships difficult to understand. This complexity can lead to misunderstanding. However, current studies are attempting to clarify and simplify many areas.

MEASUREMENT TOOLS. Tools should "not become the focus of nursing practice because they are time limited and can detract from the patient."[15:19] The lack of precise instrumentation to measure the concepts and relationships of Rogers' theory has been noted by several authors, but new tools have been and are being developed and are in use.

Rogers[10,11,13] has frequently identified the need for adequate measuring instruments. She states, "New tools of measurement are necessary adjuncts to studying questions arising out of a world view that is different from the prevalent view."[13:4]

The development of adequate and precise instruments to measure concepts and relationships remains a real need. It should be a high priority of nurse researchers.

STYLE. Anderson[1:541] wrote that Rogers' "style may discourage readers from seeking out the germinal concepts in the book which are worthy of consideration." Rogers' style is philosophical, but it is the complexity of her theory that makes reading the material slow and laborious.

CRITIQUE
Simplicity

Rogers' theory is not simple. It is complex. She uses multiple concepts that are not easily understood. She relates these concepts in her theory of homeodynamics.

Generality

Rogers' theory is abstract, and is therefore generalizable and powerful. It is usually considered a grand theory or a macro theory. It is broad in scope and attempts to explain everything.

Empirical Precision

Rogers' theory is abstract. Many would have difficulty understanding the concepts and relationships without a strong knowledge of other fields of study. Rogers' theory is deductive in logic and "the major criticism of deductive theories is the lack of empirical support."[2:443] "The difficulty in understanding the principles, the lack of operational definitions, and inadequate tools for measurement are the major limitations to the effective utilization of this theory."[4:180-181] Rogers' early theory lacks empirical precision. However, "the model is not meant to be testable, but theories drawn from it are testable."[5:259] Rogers' theory is being developed, and this will tend to increase the empirical precision.

Derivable Consequences

Gill and Atwood[6] conducted a pilot study using hypotheses derived from Rogers' principles of helicy and reciprocy. The focus was on the mutual interaction of the human and environmental field in wound healing. The study supported the homeodynamic principle of reciprocy.

Whelton[12] relates Rogers' theory to the nursing process using patients with decreased cardiac output and neurological functioning. The theory becomes a focus for applying nursing interventions and predicting outcomes.

Falco and Lobo tied the principles of homeodynamics to the nursing process (see Appendix A). They reported that "health will not be achieved by promoting homeostasis and equilibrium, but rather by taking steps to enhance dynamism and complexity within the individual."[4:175]

Many other research studies have been done (see Appendix C). All these studies have implications for guiding nursing practice and education and suggest further research.

Rogers sees the nurse as an integral part of the patient's environment. She also sees nursing as a unique science that deals with "unitary human beings" who are different from the sum of their parts.[11:13] This differentiates nursing from other service professions.

Many ideas for future study have been suggested by Rogers.[11:103-120] Based on this, it can be said that Rogers' theory is a useful theory.

CONCLUSION

Rogers is a brilliant nursing theorist. She is years ahead of her time. Understanding of her concepts and principles requires a knowledge of other fields of study, a willingness to let go of the traditional, and an ability to perceive the world in a new and creative way.

Rogers[13:1] said it well when she quoted Capra as saying, "We are trying to apply concepts of an out-dated world view to a reality that can no longer be understood in terms of these concepts." She continues:

> A science of unitary human beings basic to nursing requires a new world view and a conceptual system specific to nursing's phenomenon of concern. . . . Seeing the world from this viewpoint requires a new synthesis, a creative leap, and the inculcation of new attitudes and values. . . . A science of unitary human beings identifies nursing's uniqueness and signifies the potential of nurses to fulfill their social responsibility in human service.[13:1,4]

REFERENCES

1. Anderson, E.H. (1970, Nov.-Dec.). Researchers' bookshelf. *Nursing Research, 19*(6):541.
2. Chaska, N.L. (Ed.). (1983). *The nursing profession: A time to speak.* New York: McGraw-Hill.
3. Chinn, P.L. & Jacobs, M.K. (1983). *Theory and nursing: A systematic approach.* St. Louis: C.V. Mosby.
4. Falco, S.M., & Lobo, M.L. (1980). Martha Rogers. In Nursing Theories Conference Group, J.B. George, Chairperson, *Nursing theories: The base for professional practice.* Englewood Cliffs, N.J.: Prentice-Hall.
5. Fitzpatrick, J.J., & Whall, A.L. (1983). *Conceptual models of nursing: Analysis and application.* Bowie, Md.: Robert J. Brady.
6. Gill, B.P., & Atwood, J.R. (1981, March-April). Reciprocy and helicy used to relate in EGF and wound healing. *Nursing Research, 30*:68-72.

7. Newman, M.A. (1979). *Theory development in nursing.* Philadelphia: F.A. Davis.
8. Reynolds, P.D. (1971). *A primer in theory construction.* Indianapolis, Ind.: Bobbs-Merrill.
9. Riehl, J.P., and Roy, C. (Eds.). (1980). *Conceptual models for nursing practice* (2nd ed.). New York: Appleton-Century-Crofts.
10. Rogers, M.E. (1961). *Educational revolution in nursing.* New York: Macmillan.
11. Rogers, M.E. (1970). *An introduction to the theoretical basis of nursing.* Philadelphia: F.A. Davis.
12. Rogers, M.E. (1972). *Challenge to nursing . . . professional nursing practice . . . evaluation.* NLN Publication #15-1456. Dept. Baccalaureate Higher Education Degree Programs. pp. 62-65.
13. Rogers, M.E. (1983). Science of unitary human beings: A paradigm for nursing. In I.W. Clements, & F.B. Roberts, *Family health: A theoretical approach to nursing care.* New York: John Wiley & Sons.
14. Webster's Ninth New Collegiate Dictionary (1983). Springfield, Mass.: Merriam-Webster.
15. Whelton, B.J. (1979). An operationalization of Martha Rogers' theory throughout the nursing process. *International Journal of Nursing Studies, 16:*7-20.

BIBLIOGRAPHY
Primary Sources
Books

Rogers, M.E. (1961). *Educational revolution in nursing.* New York: McMillan.
Rogers, M.E. (1964). *Reveille in nursing.* Philadelphia: F.A. Davis.
Rogers, M.E. (1970). *An introduction to the theoretical basis of nursing.* Philadelphia: F.A. Davis.

Book Chapters

Rogers, M.E. (1983). Beyond the horizon. In N.L. Chaska, *The nursing profession: A time to speak.* New York: McGraw-Hill.
Rogers, M.E. (1983). Science of unitary human beings: A paradigm for nursing. In Imelda W. Clements, & Florence B. Roberts, *Family health: A theoretical approach to nursing care.* New York: John Wiley & Sons.

Articles

Rogers, M.E. (1953). Responses to talks on menstrual health. *Nursing Outlook, 1*(5):272-274.
Rogers, M.E. (1963). Building a strong educational foundation. *American Journal of Nursing, 63:*94-95.
Rogers, M.E. (1963, June-July). The clarion call. *Nursing Science, 1:*134-135.
Rogers, M.E. (1963). Some comments on the theoretical basis of nursing practice. *Nursing Science, 1:*11-13, 60-61.
Rogers, M.E. (1964, Feb.). Professional standards: Whose responsibility? *Nursing Science, 2:*71-73.
Rogers, M.E. (1965, Jan.). What the public demands of nursing today. *RN, 28:*80.
Rogers, M.E. (1965). Legislative and licensing problems in health care. *Nursing Administration Quarterly, 2:*71-78.
Rogers, M.E. (1965, Oct.). Editorial: Collegiate education in nursing. *Nursing Science, 3*(5):362-365.
Rogers, M.E. (1965, Dec.). Editorial: Higher education in nursing. *Nursing Science, 3*(6):443-445.
Rogers, M.E. (1966). Doctoral education in nursing. *Nursing Forum, 5*(2):75-82.
Rogers, M.E. (1966). New designs: Experiments in action. *National League Nursing Conference Paper, 20:*23-26.
Rogers, M.E. (1966, Winter). Quality nursing: Cliche or challenge. *Maine Nurse, 9*(1):2-4.
Rogers, M.E. (1967, March). Teacher preparation. *NLN Department of Associate Degree Programs, 2:*20-36.
Rogers, M.E. (1968, Feb.). Nursing science: Research and researchers, *Record, 69:*469.
Rogers, M.E. (1969, March). Nursing research: Relevant to Practice? *Nursing Research Conference, 5:*352-359.
Rogers, M.E. (1969). Nursing education for professional practice. *Catholic Nurse, 18:*28-37, 63-64.
Rogers, M.E. (1969, Nov.-Dec.). Preparation of the baccalaureate degree graduate. *New Jersey State Nurses Association Newsletter, 25*(5):32-37.
Rogers, M.E. (1970). Yesterday a nurse, today a manager: What now? *Journal of New York State Nurses Association, 1:*15-21.
Rogers, M.E. (1972). *Challenge to nursing . . . professional nursing practice . . . evaluation.* NLN Publication #15-1456. Dept. Baccalaureate Higher Education Degree Programs. pp. 62-65.

Rogers, M.E. (1972, Jan.). Nursing: To be or not to be? *Nursing Outlook, 29*(1):42-46.

Rogers, M.E. (1972, Dec.). Nursing's expanded role . . . and other euphemisms. *Journal of New York State Nurses Association, 3*(4):5-10.

Rogers, M.E. (1975). Yesterday a nurse, today a manager: What now? *Image, 2*:12-13.

Rogers, M.E. (1975). Forum: Professional commitment in nursing. *Image, 2*:12-13.

Rogers, M.E. (1975). Euphemisms in nursing's future. *Image, 7*:3-9.

Rogers, M.E. (1975, Aug.). Reactions to the two foregoing presentations, in challenge to nursing . . . professional nursing practice . . . evaluation. NLN Publication #15-1456. *Nursing Outlook, 20*:436.

Rogers, M.E. (1975, Aug.). Research is a growing word. *Nursing Science, 31*:283-294.

Rogers, M.E. (1975, October). Nursing is coming of age . . . Through the practitioner movement. *American Journal of Nursing, 75*(10):1834-43, 1859.

Rogers, M.E. (1977). Legislative and licensing problems in health care. *Nursing Administration Quarterly, 2*:71-78.

Rogers, M.E. (1978, Jan.-Feb.). Peer Review: A 1985 dissent. *Health PAC Bulletin, 80*:32-35.

Rogers, M.E. (1979, Dec.). Contemporary american leaders in nursing; an oral history. An interview with Martha E. Rogers. *Kanso-Tenbo, 4*(12):1126-1138.

Fulp, E.M., Rogers, M.E. (1982, Nov.-Dec.). N.C. Nurses visit China health services for a billion people. *Tar Heel Nurse, 44*(6):5, 8.

Lambertsen, E., et al. (1966, May). Action, reaction: Four New York State Nurses Association members react to the American Nurses Association position paper on education. *New York State Nurse, 38*(3):6-8.

Audiotape

Rogers, M.E. (1978, Oct. 20). *Nursing science: A science of unitary man*. Distinguished Lecture Series, Wright State University, Dayton, Ohio.

Rogers, M.E. (1978, Dec.). Paper presented at the Second Annual Nurse Educator Conference, New York. Audiotape available from Teach 'em Inc., 160 E. Illinois Street., Chicago, Ill. 60611.

Rogers, M.E. (1980). *The science of unitary man*. Media For Nursing. New York.

Rogers, M.E. (1984, May). Paper presented at Nurses Theorist Conference, Edmonton, Alberta, Canada. Audiotape available from Kennedy Recordings, R.R. 5, Edmonton, Alberta, Canada T5P 4B7. (4030 470-0013).

Videotape

Rogers, M.E. (1984, Oct.). The science of unitary man: An interview with Martha Rogers with E. Donnelly at Indiana University School of Nursing.

Lectures

Rogers, M.E. (1955). *Prenatal and perinatal factors in the development of childhood behavior disorders by Martha E Rogers and others*. John Hopkins University, School of Hygiene and Public Health, Baltimore.

Rogers, M.E. (1962). *Viewpoints—Critical areas for nursing education in baccalaureate and higher degree programs*. An address given at the meeting of the Council of Member Agencies of the Department of Baccalaureate and Higher Degree Programs, Williamsburg, Virginia. New York National League for Nursing, Department of Baccalaureate and Higher Degree Programs.

Rogers, M.E. (1984, Sept. 28.). *Current issues for nursing in the next decade*. Indiana Central University, Indianapolis.

Abstract

Rogers, M.E. (1954). *The association of maternal and fetal factors with the development of behavior problems among elementary school children*. The Johns Hopkins University PhD.

Secondary Sources
Book Review

Anderson, E.H. (1970, Nov.-Dec.). Researchers' bookshelf. *Nursing Research, 19*(6):541.

Books

Argyris, C., & Schon, D. (1974). *Theory in practice*. San Francisco: Jossey-Bass.

Bertalanffy, L. von (1960). *Problems of life*. New York: Harper Torch.

Bertalanffy, L. von (1960). *General systems theory: Foundations, developments, application*. New York: George Braziller.

Chardin, T. (1961). *The phenomenon of man*. New York: Harper Torch.

Chaska, N.L. (1983). *The nursing profession: A time to speak*. New York: McGraw-Hill.

Chinn, P.L., & Jacobs, M.K. (1983). *Theory and nursing: A systematic approach*. St. Louis: C.V. Mosby.

Dossey, L. (1982). *Space, time, and medicine*. Boulder, Col.: Shambhala Publications.

Einstein, A. (1961). *Relativity*. New York: Crown.

Fitzpatrick, J.J., & Whall, A.L. (1983). *Conceptual models of nursing: Analysis and application*. Bowie, Md.: Robert J. Brady.

Goldstein, K. (1939). *The organism*. New York: American Book.

Hanchett, E.S. (1979). *Community health assessment: A conceptual tool kit*. New York: John Wiley & Sons.

Herrick, C.J. (1956). *The evolution of human nature*. Austin: University of Texas Press.

King, I.M. (1971). *Toward a theory for nursing*. New York: John Wiley & Sons.

Lewin, K. (1964). *Field theory in the social sciences*. New York: Harper Torch.

Newman, M.A. (1979). *Theory development in nursing*. Philadelpia: F.A. Davis.

Parse, R.R. (1981). *Man-living-health. A theory of nursing*. New York: John Wiley & Sons.

Polanyi, M. (1958). *Personal knowledge*. Chicago: University of Chicago Press.

Reynolds, P.D. (1971). *A primer in theory construction*. Indianapolis, Ind.: Bobbs-Merrill.

Riehl, J.P., & Roy, C. (Eds.). (1980). *Conceptual models for nursing practice* (2nd ed.). New York: Appleton-Century-Crofts.

Safier, G. (1977). *Contemporary American leaders: An oral history*. New York: McGraw-Hill.

Stevens, B.J. (1979). *Nursing theory: Analysis, application, evaluation*. Boston: Little, Brown.

Toffler, A. (1970). *Future shock*. New York: Random House

Toffler, A. (1980). *The third wave*. New York: William Morrow.

Walker, L.O., and Avant, K.C. (1983). *Strategies for theory construction in nursing*. Norwalk, Conn.: Appleton-Century-Crofts.

Webster's Ninth New Collegiate Dictionary. (1983). Springfield, Mass.: Merriam-Webster

Book Chapters

Falco, S.M., & Lobo, M.L. (1980). Martha Rogers. In Nursing Theories Conference Group, J.B. George, Chairperson, *Nursing theories: The base for professional practice*. Englewood Cliffs, N.J.: Prentice-Hall.

Fawcett, J. (1984). Rogers life process model. In J. Fawcett, *Analysis and evaluation of conceptual models of nursing*. Philadelphia, F.A. Davis.

Field, L., & Newman, M. (1982). Clinical application of the unitary man framework: Case study analysis (1980). In M.J. Kim, & D.A. Moritz (Eds.), *Classification of nursing diagnosis: Proceedings of the third and fourth national conference*. New York: McGraw-Hill.

Martha Rogers. (1985). In A.I. Meleis, *Theoretical nursing: Development and progress*. Philadelphia: J.B. Lippincott.

Articles

Anderson, M. (1980). A psychosocial screening tool for ambulatory health-care clients: A pilot study of validity. *Nursing Research, 29*(6):347-351.

Atwood, J.R., & Gill-Rogers, B.P. (1984). Metatheory, methodology, and practicality: Issues in research uses of Rogers' science of unitary man. *Nursing Research, 33*(2):88-91.

Barnard, K.E. (1977). Maternal-child nursing research: Review of past and strategies for future. *Nursing Research, 26*(3):193-200.

Barnard, K.E. (1980). Knowledge for practice: Directions for the future. *Nursing Research, 29*(4):208-212.

Blair, C. (1979). Hyperactivity in children: Viewed within the framework of synergistic man. *Nursing Forum, 18*:293-303.

Bullough, B. (1975). Barriers to nurse practitioner movement: Problems of women in a womens field. *International Journal of Health Services, 5*(2):225-233.

Bullough, B. (1976). Influences on role expansion. *American Journal of Nursing, 76*(9):1476-1481.

Burr, H.S., & Northrop, F.S.E. (1935). The electrodynamic theory of life. *Quarterly Review of Biology, 10*:322-333.

Cooperative nursing investigations: Role for everyone. (1974). *Nursing Research, 23*(6):452-456.

Craig, S.L. (1980). Theory development and its relevance for nursing. *Journal of Advanced Nursing, 5*(4):349-355.

Cronenwett, L.R. (1983). Helping and nursing models. *Nursing Research, 32*(6):342-346.

Duffey, M., & Muhlenkamp, A.F. (1974, Sept.). Framework for theory analysis. *Nursing Outlook, 22*:570-574.

Ellis, R. (1968, May-June). Characteristics of significant theories. *Nursing Research, 17*:217-222.

Fawcett, J. (1975). Family as a living open system: Emerging conceptual framework for nursing. *International Nursing Review, 22*(4):113-116.

Fawcett, J. (1977). Relationship between identification and patterns of change in spouses body images during and after pregnancy. *International Journal of Nursing Studies, 14*(4):199-213.

Fawcett, J. (1984). The metaparadigm of nursing: Present status and future refinements. *Image, 16*(3):84-87.

Floyd, J.A. (1983). Research using Rogers' conceptual system: Development of a testable theorem. *Advances in Nursing Science, 5*(2):37-38.

Gill, B.P., & Atwood, J.R. (1981, March-April). Reciprocy and helicy used to relate in EGF and wound healing. *Nursing Research, 30*:68-72.

Goldberg, W.G., & Fitzpatrick, J.J. (1980). Movement therapy with the aged. *Nursing Research, 29*(6):339-346.

Greaves, F. (1980). Objectively toward curriculum improvement in nursing: Education in England and Wales. *Journal of Advanced Nursing, 5*(6):591-599.

Gresham, F.M. (1981). Assessment of children's social skills. *Journal of Psychology, 19*(2):120-133.

Gunter, L.M., & Miller, J.C. (1977). Toward a nursing gerontology. *Nursing Research, 26*(3):208-221.

Hardy, M.F. (1974, March-April). Theories: Components, development, evaluation. *Nursing Research, 23*:100-107.

Hardy, M.F. (1978). Perspectives on nursing theory. *Advance in Nursing Science, 1*:37-48.

Heidt, P. (1981). Effects of therapeutic touch on anxiety level of hospitalized patients. *Nursing Research, 30*(1):196-201.

Impact of physical-physiological activity on infants growth and development. (1972). *Nursing Research, 21*(3):210-219.

Johnson, D.E. (1974, Sept.-Oct.). Development of a theory: A requisite for nursing as a primary health profession. *Nursing Research, 23*:372-377.

Johnson, M. (1983). Some aspects of the relation between theory and research in nursing. *Journal of Advanced Nursing, 8*(1):21-28.

Johnson, R.L., Fitzpatrick, J.J., & Donovan, M.D. (1982). Developmental stage: Relationship to temporal dimensions. *Nursing Research, 31:*120. (Abstract).

Jones, P.S. (1978). Adaptation model for nursing practice. *American Journal of Nursing, 78*(11):1900-1906.

Katz, V. (1971) Auditory stimulation and developmental behavior of the premature infant. *Nursing Research, 20*(3):196-201.

Ketefish, S. (1981). Critical thinking educational preparation, and development of moral judgment among selected groups of practicing nurses. *Nursing Research, 30*(2):98-103.

Ketefish, S. (1981). Moral reasoning and moral behavior among selected groups of practicing nurses. *Nursing Research, 30*(3):171-176.

Ketefish, S. (1976). Curriculum change in nursing education: Sources of knowledge utilized. *International Nursing Review, 23*(4):107-115.

Kim, H.S. (1983). Use of Rogers' conceptual system in research: Comments. *Nursing Research, 32* (2):89-91.

Krieger, D. (1976). Healing by laying on of hands as a facilitator of bioenergetic change: The response of in vivo human hemoglobin. *International Journal of Psychoenergetic Systems, 1*:121-129.

Lanara, V.A. (1976). Philosophy of nursing and current nursing problems. *International Nursing Review, 23*(2):48-54.

Levine, N.H. (1976). A conceptual model for obstetric nursing. *Journal of Obstetrics, Gynecologic, and Neonatal Nursing, 5*(2):9-15.

McCrae, J. (1979). Therapeutic touch in practice. *American Journal of Nursing, 79*:664-665.

Majesky, S.J., Brester, M.H., & Nishio, K.T. (1978). Development of a research tool: Patient indicators of nursing care. *Nursing Research, 27*(6):365-371.

McFarlane, E.A. (1980). Nursing theory: Compassion of four theoretical proposals. *Journal of Advanced Nursing, 5*(1):3-19.

Miller, L.A. (1979). An explanation of therapeutic touch using the science of unitary man. *Nursing Forum, 18*:278-287.

Moore, G. (1982). Perceptual complexity, memory and human duration experience. *Nursing Research, 31*:189. (Abstract).

Porter, L.S. (1972). The impact of physical-physiological activity on infant growth and development. *Nursing Research, 21*(3):210-219.

Reed, P.G., et al. (1982). Suicidal crises: Relationship to the experience of time. *Nursing Research, 31:*122. (Abstract).

Rehabilitation workshops: Change in attitudes of nurses. (1972). *Nursing Research, 21*(2):132-137.

Reiner, D.K. (1977). Persons in process: Model for professional education. *Archives of the Foundation of Thanatology, 6*(3):24.

Rejoinder to commentary: Toward a clearer understanding of concept of nursing theory. (1972). *Nursing Research, 21*(1):59-62.

Roy, C., & Obloy, M. (1978). Practitioner movement: Toward a science of nursing. *American Journal of Nursing, 78*(10):1698-1702.

Schoen, D.C. (1975). Comparing body systems and conceptual approaches to nursing education. *Nursing Research, 24*(5):383-387.

Sheahan, J. (1980). Some aspects of the teaching and learning in nursing. *Journal of Advanced Nursing, 5*(5):491-511.

Taylor, S.D. (1975). Bibliography on nursing research: 1950-1974. *Nursing Research, 24*(3):207-255.

Theiss, B.E. (1976). Investigation of perceived role functions and attitudes of nurse practitioner role in a primary care clinic. *Military Medicine, 141*(2):85-89.

Walker, L.O., & Nicholson, R. (1980). Criteria for evaluating nursing process models. *Nurse Educator, 5*(5):8-9.

Whall, A.L. (1981). Nursing theory and the assessment of families. *Journal of Psychiatric Nursing and Mental Health Services, 19*(1):30-36.

Whelton, B.J. (1979). An operationalization of Martha Rogers' theory throughout the nursing process. *International Journal of Nursing Studies, 16:* 7-20.

Dissertation

Rawnsley, M.M. (1977). *Perception of the speed of time in aging and in dying: An empirical investigation of holistic theory of nursing proposed by Martha Rogers.* Doctoral dissertation. Boston University.

Appendix A

RELATIONSHIP OF THE PRINCIPLES OF HOMEODYNAMICS TO THE NURSING PROCESS FOR JANIE

Components of the Nursing Process	Principles of Homeodynamics		
	Complementarity	Resonancy	Helicy
Nursing assessment component	1. How does Janie see her environment? 2. What kind of differences are there between the hospital and her home? 3. How is she reacting to the changes in her environment? 4. How does her health problem and the environment affect each other?	1. What is Janie's past history? 2. What kind of deviations from the expected norms have there been? 3. Were these deviations individually or environmentally related? 4. What is the reason for the hospitalization? 5. How will this affect her life?	1. What are Janie's normal behavior patterns and routine? 2. Were the behaviors or routines undergoing a change prior to her admission? 3. What kinds of activities can she perform? 4. What kinds of past experiences has she had? 5. How might those experiences influence her current situation? 6. What is Janie's developmental level?

Used with permission from Falco, S.M., & Lobo, M.L. (1980). Martha Rogers. In Nursing Theories Conference Group, J.B. George, Chairperson, *Nursing theories: The base for professional practice.* Englewood Cliffs, N.J.: Prentice-Hall.

Continued.

RELATIONSHIP OF THE PRINCIPLES OF HOMEODYNAMICS TO THE NURSING PROCESS FOR JANIE—cont'd

Components of the Nursing Process	Principles of Homeodynamics		
	Complementarity	Resonancy	Helicy
Nursing assessment component—cont'd			7. Will the hospital environment support or retard developmental progress? 8. What are Janie's goals?
Nursing diagnosis component	1. What is the nature of the interaction between Janie and the hospital?	1. What is the interference this hospitalization will make in Janie's life?	1. What are the rhythmic patterns that are being exhibited?
Nursing plan for implementation component	1. How can the hospital environment be modified to reduce the differences identified? 2. How can Janie be helped to understand the differences that cannot be eliminated? 3. How can her health potential be improved by manipulating the environment?	1. How can Janie's normal development be promoted? 2. How can the effects of the interferences be minimized?	1. How can Janie's normal behavioral patterns and routines be promoted in the hospital? 2. What kind of modifications can be made to promote her normal behavioral patterns and routines? 3. What kind of provisions can be made to promote her normal growth and development? 4. How can Janie be helped to develop successful rhythmic behavioral patterns within the hospital environment? 5. How can Janie be helped to reach her goals?
Nursing evaluation component	1. Has Janie's behavior changed as a result of environmental modification? 2. What kind of new reactions are now taking place?	1. Is Janie developing normally, based on theorists? 2. Has the interference with development been minimized?	1. What kind of rhythmic repatterning has taken place? 2. Is Janie's development being supported? 3. Is she moving toward her goals?

Appendix B

GLOSSARY

Learned Profession:	A science and an art.
Science:	An organized body of abstract knowledge arrived at by scientific research and logical analysis.
Art:	The imaginative and creative use of knowledge.
Negentropy:	Increasing heterogeneity, differentiation, diversity, complexity of pattern.
Energy Field:	The fundamental unit of the living and the non-living. Field is a unifying concept. Energy signifies the dynamic nature of the field. Energy fields are infinite.
Pattern:	The distinguishing characteristic of an energy field perceived as a single wave.
Four Dimensional:	A non-linear domain without spatial or temporal attributes.
Conceptual System:	An abstraction. A representation of the universe or some portion thereof.
Unitary Man: (Human field)	An irreducible, four dimensional energy field identified by pattern and manifesting characteristics that are specific to the whole and which cannot be predicted from knowledge of the parts.
Environment:	An irreducible, four dimensional energy field identified by pattern and integral with the human field.

Appendix C

SELECTED DOCTORAL DISSERTATIONS BASED ON *NURSING: SCIENCE OF UNITARY HUMAN BEINGS*

Barrett, Elizabeth Ann. (1983). *An Empirical Investigation of Rogers' Principle of Helicy: The Relationship of Human Field Complexity, Human Field Motion, and Power.* New York University.

Cowling, W. Richard. (1982). *The Relationship of Mystical Experience, Differentiation, and Creativity in College Students: An Empirical Investigation of the Principle of Helicy in Rogers' Science of Unitary Man.* New York University.

Ference, Helen. (1979). *The Relationship of Time Experience, Creativity Traits, Differentiation, and Human Field Motion.* New York University.

Gueldner, Sarah H. (1983). *A Study of the Relationship Between Imposed Motion and Human Field Motion in Elderly Individuals Living in Nursing Homes.* University of Alabama in Birmingham.

Ludomirski-Kalamin, Betty. (1984). *Relationship Between the Environmental Energy Wave Frequency Pattern Manifest in Red Light and Blue Light and Human Field Motion in Adult Individuals with Visual Sensory Perception and Those With Total Blindness.* New York University.

Macrae, Janet A. (1982). *A Comparison Between Meditating Subjects and Non-Meditating Subjects on Time Experience and Human Field Motion.* New York University.

Available through Dissertation Abstracts.

Malinski, Violet. (1980). *The Relationship Between hyperactivity in Children and Perception of Short Wave Length Light: An Investigation into the Conceptual System Proposed by Martha E. Rogers*. New York University.

Miller, Fay. (1984). *The Relationship of Sleep, Wakefulness, and Beyond Waking Experience: A Descriptive Study of M. Rogers Concept of Sleep-Wake Rhythm*. New York University.

Raile, Martha M. (1982). *The Relationship of Creativity, Actualization, and Empathy in Unitary Human Development: A Descriptive Study of Rogers' Principle of Helicy*. New York University.

Rawnsley, Marilyn. (1977). *Relationships Between the Perception of the Speed of Time and the Process of Dying: An Empirical Investigation of the Holistic Theory of Nursing Proposed by Martha Rogers*. Boston University.

Reeder, Francelyn. (1984). *Nursing Research, Holism, and Philosophies of Science: Points of Congruence Between Edmund Husserl and Martha E. Rogers*. New York University.

Sarter, Barbara. (1984). *The Stream of Becoming: A Metaphysical Analysis of Rogers' Model of Unitary Man*. New York University.

Joyce J. Fitzpatrick

29

Life Perspective Model

Sarah J. Beckman, Patricia Chapman-Boyce, Sydney Coleman-Ehmke,
Cheryl A. Hailway, Rosalyn A. Pung

CREDENTIALS AND BACKGROUND OF THE THEORIST

Joyce J. Fitzpatrick was born May 4, 1944. She received her B.S.N. in 1966 from Georgetown University, in Washington, D.C., and her M.S. in Psychiatric Mental Health from Ohio State University, in Columbus in 1967. She took post master's courses in Community Health at Ohio State in 1971 to 1972, and achieved a

The authors wish to express appreciation to Dr. Joyce J. Fitzpatrick for critiquing the chapter.

Ph.D. in nursing from New York University in 1975.

Fitzpatrick has held many positions including staff nurse, public health nurse, instructor, and the director of training for suicide prevention, all in Columbus, Ohio. She has served as an assistant professor at New York University and Associate Professor at Wayne State University. In addition, she has also been the chairperson for the Department of Nursing Systems at Wayne State and the director of the Center for Health Research at Wayne State. Fitzpatrick has been Visiting Professor at Rutgers—The State University, College of Nursing. In 1982

Fitzpatrick became Professor and Dean of Nursing at Case Western Reserve University in Cleveland, Ohio, and Administrative Associate at University Hospitals of Cleveland.

Since 1974 Fitzpatrick has worked as a consultant in such areas as faculty development, research development, and development of master's and doctoral programs in nursing with several institutions, including Indiana University, Michigan State University, The Ohio State University, Rutgers University, University of Kansas, University of Virginia, Vanderbilt University, and Wright State University.

Fitzpatrick has received honoraries and is affiliated with several organizations. Professional activities have been numerous. She has presented workshops on community health, current issues in health, stress, crisis intervention, dying and death, suicidology, and theory development. She has been the investigator and director for several research grants, has done numerous paper and research presentations, and has published extensively.[5]

THEORETICAL SOURCES FOR THEORY DEVELOPMENT

Fitzpatrick is a well-known, published scholar among nursing professionals. She constructed her theory model based on the ideas and work of Martha Rogers. Fitpatrick* used rhythm patterns, which are operational modes specifying the pattern of person and environment that were explicated by Rogers. In addition, Fitzpatrick[5:310] incorporated the peak and wave pattern ideas of E. Haus and G.G. Luce. To round out the model, she drew from G. Caplan's crisis theory.†

USE OF EMPIRICAL EVIDENCE

Fitzpatrick's Life Perspective Model is synthesized from interpretations made from Rogers'

theory work. Colleagues consider Rogers one of the most original thinkers in nursing who capitalizes on knowledge from other disciplines such as anthropology, sociology, astronomy, religion, philosophy, history, and mythology. The model's concept of environment is drawn from von Bertalanffy and others who question the failure of physical laws to explain evolution of life. According to S.M. Falco and M.L. Lobo, "There is a strong parallel between Rogers' basic assumptions and general systems theory."[2:167] Rogers also draws from Einstein in using the concept of four dimensionality.

MAJOR CONCEPTS AND DEFINITIONS

The four major concepts in this model are *nursing, person, health,* and *environment.* "The ontogenetic and phylogenetic interactions among person and health are looked upon as the essence of nursing."[7:306] Person is seen as an open system, a unified whole characterized by a basic human rhythm. Health is viewed as a human dimension under continuous development—a heightened awareness of the meaningfulness of life.[7:306] According to J.L. Pressler,[7] Fitzpatrick mirrors Rogers' definition of environmental field.

MAJOR ASSUMPTIONS

Fitzpatrick repeats the five basic assumptions proposed by Rogers in her theory of unitary man:

1. Man is a unified whole possessing his own integrity and manifesting characteristics that are more than and different from the sum of his parts.
2. Man and environment are open systems, continually exchanging matter and energy with each other.
3. The life process evolves irreversibly and unidirectionally along the space time continuum.
4. Pattern and organization identify man and reflect his innovative wholeness.

---

*References 4; 5:299-301.
†References 4:23-24; 7:310.

5. Man is characterized by the capacity for abstraction and imagery, language and thought, sensation and emotion.[3:299-300]

According to Pressler, four implicit assumptions pertinent to understanding Fitzpatrick's model were previously identified. These are:
1. Differences in behavioral manifestations are more easily identified during the peaks of wave patterns.
2. Identified by congruency, consistency, and integrity of rhythmic patterns, health is to the manifestations of symphonic interaction of persons and their environments.
3. Emphasized through selected research on temporality, the meaning attached to life is a central concern of nursing.
4. Nursing is a philosophy, a science, and an art.*

THEORETICAL ASSERTIONS

The Life Perspective Model is a developmental model that proposes that the process of human development is characterized by rhythms. The person is treated as an open, holistic, rhythmic system that can best be described by temporal, motion, consciousness, and perceptual patterns. It is possible to identify peaks and troughs of particular human rhythms throughout the developmental process. There are patterns within a pattern or overall life patterns. Life's pattern continues toward timelessness, becoming more dominant as one's development occurs. This may best be described as patterns within a pattern or rhythms within an overall life rhythm. Health is viewed as a continuously developing characteristic of humans with the full life potential that may characterize the process of dying, as the heightened awareness of the meaningfulness of life, and as representing a more fully developed dimension of health. Health is seen as the interactions of persons with their environment. Nursing's central concern is focused on

the person in relation to health, with the goal of enhancing the developmental process toward health so people may develop their potential as human beings. "The meaning attached to life, the basic understanding of human existence, is a central concern of nursing as science and profession."[3:301] The hypothesis is that "individuals experiencing crisis had difficulty integrating the present situation within their life perspective."[3:295]

A conceptual model was developed to depict the essential theoretical representation of person, environment, health, and nursing as if one were looking through a Slinky. Fitzpatrick, expanded the Slinky concept to symbolize her view of man. The representation helps in picturing the relationships found in the Life Perspective Model (Figure 29-1).

LOGICAL FORM

Fitzpatrick developed the Life Perspective Model using a deductive logical approach. That is, the author uses empirical findings to support a proposed developmental model. This model indicates that human development is characteristic of temporal, motion, perceptual, and consciousness rhythms. These patterns show the continuous person-environment interaction in relation to one's personal development.

An individual's progression through life contains varying high and low intervals, but the general direction represents rapidity. While explaining the broadness in life, such progression relates life and health. In this model health represents a basic human element that is a continuous development from birth to death. Understandably, the meaning one attaches to life and health or humanness is significant in this model. Accordingly, health or potentiating health is considerably influential to one's meaning in life.

Because of Fitzpatrick's extensive work and study under Rogers, Fitzpatrick bases the Life Perspective Model on Rogers' unitary man assumptions and model concepts in addition to

---

*References 4; 7:309-310.

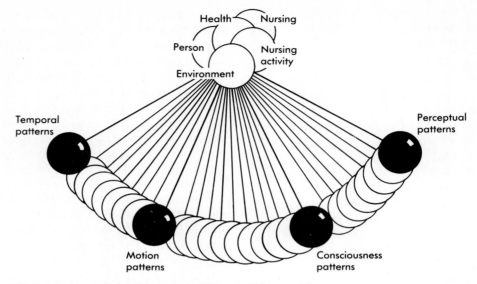

Figure 29-1. Relationships within life perspective model.

Used with permission from Pressler, J.L. (1983). Fitzpatrick's Rhythm Model: Analysis for Nursing Science. In J.J. Fitzpatrick, & A. Whall, *Conceptual models of nursing: Analysis and application.* Bowie, Md.: Robert J. Brady.

expanding the Slinky representation in her own model. To add further merit to this model's development, Fitzpatrick drew from the biological rhythm theory and also from Caplan's crisis theory. Fitzpatrick also used her own personal interests and professional experience in crisis in the model's development. The model's hypothesis was derived based on these aspects. It states, "Individuals experiencing crisis had difficulty integrating the present situations within their life perspective."[3:295]

The next logical step is empirical testing, which is imperative in any model's development and future. Much of the testing of this model has related only to the temporal pattern with a selective population focus on the elderly in nursing homes and during hospitalization. Recent studies have dealt with terminally ill cancer patients and with suicidal individuals. Using results from the completed investigations, Fitzpatrick continues to broaden the model, such as in her meaning attached to life and death. But

she acknowledges that the limitations of the empirical investigations hold back the model's developmental progress and the gathering of further logical support.

ACCEPTANCE BY THE NURSING COMMUNITY
Practice

Because her model is still in the developmental stage, Fitzpatrick encourages further study and ongoing empirical testing. With more involvement by the nursing community, progress will be made. The model is not currently being used in practice.

Education

The majority of testing has been completed by graduate students studying with Fitzpatrick. The model has not been incorporated into any nursing curriculum, but critics feel the theory is potentially adoptable for educational purposes.

Fitzpatrick has incorporated her theory and conceptualization into her graduate-level theory and nursing research courses.

Research

Fitzpatrick is active in current nursing research. Since 1976 she has received research grants totaling more than 1 million dollars. Her research projects have dealt with temporal experiences of the terminally ill cancer patients, the aging process, temporal experiences of the suicidal, the advancement of doctoral programs, and interpretations of life and death. Fitzpatrick's proposals are initiating new ideas and research that is useful for the advancement of nursing science.

FURTHER DEVELOPMENT

As previously discussed, the Life Perspective Model is in a beginning developmental stage. The multiple definitions given to nursing and health in the model are problematic. The vast interrelationship between person and environment is highly complex and not easily understood. Because most of the completed research focuses on the temporal pattern, the other patterns still need to be researched. But even the completed temporal pattern research shows that operational measurement is problematic and raises other considerations for future research. Until significant investigation is completed in all rhythms, this model cannot be addressed holistically. Although the model's individual components may have merit and nursing support, the complete model still needs to be tested. Therefore this model's future place in a creative nursing science, in nursing practice, and in nursing theory consideration is uncertain.

CRITIQUE
Clarity

Fitzpatrick consistently follows theoretical form by stating a hypothesis and listing assumptions.

She continues by stating relationships of concepts and displays her theory in a four dimensional Slinky model, representing the relationship statements. Most of the empirical testing has occurred with temporal patterns, but plans are in process to develop the theory, and to empirically test the conscious rhythm, perceptual rhythms, motion rhythms, and their relationships with the meaning attached to life and life perspective.

Simplicity

This model is complex in its concepts and interrelationships. Sufficiently understanding and explaining the interrelationships between health, nursing, person, environment, and nursing activity in respect to the temporal, motion, consciousness, and perceptual patterns are highly complex and involved undertakings. Such interrelationships are not easily taken from concept to operational measurement.

Generality

Most of the empirical investigations relate to the elderly, terminally ill cancer patients, and suicidal individuals and contain a heavy psychosocial orientation. Fitzpatrick acknowledges that the model needs testing in other populations, such as the young and infants.

Empirical Precision

Fitzpatrick and her researchers have been successful in scientifically testing and evaluating several of the relationships presented in the Life Perspective Rhythm Model. But the current literature indicates that only some educators and students are in the process of empirically testing relationships in this projected model. Interested researchers and practitioners are encouraged to become involved in the efforts to further develop the Life Perspective Rhythm Model.

Derivable Consequences

The derivable consequences connect the theory with achievable nursing outcomes. Because this model is at the beginning development stage, its application and usefulness in nursing practice and science have been limited. The concepts, and some of the research, are stimulating and warrant further work and additional development. Conceivably, some concepts of the model may in the future help broaden perspectives in relation to humanness and move nursing closer to holistic nursing practice.[1:133-143]

REFERENCES

1. Chinn, P.L., & Jacobs, M.K. (1983). *Theory and nursing: A systematic approach.* St. Louis: C.V. Mosby.
2. Falco, S.M., & Lobo, M.L. (1980). Martha Rogers. In Nursing Theories Conference Group, J.B. George, Chairperson, *Nursing theories: The base for professional nursing practice.* Englewood Cliffs, N.J.: Prentice-Hall.
3. Fitzpatrick, J.J., & Whall, A.L. (1983). *Conceptual models of nursing: Analysis and application.* Bowie, Md.: Robert J. Brady.
4. Fitzpatrick, J.J. (1982). The crisis perspective: Relationship to nursing. In J.J. Fitzpatrick, et al., (Eds.), *Nursing models and their psychiatric mental health applications.* Bowie, Md.: Robert J. Brady.
5. Fitzpatrick, J.J. (1984). Curriculum vitae.
6. Goldberg, W.G., & Fitzpatrick, J.J. (1980, Nov.-Dec.). Movement therapy with the aged. *Nursing Research, 29*(6):339-346.
7. Pressler, J.L. (1983). Fitzpatrick's rhythm model: Analysis for nursing science. In J. Fitzpatrick & A. Whall, *Conceptual models of nursing: Analysis and application.* Bowie, Md.: Robert J. Brady.

BIBLIOGRAPHY
Primary Sources
Books

Fitzpatrick, J.J., Johnston, A.L., & Floyd, J.A. (1982). *Nursing models and their psychiatric mental health applications.* Bowie, Md.: Robert J. Brady.

Fitzpatrick, J.J., & Whall, A.L. (1983). *Conceptual models of nursing: Analysis and application.* Bowie, Md.: Robert J. Brady.

Werley, H.H., & Fitzpatrick, J.J. (Eds.). (1984). *Annual review of nursing research* (Vol. I). New York: Springer.

Werley, H.H., & Fitzpatrick, J.J. (Eds.). (1984). *Annual review of nursing research* (Vol. II). New York: Springer.

Chapters and Proceedings

Fitzpatrick, J.J. (1976). Repatterning alcoholic behaviors: Nursing strategies. In J. Chodil (Ed.), *Proceedings of the 8th Annual Clinical Sessions.* New York: New York University.

Fitzpatrick, J.J. (1982). The path of nursing, the path of science? In V. Engle, *Proceedings of the Fourth Annual Research Symposium of the Michigan Sigma Theta Tau Consortium.* Indianapolis, Ind.: Sigma Theta Tau.

Fitzpatrick, J.J. (1983). Integrating the domains of nursing. In *Proceedings of the 1982 Forum on Doctoral Education in Nursing.* Cleveland, Ohio: Case Western Reserve University.

Fitzpatrick, J.J. (1983). Techniques of gerontological counseling. In S. Lego (Ed.), *Lippincott manual of psychiatric nursing.* Philadelphia: J.B. Lippincott.

Fitzpatrick, J.J. (1982). The crisis perspective: Relationship to nursing. In J.J. Fitzpatrick, et al., *Nursing models and their psychiatric mental health applications.* Bowie, Md.: Robert J. Brady.

Fitzpatrick, J.J. (1983). A life perspective rhythm model. In J.J. Fitzpatrick, & A.L. Whall (Eds.), *Conceptual models of nursing: Analysis and application.* Bowie, Md.: Robert J. Brady.

Fitzpatrick, J.J., & Whall, A.L. (1983). Nursing models: Summary and future projections. In J.J. Fitzpatrick, & A.L. Whall (Eds.). *Conceptual models of nursing: Analysis and application.* Bowie, Md.: Robert J. Brady.

Fitzpatrick, J.J., & Whall, A.L., (1983). Overview of nursing models and nursing theories. In J.J. Fitzpatrick, & A.L. Whall (Eds.), *Conceptual models of nursing: Analysis and application.* Bowie, Md.: Robert J. Brady.

Johnston, R.L., & Fitzpatrick, J.J. (1982). Relevance of psychiatric mental health nursing theories to nursing models. In J.J. Fitzpatrick, et al., *Nursing models and their psychiatric mental health applications.* Bowie, Md.: Robert J. Brady.

Roy, C., et al. (1981). Theoretical framework for classification of nursing diagnosis: Panel discussion. In M.J. Kim, & D. Moritz (Eds.), *Classification of nursing diagnosis: Proceedings of the third and fourth national conferences.* New York: McGraw Hill.

Articles

Downs, F.S., & Fitzpatrick, J.J. (1976, Nov.-Dec.). Preliminary investigation of the reliability and validity of a tool for the assessment of body position and motor activity. *Nursing Research, 25:*404-408.

Fitzpatrick, J.J. (1970, Feb.). Aging and institutionalization as determinants of temporal and motor phenomena. *Image, 1:*24.

Fitzpatrick, J. (1970). Learning is . . . . *Capital, 54:*7-9.

Fitzpatrick, J. (1978). Aging and institutionalization as determinants of temporal and motor phenomena. *Image, 10:*24.

Fitzpatrick, J.J. (1980, Sept.-Oct.). Patients' perceptions of time: Current research. *International Nursing Review, 5:*143-153, 160.

Fitzpatrick, J.J. (1983, May). Suicidology and suicide prevention: Historical perspectives from the nursing literature. *Journal of Psychosocial Nursing and Mental Health Service, 5:*20-28.

Fitzpatrick, J.J., & Donovan, M.J. (1978, July). Temporal experience and motor behavior among the aging. *Research in Nursing and Health, 2:* 60-68.

Fitzpatrick, J.J., & Donovan, M.J. (1979, May-June). A follow-up study of the reliability and validity of the motor activity rating scale. *Nursing Research, 3:*179-181.

Fitzpatrick, J.J., Donovan, M.J., & Johnston, R.L. (1980, June). Experience of time during the crisis of cancer. *Cancer Nursing, 3:*191-194.

Fitzpatrick, J.J., & Reid, P.G. (1980, Dec.). Stress in the crisis experience: Nursing interventions. *Occupational Health Nursing, 28:*19-21.

Flagherty, G.G., & Fitzpatrick, J.J. (1978, Nov.-Dec.). Use of a relaxation technique to increase comfort level of postoperative patients: A preliminary study. *Nursing Research, 6:*352-355.

Goldberg, W.G., & Fitzpatrick, J.J. (1980, Nov.-Dec.). Movement therapy with the aged. *Nursing Research, 6:*339-346.

Horowitz, B., Fitzpatrick, J.J., & Flaherty, G. (1984). Relaxation techniques to relieve pain in postoperative open heart surgery patients: A clinical study, *Dimensions of Critical Care Nursing Journal. 3*(6):364-371.

Kiley, M., et al. (1983). Computerized nursing information systems (NIS). *Nursing Management, 14:*26-29.

Pacini, C.M., & Fitzpatrick, J.J. (1982, June). Sleep patterns of hospitalized aged individuals. *Journal of Gerontological Nursing, 6:*327-332.

Roberts, B.L., & Fitzpatrick, J.J. (1983, March).

Improving balance. Therapy of movement. *Journal of Gerontological Nursing, 3:*150-156.

Roslaniec, A., & Fitzpatrick, J.J. (1979, Dec.). Changes in mental status in older adults with four days of hospitalization. *Research in Nursing and Health, 2:*177-187.

Study Group on Nursing Information Systems (1983). Special report computerized nursing information systems: An urgent need. *Research in Nursing and Health, 6:*101-105.

Wilson, L.M., & Fitzpatrick, J.J. (1984). Dialectic thinking as a means of understanding systems-in-development: Relevance to Rogers' principles. *Advances in Nursing Science, 6*(2):24-41.

Thesis

Fitzpatrick, J.J. (1967). *A study of staff nurses' perceptions of the importance of selected nursing activities in carrying out their nursing role.* Unpublished master's thesis. The Ohio State University.

Dissertation

Fitzpatrick, J.J. (1975). *An investigation of the relationship between temporal orientation, temporal extension, and time perception.* Unpublished doctoral dissertation. New York University.

Abstracts, Book Reviews, Editorials

Downs, F.S., & Fitzpatrick, J.J. (1977). Preliminary investigation of the reliability and validity of a tool for the assessment of body position and motor activity. *Psychological Abstracts.* Washington, D.C.: American Psychological Association. (Research abstract).

Fitzpatrick, J. (1978). Temporal experiences among hospitalized individuals: A pilot study. In R. Williams, & C. Wrotny (Eds.), *Health promotion: In health and illness: Proceedings of the First Annual Research Symposium of the Michigan Sigma Theta Tau Consortium.* Indianapolis, Ind.: Sigma Theta Tau (Abstract).

Fitzpatrick, J. (1980). Review of *Nursing theory: Analysis, application, evaluation* by Barbara J. Stevens, *Nursing Research, 29:*114.

Fitzpatrick, J. (1980). Why a newsletter? *Center for Health Research NEWS, 1*(1):1.

Fitzpatrick, J. (1980). Time is relevant. *Center for Health Research NEWS, 1*(2):1.

Fitzpatrick, J. (1980). Identity crisis resolved. *Center for Health Research NEWS, 2*(1):1.

Fitzpatrick, J. (1981). Is nursing the science of health? *Center for Health Research NEWS, 2*(2):1.

Fitzpatrick, J. (1981). Toward the future . . . . *Center for Health Research NEWS, 2*(3):1.

Fitzpatrick, J. (1981). *Review of The many faces of suicide: Indirect self-destructive behavior* by N.L. Farberow (Ed.). *Nursing Outlook, 29:*435.

Fitzpatrick, J. (1981). Answer 2 to research replication: Questions and answers. *Western Journal of Nursing Research, 3:*96-97.

Fitzpatrick, J. (1982). Review of *Readings on the research process in nursing* by D.J. Fox, & I.R. Leeser (Eds.). *Nursing Research, 31:*158.

Fitzpatrick, J.J. (1982). Preface in *Creating research environments for the 1980's (MNRS).* Indianapolis: Midwest Alliance in Nursing.

Fitzpatrick, J.J. (1983). Review of *Suicide intervention for nurses* by M. Miller (Ed.). *Journal of Psychosocial Nursing, 21*(2):39.

Fitzpatrick, J.J., Donovan, M.J., & Johnston, R. (1979). Temporal experiences among terminally ill cancer patients: An exploratory study. *Proceedings of the Second Annual Research Symposium, Michigan Sigma Theta Tau Consortium.* Indianapolis, Ind.: Sigma Theta Tau (Abstract).

Fitzpatrick, J.J., Johnston, R.L., & Donovan, M.J. (1980). Hospitalization as a crisis: Relation to temporal experience, in WICHE proceedings. *Communicating Nursing Research Directions for the 1980's, 13:*48 (Abstract).

Johnston, R.L., Fitzpatrick, J.J., & Donovan, M.J. (1982). Developmental stage: Relationship to the experience of time. *Nursing Research, 31:*120 (Abstract).

Reed, P.G., et al. (1982). Suicidal crises: Relationship to the experience of time. *Nursing Research, 31:*122, (Abstract).

Sills, G.M., & Fitzpatrick, J.J. (1979). Women: Psychotropic drug use and eclectic relaxation therapy. In *Nursing Research: Synopses of selected clinical studies.* Kansas City: American Nurses' Association. (Abstract).

Correspondence

Fitzpatrick, Joyce (1984). Personal correspondence.

Interview

Fitzpatrick, J.J. (1984, March 22). Telephone interview.

Fitzpatrick, J.J. (1985). Telephone interviews.

Secondary Sources
Book Reviews

Fitzpatrick, J.J., Whall, A.L., & Johnston, R.L. (1982). *Nursing models and their psychiatric mental health applications.*
*American Journal of Nursing, 1:*102-103, January 1983.
*Nursing Outlook, 3:*148, May-June 1983.
*Research in Nursing and Health, 1:*41, March 1983.

Chapters

Pressler, J.L. (1983). Fitzpatrick's rhythm model: Analysis for nursing science. In J. Fitzpatrick, & A. Whall, *Conceptual models of nursing: Analysis and application.* Bowie, Md.: Robert J. Brady.

Biographical Sources

Fitzpatrick, J.J. (1980, Aug.). *Directory of nurses with doctoral degrees* (Vol. 1). Kansas City: American Nurses Association.

Fitzpatrick, J.J. (1984, Jan.). *The National Faculty Directory* (Vol. 1). Detroit: Gale Research.

Other Sources

Caplan, G. (1961). *An approach to community mental health.* New York: Grune & Stratton.

Caplan, G. (1964). *Principles of preventive psychiatry.* New York: Basic Books.

Chinn, P.L., & Jacobs, M.K. (1983). *Theory and nursing: A systematic approach.* St. Louis: C.V. Mosby.

Falco, S.M., & Lobo, M.L. (1980). Martha Rogers. In Nursing Theories Conference Group, J.B. George, Chairperson, *Nursing theories: The base for professional nursing practice.* Englewood Cliffs, N.J.: Prentice-Hall.

Haus, E. (1978). Perspectives on nursing theory. *Advances in Nursing Science, 1:*37-48.

Luce, G.G. (1970). *Biological rhythms in psychiatry and medicine.* National Institute of Mental Health. Washington, D.C.: U.S. Dept. of Health, Education, and Welfare.

Rogers, M.E. (1967). The theoretical basis of nursing. Philadelphia: F.A. Davis.

Margaret A. Newman

30

Model of Health

DeAnn M. Hensley, Kimberly A. Kilgore, Jill Vass Langfitt, LaPhyllis Peterson

CREDENTIALS AND BACKGROUND OF THE THEORIST

Margaret A. Newman was born October 10, 1933,[25:588] in Memphis, Tennessee. She earned her first bachelor's degree in home economics and English from Baylor University, in Waco, Texas, in 1954, and her second in nursing from the University of Tennessee in Memphis in 1962. She received her master's degree in med-

ical-surgical nursing and teaching from the University of California at San Francisco in 1964 and her Ph.D. in nursing science and rehabilitation nursing from New York University in New York City in 1971.

Newman progressed through the academic ranks at the University of Tennessee, New York University, The Pennsylvania State University, and is currently, professor at the University of Minnesota in Minneapolis. In addition, she has been the director of nursing for the Clinical Research Center at the University of Tennessee, the acting director of the Ph.D. program in the Division of Nursing at New York University,

The authors wish to express appreciation to Dr. Margaret A. Newman for critiquing the chapter.

and Professor-in-Charge of the Graduate Program and Research at The Pennsylvania State University.

Newman was admitted to the American Academy of Nursing in 1976. She received the Outstanding Alumnus Award from the University of Tennessee College of Nursing in Memphis in 1975 and the Distinguished Alumnus Award from the Division of Nursing at New York University in 1984.[18:1-2] She was a Latin American Teaching Fellow in 1976-1977 and an American Journal of Nursing Scholar in 1979. She was a Distinguished Faculty at the Seventh International Conference on Human Functioning at Wichita, Kansas, in 1983 and is listed in *Who's Who in American Women*.[18]

THEORETICAL SOURCES

Newman uses many fields of inquiry as sources for theory development. Central to her assumptions is the use of Hegel's theory of synthesis of opposites from the field of philosophy.[15:56] The rationale for drawing broad conclusions from the use of a limited number of concepts comes from Capra, an eastern physicist. Capra's position is that many phenomena can be explained in terms of a few. Newman[15:59] draws from Capra in general, and Bentov in particular, for her position on the importance of holistic health and expansion of consciousness. "Bentov has postulated that time is a measure of consciousness."[15:64] Newman[18:1] states, "From the standpoint of nursing theorists, those who were most influential on my thinking were Dorothy Johnson, during my undergraduate studies, and Martha Rogers, in a more extensive way during my graduate study."

EMPIRICAL EVIDENCE

Research has been conducted on the theoretical sources used. Newman[15:23] writes that "in order for nursing research to have meaning in terms of theory development, it must (1) have as its purpose the testing of theory, (2) make explicit the theoretical framework upon which the testing relies, and (3) reexamine the theoretical underpinnings in light of the findings." To Newman,[15:73] "The expansion of knowledge related to man's health and the development of practice based on that knowledge are the responsibility, and perhaps the 'rightful heritage,' of nursing."

MAJOR CONCEPTS AND DEFINITIONS

Newman's major concepts are *movement, time, space,* and *consciousness*. These are all interrelated—movement is a reflection of consciousness; time is a function of movement; time is a measure of consciousness and movement is a means whereby space and time become a reality (Figure 30-1).[15:60]

Newman[13:23] emphasizes that "movement through space is integral to the development of a concept of time in man and is utilized by man as a measure of time." She maintains that "movement brings about change, without which there is no manifest reality."[15:61] To further explain this concept Newman[13:1] uses the example of "the person restricted in his mobility by structural or psychological pathology [who] must adapt to an altered rate of movement."

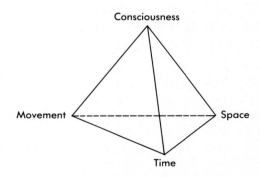

Figure 30-1. Newman's Model of Health.
Used with permission from Newman, M. (1979). *Theory development in nursing.* Philadelphia: F.A. Davis.

Time and space have a complementary relationship.[15:61] "The concept of space is inextricably linked to the concept of time. . . . When one's life space is decreased, as by either physical or social immobility, one's time is increased."[13:61]

Time in Newman's model includes a sense of time perspective, that is, orientation to past, present, and future, but it centers primarily on time as perceived duration. Perceived duration is defined as the ratio of the individual's awareness to content.

$$\text{Perceived duration} = \frac{\text{Awareness}}{\text{Content}}$$

Perceived duration is used synonymously with subjective time as defined by Bentov.* "Factors related to the awareness component include emotional state and attention to a task; factors related to content are external events, body movement, and metabolism."[16:137]

$$\text{Subjective time} = \frac{\text{Awareness}}{\text{Content}}^{21:137}$$

Newman uses the theories of time perception, modified by Bentov's conceptualization of time and consciousness. "He calculates an index of consciousness by establishing a ratio of subjective time (the number of seconds judged to have elapsed) to objective time (actual clock time)."[15:64]

$$\text{Index of consciousness} = \frac{\text{Subjective time}}{\text{Objective time}}^{16:291}$$

Consciousness, the fourth and final concept, is defined as the informational capacity of the system and is manifested in the quantity and quality of interaction with the environment.[17] The life process is seen as progressing toward higher levels of consciousness.[15,17] "The expansion of consciousness is what life, and therefore health, is all about."[15:66] Newman refers to the time sense as a factor altered in the changing level of consciousness. Thus, the perception of time is an indicator of man's health status.[13:6]

MAJOR ASSUMPTIONS

The foundation for Newman's assumptions[15:56] is her definition of health, which is rationalized through the Hegelian dialectical process of thesis, antithesis, and synthesis. Another influential component is Rogers' 1970 model for nursing that focuses on wholeness, person/environment, life process, pattern/organization, and man's capacity for the higher, complex processes of the mind.[15:57;15] From this Newman[15:57-58] developed the following assumptions:

1. Health encompasses conditions heretofore described as illness, or in medical terms, pathology.
2. These "pathological" conditions can be considered a manifestation of the total pattern of the individual.
3. The pattern of the individual that eventually manifests itself as pathology is primary and exists prior to structural or functional changes.
4. Removal of the pathology in itself will not change the pattern of the individual.
5. If becoming "ill" is the only way an individual's pattern can manifest itself, then that is health for that person.

Newman developed her central premise based on these assumptions. She states, "Health is the expansion of consciousness."[13:58] The "process of unfolding consciousness will occur regardless of what we as nurses do. We can, however, assist clients in getting in touch with what is going on, and in that way facilitate the process."[18]

THEORETICAL ASSERTIONS

Newman has developed five interrelationships between her major concepts.

"Time and space have a complementary relationship."* Newman gives examples of this

---

*References 14:290-291.

*References 15:60; 17:165.

relationship at the macrocosmic, microcosmic, and humanistic (everyday) levels. She states that at the humanistic level "the highly mobile individual lives in a world of expanded space and compartmentalized time. When one's life space is decreased, as by either physical or social immobility, one's time is increased."[17:61]

"Movement is a means whereby space and time become a reality."* Man is in a constant state of motion and is constantly changing. This occurs both internally, at the cellular level, and externally through body movement and interaction with the environment. This movement through time and space is what gives man his own unique perception of reality. Movement brings change and enables the individual to experience the world around him.[15:61-63]

"Movement is a reflection of consciousness."* Movement not only is the means of experiencing reality, but it is also the means by which one expresses his thoughts and feelings about the reality he experiences. An individual conveys his awareness of self through the movement involved in language, posture, and body movement.[15:62] "The rhythm and pattern which are reflected in movement are an indication of the internal organization of the person and his perception of the world. Movement provides a means of communication beyond that which language can convey."[15:62]

"Time is a function of movement."* This assertion is supported by Newman's previous studies regarding the experience of time as related to movement and gait tempo. Newman's research shows that the slower one walks, the less subjective time one experiences. When compared with clock time, however, time seems to "fly." Although the individual who is moving quickly subjectively feels he is "beating the clock," he finds when checking a clock that time seems to be dragging.[15:63; 13:1]

"Time is a measure of consciousness."[15:60] This assertion was first proposed in 1977 by Bentov, who measured consciousness with a ra-tio of subjective to objective time. Newman applied this measure of consciousness to the subjective and objective data compiled in her research. She found that the consciousness index increased with age. Some of her most recent research has also supported the finding of increasing consciousness with age.[16:293] Newman[13:64] cites this evidence as support for her position that the life process evolves toward consciousness expansion. "However, certain moods, such as depression, may be accompanied by a diminished sense of time."[21:139]

LOGICAL FORM

Newman uses both inductive and deductive logic. Inductive logic is based on observing particular instances and then relating those instances to form a whole. Newman's theory development was derived from her earlier research on time perception and gait tempo. Time and movement, along with space and consciousness, are subsequently used as central components in her conceptual framework. These concepts help explain "the phenomena of the life process, and therefore of health."[15:59]

But Newman's theory also uses deductive logic.

> A holistic approach is not to be confused with, or construed to mean a multivariate approach. It is not the summing up of many factors . . . to make a whole. It is the identification of patterns which are reflective of the whole. What these parameters are will vary according to one's ability to see the whole. For some, the universe can be seen in a grain of sand. For others, characteristics which present identifiable patterns of the individual, e.g., the way a person walks or the way he talks, are a good place to start.[15:70]

ACCEPTANCE BY THE NURSING COMMUNITY
Practice

Newman's model of health is potentially useful in the practice of nursing because it uses con-

*References 15:60; 17:165.

cepts employed by the nursing profession. Movement and time are an intrinsic part of nursing intervention, that is, range-of-motion, ambulation, turning, coughing, and deep breathing. These parameters are used each day by the nurse in practice.[4:271-272]

Barbara Doberneck, a graduate student at The Pennsylvania State University, used Newman's model to work with caregivers of chronically ill people. She was helped by Newman's discussion of application of the model to practice in her chapter in the Clements and Roberts book on *Family Health* and her further elaboration at the May 1984 Edmonton Conference. Doberneck believes Newman's model addresses issues intrinsic to caring that other theories omit, such as unconditionally being with another person and noncommitment to specific predetermined outcomes.[5]

Education

Roy states,

> The function of nursing education [is] the development and sharing of knowledge concerning the theories about the phenomena of nursing and the knowledge and skills related to the theories of the practice of nursing. Since theories describe and predict nursing practice, then nursing education must develop and promote them in such a way that students become nurses who use and develop theory.[22:17]

Newman[18] does "not advocate one model as the sole basis for a curriculum. . . . Students should have the opportunity to study various approaches to health and nursing and to choose what is relevant to them in their practice and research."

Newman has consulted with faculty and students from several universities including Indiana University, Louisiana State University, Medical College of Virginia, New York University, The Pennsylvania State University, University of Akron, University of Alabama, University of California at San Francisco, University of Colorado, University of Minnesota, University of Oregon, University of Southern Florida,

University of Tennessee, and Wayne State University.[20] Faculty at the University of Akron have incorporated Newman's work into the philosophical and conceptual framework of their master's program. They define health as the expansion of consciousness.[12] At some institutions, Newman's model is presented in classes about theoretical models in nursing, and some graduate students conduct research based on it at various institutions.

Research

Research has a dual role: to test theory and establish a scientific knowledge base from which to practice professional nursing. In addition to Newman, several researchers have done research about time, space, or movement. They include Barnard,[1] Chapman,[2] Downs and Fitzpatrick,[6] Engle,[7] Fitzpatrick and Donovan,[9] Goldberg and Fitzpatrick,[10] Smith,[23] and Tompkins.[24] Several of these researchers, including Newman, were influenced by Rogers. By using similar methodology, a cohesive body of knowledge is being developed on the relationship between movement and time across different age groups. "Traditional methodologies may not be sufficient to examine the [relationships], because the model is future-oriented and visionary."[8:270-271]

FURTHER DEVELOPMENT

Newman[17] is progressing toward a theory. She uses Popper's definition that a theory is a powerful, unifying idea to guide the development of her theory. But, Newman[13:6-7] believes that a theory must also provide for "new relationships [that] may be deduced and tested, and the data therefrom then will either strengthen or weaken the theoretical system from which the tested relationship is drawn."

Newman's concepts are being operationally defined to allow for empirical testing. The interrelationships between the concepts need to be further developed with greater focus directed toward the usefulness within applied nursing practice. Several researchers, including a number of students, are operationalizing and testing aspects of the theory. Further development of the theory is expected in Newman's book *Health as Expanding Consciousness* scheduled to be published in 1986 by C.V. Mosby.

CRITIQUE
Simplicity

Newman's theory includes four major concepts. She has developed five interrelationships between these concepts.

Generality

The concepts in Newman's theory are broad in scope because they all relate to health. This renders her theory generalizable. The broad scope provides a focus for future theory development.

Empirical Precision

Aspects of the theory have been operationalized and tested within a traditional scientific mode. However, quantitative methods are limited in capturing the dynamic, changing nature of this model. Qualitative approaches are needed for a full explication of its meaning and application.

Derivable Consequences

Newman's theory is potentially useful in nursing practice because it uses concepts already familiar to nursing, such as time and movement. It has received increased recognition regarding application to practice in recent publications and presentations at conferences.[5,15]

REFERENCES

1. Barnard, R. (1973). *Field-dependence/independence and selected motor abilities.* Unpublished doctoral dissertation. New York University.
2. Chapman, J. (1978). The relationship between auditory stimulation and gross motor activity of short-gestation infants. *Research in Nursing and Health, 1*:29-36.
3. Chinn, P.L. (1983). Nursing theory development: Where we have been and where we are going. In N.L. Chaska (Ed.), *The nursing profession: A time to speak.* New York: McGraw-Hill.
4. Chinn, P.L., & Jacobs, M.K. (1983). *Theory and nursing: A systematic approach.* St. Louis: C.V. Mosby.
5. Doberneck, B. (1985). Graduate student at Pennsylvania State University. Telephone interview.
6. Downs, F., & Fitzpatrick, J. (1976). Preliminary investigation of the reliability and validity of a tool for the assessment of body position and motor activity. *Nursing Research, 25*:404-408.
7. Engle, V. (1981). *A study of the relationship between self-assessment of health, function, personal tempo and time perception in elderly women.* Unpublished doctoral dissertation. Detroit: Wayne State University.
8. Engle, V. (1983). Newman's model of health. In J.J. Fitzpatrick, & A.L. Whall (Eds.), *Conceptual models of nursing: Analysis & application.* Bowie, Md.: Robert J. Brady.
9. Fitzpatrick, J., & Donovan, M., (1978). Temporal experience and motor behavior among the aging. *Research in Nursing and Health, 1*:60-68.
10. Goldberg, W., & Fitzpatrick, J. (1980). Movement theory and the aged. *Nursing Research, 29*:339-346.
11. Kim, H.S. (1983). *The nature of theoretical thinking in nursing.* Norwalk, Conn.: Appleton-Century-Crofts.
12. Marchione, J. (1985). Associate professor at the University of Akron, Telephone interview.
13. Newman, M.A. (1971). *An investigation of the relationship between gait tempo and time perception.* Unpublished doctoral dissertation. New York University.
14. Newman, M.A. (1978). *Second Annual Nurse Educator's Conference.* Held in New York City, December 4-6, 1978. (Audiotape).
15. Newman, M.A. (1979). *Theory development in nursing.* Philadelphia: F.A. Davis.
16. Newman, M.A. (1982, Sept.-Oct.). Time as an index of expanding consciousness with age. *Nursing Research, 31*:290-293.
17. Newman, M.A. (1983). Newman's health theory. In I.W. Clements, & F.B. Roberts, *Family health: A theoretical approach to nursing care.* New York: John Wiley & Sons.
18. Newman, M.A. (1984). Personal correspondence.
19. Newman, M.A. (1985). Personal correspondence.

20. Newman, M.A. (1985) Telephone interview.
21. Newman, M.A., & Gaudiano, J.F. (1984, May-June). Depression as an explanation for decreased subjective time in the elderly. *Nursing Research, 33:*137-139.
22. Roy, C. (1979, March-April). Relating nursing theory to education: A new era. *Nurse Educator, 29:*16-21.
23. Smith, M. (1979). Duration experience for bed-confined subjects: A replication and refinement. *Nursing Research, 28:*139-144.
24. Tompkins, E. (1980). Effect of restricted mobility and dominance in perceived duration. *Nursing Research, 29:*333-338.
25. *Who's Who of American women.* (1983-1984). Chicago: Marquis.

BIBLIOGRAPHY
Primary Sources
Books

Downs, F.S., & Newman, M.A. (Eds.). (1977). *A source book of nursing research.* Philadelphia: F.A. Davis.
Newman, M.A. (1980). *Theory development in nursing.* Philadelphia: F.A. Davis.

Book Chapters

Feild, L., & Newman, M. (1982). Clinical application of the unitary man framework: Case study analysis. In M.J. Kim & D.A. Morita (Eds.), *Classification of nursing diagnosis.* New York: McGraw-Hill.
Newman, M.A. (1973). Identifying patient needs in short-span nurse-patient relationships. In M.E. Auld, & L.H. Birum (Eds.), *The challenge of nursing.* St. Louis: C.V. Mosby.
Newman, M.A. (1981). The meaning of health. In G.E. Laskar (Ed.), *Applied systems research and cybernetics: Vol. 4. Systems research in health care, biocybernetics and ecology.* New York: Pergamon.
Newman, M.A. (1983). The continuing revolution: A history of nursing science. In N.L. Chaska (Ed.), *The nursing profession: A time to speak.* New York: McGraw-Hill.
Newman, M.A. (1983). Nursing's theoretical evolution. In T.A. Duespohol (Ed.), *Nursing in transition.* Rockville, Md.: Aspen Systems.
Newman, M.A. (1983). Newman's health theory. In I. Clements & F. Roberts (Eds.), *Family health: A theoretical approach to nursing care.* New York: John Wiley & Sons.

Newman, M.A. (1983). Health as expanding consciousness. *In Proceedings of Seventh International Conference on Human Functioning.* Wichita, Kan.: Biomedical Synergistics Institute.
Roy, C., et al. (1982). Nursing diagnosis and nursing theory. In M.J. Kim, & D.A. Moritz (Eds.), *Classification of nursing diagnosis.* New York: McGraw-Hill.

Articles

Newman, M.A. (1966). Identifying and meeting patient's needs in short-span nurse-patient relationships. *Nursing Forum, 5:*76-86.
Newman, M.A. (1972). Time estimation in relation to gait tempo. *Perceptual and Motor Skills, 34:*359-366.
Newman, M.A. (1972, July). Nursing's theoretical evolution. *Nursing Outlook, 20:*449-453.
Newman, M.A. (1975, Nov.). The professional doctorate in nursing: A position paper. *Nursing Outlook, 23:*704-706.
Newman, M.A. (1976, Aug.). Movement, tempo and the experience of time. *Nursing Research, 25:*273-279.
Newman, M.A. (1982, Sept.-Oct.). Time as an index of expanding consciousness with age. *Nursing Research, 31:*290-293.
Newman, M.A. (1982, Oct.). What differentiates clinical research? *Image, 14:*86-88.
Newman, M.A. (1983). Editorial. *Advances in Nursing Science, 5:*x-xi.
Newman, M.A. (1984, Dec.). Nursing diagnosis: Looking at the whole. *American Journal of Nursing, 84*(12):1496-1499.
Newman, M.A., & Gaudiano, J.K. (1984, May-June). Depression as an explanation for decreased subjective time in the elderly. *Nursing Research, 33:*137-139.
Newman, M.A., & O'Brien, R.A. (1978, Feb.). Experiencing the research process via computer simulation. *Image, 10:*5-9.

Dissertation

Newman, M.A. (1971). An investigation of the relationship between gait tempo and time perception. Unpublished doctoral dissertation. New York University, School of Education.

Reports

Newman, M.A. (1977). Nursing course content in doctoral education. *Proceedings of National Confer-*

ence on Doctoral Education in Nursing. Philadelphia: University of Pennsylvania.

Newman, M.A. (1982). What differentiates clinical research? *Proceedings of the Second Phyllis J. Verhonick Nursing Research Course.* Washington, D.C.: Nursing Research Service, Walter Reed Army Medical Center.

Newman, M.A., et al. (1980). Movement, time, and consciousness: Parameters of health. (Symposium). Proceedings of Western Society for Research. *Nursing Research, 13:*45-49.

Newman, M.A., & Gaudiano, J.K. (1983). Depression as an explanation for decreased subjective time in the elderly. In M.C. Smith (Ed.)., *Proceedings of the Second Annual Research Conference of the Southern Council on Collegiate Education in Nursing.*

Audiotapes

Newman, M.A. (1978, Dec. 4-6). Paper presented at Second Annual Conference, New York City. Tapes available from Teach 'em Inc., 160 E. Illinois Street, Chicago, Ill. 60611.

Newman, M.A. (1984, May). Paper presented at Nursing Theory Conference, Boyle, Letourneau Conference, Edmonton, Canada. Tapes available from Ed Kennedy, Kennedy Recording, R.R. 5, Edmonton, Alberta, Canada T5P4B7 (403-470-0013).

Correspondence

Newman, M.A. (1984). Personal correspondence.
Newman, M.A. (1985). Personal correspondence.

Interview

Newman, M.A. (1985). Telephone interview.

Secondary Sources
Book Reviews

Newman, M.A. (1980). *Theory development in nursing.*
*Continuing Education in Nursing, 2:*8†, Nov.-Dec. 1979.
*Nursing Administration Quarterly, 4:*81-82, Spring 1980
*Nursing Leadership, 3:*38, March, 1980
*Nursing Research, 29:*311, Sept.-Oct., 1980
*Western Journal of Nursing Research, 2:*250-251, Spring, 1980

Books

Chinn, P.L., & Jacobs, M.K. (1983). Theory in nursing: A current overview In P.L., Chinn & M.K. Jacobs (Eds.), *Theory and nursing.* St. Louis: C.V. Mosby.

Kim, H.S. (1983). *The nature of theoretical thinking in nursing.* Norwalk, Conn.: Appleton-Century-Crofts.

Rogers, M.E. (1970). *An introduction to the theoretical basis of nursing.* Philadelphia: F.A. Davis.

Who's Who of American Women (1983-1985). Chicago: Marquis Who's Who.

Book Chapters

Chinn, P.L. (1983). Nursing theory development: Where we have been and where we are going. In N.L. Chaska (Ed.), *The nursing profession: A time to speak.* New York: McGraw-Hill.

Engle, V. (1983). Newman's model of health. In J.J. Fitzpatrick, & A.L. Whall (Eds.), *Conceptual models of nursing: Analysis and application.* Bowie, Md.: Robert J. Brady.

Articles

Engle, V.E. (1984, Oct.). Newman's conceptual framework and the measurement of older adults' health. *Advances in Nursing Science, 7*(1):24-36.

Roy, C. (1979, March-April). Relating nursing theory to education: A new era. *Nurse Educator, 29:*16-21.

Tompkins, E. (1980, Nov.-Dec.). Effect of restricted mobility and dominance in perceived duration. *Nursing Research, 29*(6): 333-338.

News Releases

Brown, N.M. (1983, Nov.). The body is not a machine. *Research/Penn State 4*(4):19-20.

M.A. Newman appointed as full tenured professor at University of Minnesota School of Nursing. (1984, March). *Nursing Outlook, 32:*2.

Abstracts

Newman, M.A. (1981). Relationship of age to perceived duration. *Abstracts of ANF funded research 1979-1980.* Kansas City: American Nurses' Foundation.

Dissertation Proposal

Page, G. (1985). *An exploration of the relationship between a person's daily patterning and weight loss:*

Maintenance or non-maintenance. Dissertation proposal. Wayne State University.

Master's Theses

Butren, J. (1983). *Differences in time perspective and hemisphericity between educated and noneducated Zairians.* Masters thesis. Pennsylvania State University.

Griscavage, D. (1982). *Relationships among state anxiety time estimation, body movement, and repression-sensitization in preoperative patients.* Master's thesis. Pennsylvania State University.

Pollard, M. (1981). *Emotional expressiveness in cancer and noncancer patients.* Master's thesis. Pennsylvania State University.

Pollock, D. (1983). *The relationship of sleep deprivation to cerebral hemisphericity and temporal orientation.* Master's thesis. Pennsylvania State University.

Zack, C. (1983). *Hospitalized patients' personal space preferences in relation to female and male nurses.* Master's thesis. Pennsylvania State University.

Other

Acton, H.B. (1967). George Wilhelm Friedrich Hegel 1770-1831. In *The encyclopedia of philosophy* (Vols. 3 & 4). New York: Macmillan & Free Press.

Barnard, R. (1973). *Field-dependence–independence and selected motor abilities.* Unpublished doctoral dissertaiton. New York University.

Bentov, I. (1977). *Stalking the wild pendulum.* New York: E.P. Dutton.

Bentov, I. (1978, Nov. 17-20). *The mechanics of consciousness.* Paper presented at the symposium on New Dimensions of Consciousness, sponsored by Sufi Order in the West. New York.

Capra, F. (1975). *The tao of physics.* Boulder, Col.: Thambhala Publications.

Chapman, J. (1978). The relationship between auditory stimulation and gross motor activity of short-gestation infants. *Research in Nursing and Health, 1:*29-36.

Downs, F., & Fitzpatrick, J. (1976). Preliminary investigation of the reliability and validity of a tool for the assessment of body position and motor activity. *Nursing Research, 25:*404-408.

Engle, V. (1981). *A study of the relationship between self-assessment of health, function, personal tempo and time perception in elderly women.* Unpublished doctoral dissertation. Wayne State University.

Fitzpatrick, J., & Donovan, M. (1978). Temporal experience and motor behavior among the aging. *Research in Nursing and Health, 1:*60-68.

Goldberg, W., & Fitzpatrick, J. (1980). Movement therapy and the aged. *Nursing Research, 29:*339-346.

Marcuse, H. (1954). *Reason and revolution: Hegel and the rise of social theory* (2nd ed.). New York: Beacon.

Rogers, M.E. (1980). Nursing, a science of unitary man. In J.P. Reihl, & C. Roy, *Conceptual models for nursing practice.* New York: Appleton-Century-Crofts.

Smith, M. (1979). Duration experience for bed-confined subjects: A replication and refinement. *Nursing Research, 28:*139-144.

Tompkins, E. (1980). Effect of restricted mobility and dominance in perceived duration. *Nursing Research, 29:*333-338.

Interviews

Doberneck, B. (1985). Graduate student at Pennsylvania State University. Telephone interview.

Marchione, J. (1985). Associate professor at the University of Akron. Telephone interview.

INDEX